HIGH ENERGY LIVING

▶ SWITCH ON THE SOURCES TO:

- Increase Your Fat-Burning Power
- Boost Your Immunity and Live Longer
- Stimulate Your Memory and Creativity
- Unleash Hidden Passions and Courage

BY ROBERT K. COOPER, PH.D.

RODALE

Cover Designer: Christopher Rhoads
Interior Designer: Richard Kershner
Illustrator: Michael Gellatly

Library of Congress Cataloging-in-Publication Data

Cooper, Robert K.
    High-energy living : switch on the sources to: increase your fat-burning power, boost your immunity and live longer, stimulate your memory and creativity, unleash hidden passions and courage / by Robert K. Cooper.
        p.   cm.
    Includes index.
    ISBN 1–57954–126–7   hardcover
    1. Health.   2. Vitality.   I. Title.
    RA776.5 .C67   2000
    613—dc21   00–033310

Distributed to the book trade by St. Martin's Press

2   4   6   8   10   9   7   5   3   1   hardcover

Visit us on the Web at www.preventionbookshelf.com, or call us toll-free at (800) 848-4735.

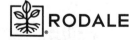

RODALE

WE INSPIRE AND ENABLE PEOPLE TO IMPROVE
THEIR LIVES AND THE WORLD AROUND THEM

To everyone who dreams of being 100 percent alive
and has the courage to explore uncommon ways
to turn the dream into reality.

To Leslie, my wife and best friend,
To each of you, my children,
Chris,
Chelsea,
Shanna,
And to my grandparents and parents.

One at a time or all together,
Over the years
You have helped open my eyes and heart
To a universe of energy and love I never knew.

Contents

Part 4: Sensory Energy

Part 5: Heartfelt Energy

Part 6: Conclusion

Resources

Acknowledgments

Every morning of our lives, we awaken and turn from unconsciousness to consciousness, from dreaming to being. It is energy—and people—that make this possible.

To my beautiful wife and dearest friend, Leslie: I thank you for all that you are and do. From the very first moment, your love has uplifted my heart and spirit.

To our children, Chris, Chelsea, and Shanna: I thank you for the joy, laughter, learning, and love that you have brought into my life. The capacity in each of you is new in nature, and so is your unique potential to make a difference in the world.

To my parents, Hugh and Margaret Cooper: Whether near or far, I have felt your support and encouragement every day of my life. I honor the greatness in each of you.

To my sister, Mary, and brother, David: I thank you for the many times we have laughed together and faced challenges along the way.

To my grandparents, Hugh and Nora Cooper and Wendell and Marion Downing: I will be forever grateful for the way you urged me forward and intensified my curiosity about the untapped possibilities in shaping a life worth leading.

To Larry and Lynn Taylor: I am grateful for the gift of your exceptional friendship.

To Stephanie Tade, my literary agent and friend: Thank you for being second to none in your field and adding your unique brilliance to my work.

To my superb editor, Ed Claflin, who loved this book from the start and added much to its completion.

To many others at *Prevention* Health Books and Rodale who have worked on this project and left their unique imprints on it. My heartfelt thanks to Pat Corpora, Brian Carnahan, Karen Arbegast, Denyse Corelli, Susan Massey, Cindy Ratzlaff, Mary Lengle, Gary Krebs, Kathryn C. LeSage, Richard Kershner, Christopher Rhoads, and Donna G. Rossi.

This book has also been influenced by the pioneering work or enduring support of many other individuals. Thank you to Bob Arnot, M.D.; Steven N. Blair; Ken Blanchard, Ph.D.; Harold Bloomfield, M.D.; Guy Brown, Ph.D.; René Cailliet, M.D.; Michael D. Chafetz, Ph.D.; Donald O. Clifton, Ph.D.; Kenneth H. Cooper, M.D.; Bruce Cryer; Mihaly Csikszentmihalyi, Ph.D.; Antonio Damasio, M.D., Ph.D.; Marian Cleeves Diamond, Ph.D.; Susan Duggan, Ph.D.; Tom Ferguson, M.D.; Etienne Grandjean, M.D., Ph.D.; Peter Hauri, Ph.D.; Sheldon Saul Hendler, M.D., Ph.D.; Mary Hershberger; Denny and Liz Hill; Larry and Bunny Holman and everyone at Wyncom; Alan Horton; Deborah Kiley, Ph.D.; John and Marcia Kulick; James E. Loehr, Ed.D.; James J. Lynch, Ph.D.; Karen and George McCown; Ashley Montagu, Ph.D.; Martin Moore-Ede, M.D., Ph.D.; Esther Orioli and everyone at Q-Metrics and Essi Systems; Dean Ornish, M.D.; Robert Ornstein, Ph.D.; Harry Paul; James Pennebaker, Ph.D.; Tom Peters; Karl H. Pribram, M.D., Ph.D.; Michael Ray, Ph.D.; Rachel Naomi Remen, M.D.; Elly Rose; Ernest Lawrence Rossi, Ph.D.; Ayman and Rowan Sawaf; Martin E. P. Seligman, Ph.D.; Sandy Stafford; Bryant A. Stamford, Ph.D.; Robert E. Thayer, Ph.D.; Karen Trocki, Ph.D.; Sirah Vettese, Ph.D.; Bob and Tina Webster; Brent and Dotty Williams; Redford Williams, M.D.; Virginia Williams, Ph.D.; Dave and Kim Williamson; and Judith J. Wurtman, Ph.D.

Part 1

The Key to Feeling 100 Percent Alive

Chapter 1

Prime Yourself for Unparalleled Energy

D o you know what it's like to feel fully alive?

Few people do.

What if you could experience your best day every day? What if you could consistently feel as alert, vibrant, confident, focused, enthusiastic, and in touch with yourself as you do when you're at the peak of your energy?

When I challenge people with those questions, their first reply, invariably, is "Yes, I'd love it! Just show me how."

But I sense that they don't really believe that it's possible.

And I understand. The truth is, most of us don't believe that we can feel fully alive. Right now, you may be wondering, "Why do I feel tense or tired so often? Why am I so often 'not there' for my spouse, my friends, or my children? What about those days that I just get through, as if I were treading water or climbing uphill?"

These are hardly unusual thoughts, especially in these times. And there are more questions like them—in fact, they're the very questions that are at the core of this book.

- Those mornings when I have to drag myself out of bed . . . why? What's making me feel so sluggish and slow?
- When I lose my temper at drivers on the road, friends, family, people at work, what's really going on? Why do I get so impatient?
- What about those times when I can't remember things, when my mind seems to drift, when I'm just overwhelmed with everything I have to do?

Sound familiar?

Warring with Tiredness

Often, our sense of tiredness and frustration is deep. It affects our outlook, our health, our work, and our most important relationships. It gets to the point where we aren't eating well or sleeping well.

We don't have the energy to get even the minimal amount of exercise—20 to 30 minutes a day—that would help us live more vigorously and many years longer. (Yes, science has proved the benefits of exercise; but knowing this and doing something about it are two different things.)

Or what about the health problems that seem to sabotage our energy just when we need it most? We can't quite put our fingers on it, but we know that we have aches, pains, and discomforts that seem to get worse, not better. And we know the tension, too—the kind of tension that invades our backs, shoulders, jaws, or necks. Sometimes, that tension is so all-encompassing that it seems to travel all through our bodies, blunt our senses, and dim our minds.

Headaches that won't go away. Stomach upsets that doctors have told us are often stress-related. In fact, we've heard and read volumes about all the damage that stress-related problems can cause. But what's the good of knowing about stress if we don't have the energy to do anything about it?

The Cost of a Shrinking World

Not surprisingly, feelings of fatigue, frustration, and lack of good health have become universal in scope. Yes, our world is getting smaller, and the problems of hectic, fast-paced techno-living are being shared nationwide and worldwide. In the hundreds of seminars that I've held with thousands of men and women in the United States and around the world, I've discovered that many of us are engaged in a common search, one that's as compelling as the search for the Holy Grail.

What are we searching for? I believe that it can be summed up in a single word: *energy*.

How do we find it? Why do we lose it? When we don't have it, where does it go?

And why is energy so fickle? Sometimes, we get a burst of energy when we feel really low and in need. But there are other times—far too many—when it seems to desert us entirely.

Like anything that behaves in seemingly mysterious ways, the quality called human energy is something that many people regard as almost magical. "I just pray for more energy," people have told me. "I'm so tired all the time. I wish this feeling would go away." I call this *if only . . .* thinking because it's as if wishing it were so would make it so.

There are those who confide in me, "I've tried everything. No matter what I do, I just don't feel like I'm 100 percent." As a 21st-century human being with all of the cares and concerns that you face every day, it's very typical for you to have these feelings.

But there's one thing that I *don't* believe about this force called human energy: I don't think that it actually does come and go in completely mysterious ways. On the contrary, my research has led me to the conclusion that human energy—yours and mine—is in many ways just as controllable as the energy that comes from an ignited spark or a burning flame.

There is extensive evidence that how energetic we feel is a major determinant of how happy, healthy, productive, and creative we are. It is surprising that, until now, so little attention has been paid to our energy levels and what drains them.

In Search of the Secret of Being 100 Percent Alive

"Compared with what we ought to be, most of us are only half-awake," said William James, M.D., Ph.D., Harvard University's noted philosopher and psychologist, at the beginning of the 20th century. "We are making use of only a small part of our possible mental and physical resources. Our energy is far below the maximum."

Life, added Dr. James, is a "mass of small choices." Whether changed or ignored, he said, "these small choices bear us irresistibly toward our destiny."

How can we use more of what Dr. James calls our mental, emotional, and physical resources? How do we find our maximum energy?

As I started searching for those answers, I found that there were other questions that needed replies. I began asking, "Where does our energy come from?" and "How can we control it?" Almost immediately, I started to examine simple, day-to-day habits and routines.

Fortunately, I did not have to perform thousands of experiments to understand the impact of these routines. The experiments have already been done, and the body of scientific evidence has become extensive. Pursuing my search, then, has been a matter of sifting through all of the reports and listening very carefully to the testimony offered by dozens of experts and thousands of men and women.

Although this undertaking began with small questions like "Where does our energy come from?" before long I was face-to-face with far bigger issues, such as:

- Why does our health often fail when our energy fails?
- Why are feelings of hopelessness, helplessness, and confusion linked to fatigue?
- How can each of us, in our own way, realize our true potential for living?

Small choices, as Dr. James pointed out, are indeed linked to our destinies. But how can we make the small changes in our habits that will lead to the kinds of positive life changes that we seek in our destinies?

In Pursuit of Alertness

How can we be 100 percent alive not once in a while but most of the time?

I believe that, remarkably enough, you'll find in this book many of the answers to that crucial question.

These discoveries are not mine alone. They emerge from the bringing together of a vast number of scientific studies. Fascinating in their own right, these studies point to similar conclusions.

It has been my goal to find out where this energy is and how we can tap into it. Based on the existing research and everything we now know about human behavior and our ability to grow and change at every age, what are the switches that will help you and me get access to our inner energy resources? What lessons can be learned from neuroscience, physiology, psychology, biology, and a host of other scientific fields that we can apply to our day-to-day lives? And what do those lessons tell us about our most valuable resource, human energy?

I have pursued these questions precisely because they have meaning for you and me and the way we relate to those who are important to us and the way we live and work at our best during our daily lives.

And because I've focused on practical strategies and everyday solutions for busy people like you, I believe that you will find in this book the answers that you need, answers to questions such as:

- After a hard day at work, how can I still have enough energy to give the best of myself to the people who are most important to me—my own family?
- I'm exhausted at the end of the day, so how can I sleep more soundly to get recharged again?
- I'm not old, but I feel tired. How can I act younger and feel younger?
- All this stress is taking a toll on my health. How can I deal with that stress so it doesn't overwhelm me?
- I eat when I'm not hungry and keep eating when I'm full! How can I eat for energy and stop feeling hungry?
- What happened to my creative power? How can I bring it back to my household and my work?
- How can I just let go and relax, without feeling guilty because I'm "giving up" or "letting people down"?

Use Skillpower, Not Willpower

This book will provide you with something far different from theory. It will give you practical tools and methods that you can use every day to gain access to your internal reserves of energy. Surprisingly enough, it will show you how to do that without working harder at *anything*. In fact, once you start a pattern of high-energy living, life often becomes easier.

There's no luck required. Just practical techniques—what I call switches. Each of these switches must be something that you and I can do easily in our daily lives to tap into the energy that is at the core of our beings. Each of these switches will take us one step closer to feeling 100 percent alive.

Chapter 2

Recognize the Four Kinds of Energy

I want to give you a quick overview of all the switches that you can use to turn on your energy. But first, I want to share some conclusions that I've come to based on an extensive review of worldwide research.

To put it in a nutshell, there isn't just *one* kind of human energy, as many scientists have contended for years. There are *four* kinds of essential energy: calm, active, sensory, and heartfelt. While these kinds of energy have much in common, they also have some distinct differences. Take a look at these complementary kinds of energy, and I think you'll agree that each is vitally necessary to our lives at work and at home and to our health and relationships.

The Concept of Calm Energy

Calm energy is the natural flow state in which you get a kick out of living.

If you have calm energy, you can work better than ever, with less strain. You don't feel like you're part of the rat race. You can make the most of your time and resources by better applying your talents, strengths, and passions.

In virtually every field of endeavor, those who achieve world records and breakthroughs are masters of calm energy. Those who achieve great acts of creativity also know the meaning of calm energy. But you don't have to be an Olympic athlete, a computer whiz, or a master composer to benefit from calm energy. It is a state that each of us can reach and sustain in our own unique way, if we choose to.

What if you could always have the most fun and the least struggle while accomplishing more of whatever matters most to you? That's the experience of calm energy.

The Opposite: Tense Energy

The opposite of calm energy is tense energy. When you have tense energy, you're under the illusion that you feel just fine and, at times, quite vigorous. But that vigor comes from a surge of adrenaline, the same jolt of energy that would make you hypervigilant and tense when walking at the edge of a cliff. Or tense energy comes from the buzz of caffeine, the temporary lift that you get from a cup of strong coffee. Or it's triggered by anger or time urgency or stress, the kinds of pressures that can actually damage your health and performance.

Tense energy is a kind of fake energy. I call it fake because it doesn't really help you stay more alert or act more effectively. In fact, it interferes with the function of neurotransmitters, the brain-messenger chemicals that help you perform at your best. When you're operating on the reserves of this fake energy, you eventually collapse in a heap, tense and tired. Along the way, tense energy breaks down health and impedes healing.

Few Americans ever experience calm energy anymore, according to Robert E. Thayer, Ph.D., professor of biological psychology at California

State University, Long Beach. Instead, we're trapped in a cycle of tense energy that leaves us falling far short of the lives that we *could* live. Not surprisingly, tense energy leads to tense tiredness, and both have become so common that they seem normal. They're not. When we're trapped by reliance on adrenaline and caffeine, we risk our health and well-being.

Where Active Energy Kicks In

Active energy is produced by motion. It is triggered and turned on by your brain's alertness switches.

Active energy is a primary source of physical pep and mental drive. It builds vital reserves of stamina and fortifies your ability to bounce back from difficult times and challenging situations.

When energy is generated by action in simple ways here and there throughout the day, you can lose excess body fat automatically, even while you sleep. As you increase active energy, you also improve your metabolism, the processes of making new energy molecules in your brain and body.

When the switches of active energy are turned on, your metabolism is naturally higher, as is your ability to burn off excess fat and stay healthier during stressful times.

The Opposite: Reserved Energy

The opposite of active energy is reserved energy. Are you driving instead of walking? If so, you're reserving your energy rather than using it. Are you sitting instead of standing? Sitting reserves energy. Are you watching sports on television instead of playing catch or gardening? Chalk that up as reserved energy rather than active energy.

Putting our time into reserved energy has become the predominant pattern for almost half of all Americans. But there are ways to change this pattern, as I will explain in this book.

From hour to hour, your active energy must be switched on. Your metabolism relies on every one of the small but crucial signals that you give it. If that energy remains in reserve, if it doesn't get switched on, your overall vigor and vitality noticeably wane.

Feeling Your Sensory Energy

Sensory energy is the primary energy that enables you to soak up more of life's richness by reaching out with your senses—not just the traditional five senses, but the dozens of others that have been discovered by scientists. Use your sensory energy, and you literally engage with life.

Do you ever feel like you're going through the motions? Tapping into sensory energy, you move beyond that zone. You savor your experiences more fully. Sunsets are richer. The stars are brighter. A child's smile means more. You notice the uniqueness in others and more fully sense the value of the efforts that they are making. You feel more present, and you're more aware of everything that's happening around you, because all of your senses are alert during every waking moment.

When you have sensory energy, you achieve a rare level of exceptional attentiveness to people and possibilities. This can help you in many ways. A child reacts immediately and positively to a parent who has sensory energy. Colleagues at work will instantly pick up on the energy. In fact, sensory energy happens to be one of the most sought-after traits for creative insights and successful leadership at work.

Sensory energy is essential to longevity and to "growing young," according to Ashley Montagu, Ph.D., professor in the department of anthropology at Rutgers University in New Brunswick, New Jersey, and

Marian Cleeves Diamond, Ph.D., neuroanatomist at the University of California, Berkeley, and author of *Enriching Heredity: The Impact of the Environment on the Anatomy of the Brain*. In essence, the more sensory energy you produce, the more you are naturally inclined to learn and to stretch your senses beyond all the boundaries that may have limited you in the past. As a result, your brain's unused or little-used pathways light up.

By living more fully, you turn back the common aging process. Over the course of a lifetime, the average person may use only $\frac{1}{10,000}$ of their brainpower (far less than the $\frac{1}{10}$ that was considered the rule of thumb for many years). Yet when you tap into sensory energy, your brainpower never stops growing—no matter what your age.

The Opposite: Routine Energy

The opposite of sensory energy is routine energy. This is, quite simply, being in a rut. Perhaps there's some pleasure and security to routine energy. But as much as you may crave it, routine energy contributes to a stunted view of life's possibilities, and, at the same time, promotes premature, accelerated aging. You may not even notice this because everyone around you may be going downhill fast too. Worse, when you operate on routine energy, a lot of the fun goes out of living.

Heartfelt Energy—Straight from the Heart

Heartfelt energy is what awakens and empowers your deepest drive for a meaningful life and for strong, mutually significant relationships. This energy is literally electric. Your body's trillions of cells are energized by huge electrical fields driving vast currents through tiny molecular structures—motors, pumps, gates, switches, and chemical factories that together make you alive. At the center of this energy dynamo is your heart.

It's natural to have heartfelt energy that's directed toward your spouse or children. But heartfelt energy has the potential to reach beyond, to all your efforts and interpersonal relationships, including those at work.

When you have heartfelt energy, you're also engaged in a profound and lasting search for your calling, for the ways that you contribute the most to the world and make the greatest difference.

With heartfelt energy comes the building of character. When heartfelt energy is absent in someone, we sense in that person a shallowness or emptiness, despite an outer semblance of fitness or success. Heartfelt energy is the primary wellspring of courage and commitment. It enables you to live your values and vision, rather than just talk about them.

Heartfelt energy is also the central factor in social-support systems that have been linked to faster healing, strengthened immunity, and longevity. Heartfelt energy prompts a heightened degree of empathy, the vital ability to be intimate and trusting with others. And the benefits of that positive trait go beyond family relationships. Empathy is the most vital practical trait in a leader, according to Peter Drucker, Ph.D., professor of social sciences at Claremont Graduate School in California. This suggests the benefits of taking this positive energy to the workplace.

Experiments show that the heart's energy, in the form of electromagnetic signals, is transmitted to every cell of the body and then emanates outward. Remarkable power and influence are generated by this energy field of the heart. Electrophysiological changes in feelings transmitted by the heart have been detected up to 5 feet away, according to studies published in the *American Journal of Cardiology*. Further studies measure the heart's energy field at 10 feet away.

It's intriguing to consider that the boundaries of our bodies aren't as clearly defined as we once thought they were. It's likely that in promising new areas of physical-science research, we'll begin to find further explanations for some of the phenomena that I call heartfelt energy.

The Opposite: Surface Energy

The opposite of heartfelt energy is surface energy. People with surface energy may be blessed with Hollywood smiles and schmoozing words, but the energy is self-centered and shallow. They pretend to care rather than actually care. They feign honesty and fake commitment. But ultimately, when there's only surface energy and no heartfelt energy, relationships are doomed to fizzle. Many people powered solely by surface energy find themselves at a loss for a sense of higher purpose and meaning in their lives and work.

Sources and Switches

Calm, active, sensory, and heartfelt energy are the kinds of energy that I have identified in my research. But just knowing about these four kinds of energy doesn't answer the question that we're all asking: "How can I automatically turn on this human energy so that I can feel 100 percent alive?"

There is a way—one that's both practical and scientifically based—to crack the code. All it takes is a willingness to test some everyday strategies and practical techniques that give you access to your deepest human-energy sources.

In fact, there are 21 switches that you can use any time, in any way, to give you more of the energy that you need. These switches are available to all of us, no matter what our ages, lifestyles, or professions.

The "ID Your Energy Blockers" quiz and guidelines on the following pages will guide you to the switches that may prove most helpful to you, personally. On the first two pages, you'll find 34 questions that will help you identify your personal energy needs. It won't take long to answer those questions. Then, turn to page 18 for specific recommendations about the parts of this book that may be most likely to help you.

ID Your Energy Blockers

In this book, you'll find 21 switches that can help you turn on the four different kinds of energy—calm, active, sensory, and heartfelt.

But which of these switches is most useful to you? What kind of energy can do you the most good? Where are your greatest energy needs?

To answer these questions, simply take the quiz below. If you don't want to mark up the book, photocopy these pages.

After you've responded to all the statements, you'll find guidelines directing you to the sections of this book that may prove most helpful to you, based on your answers.

	Often	Sometimes	Never
1. When I'm under pressure, I become flustered and anxious.	❏	❏	❏
2. By the end of the day, I can feel the stress and strain in my back, neck, or shoulders.	❏	❏	❏
3. Daily life seems humdrum and uninteresting.	❏	❏	❏
4. I'm very susceptible to colds and infections.	❏	❏	❏
5. I have trouble falling asleep.	❏	❏	❏
6. I feel cranky, jittery, and on edge.	❏	❏	❏
7. I feel older than my years.	❏	❏	❏
8. I feel uncomfortable, uneasy, and discontented.	❏	❏	❏
9. I feel physically lethargic.	❏	❏	❏
10. I get frustrated because of trying different weight-loss strategies that don't work for long.	❏	❏	❏
11. I go through times when my motivation takes a sharp nosedive.	❏	❏	❏
12. Under stress, I feel overwhelmed or out of control.	❏	❏	❏

	Often	Sometimes	Never
13. My attention drifts when I'm meeting with other people or trying to focus on my work.	❏	❏	❏
14. I have trouble facing up to daily pressures and challenges.	❏	❏	❏
15. At the end of a long workday, I go home feeling wired, tense, or tired.	❏	❏	❏
16. My energy and attention bottom out in the afternoon.	❏	❏	❏
17. I wake up in the morning feeling groggy rather than alert.	❏	❏	❏
18. My thinking is fuzzy or I have trouble remembering things.	❏	❏	❏
19. I don't feel that I'm paying enough attention to other people.	❏	❏	❏
20. I fall back on old habits when doing new things.	❏	❏	❏
21. I feel like my youthful energy is draining away.	❏	❏	❏
22. I want more intellectual challenges that are fun.	❏	❏	❏
23. Trivial problems and details seem to consume most of my time and energy.	❏	❏	❏
24. I spend too much time doing what I *have* to do and not enough time having fun.	❏	❏	❏
25. I feel that it has been a long time since I learned anything really exciting.	❏	❏	❏
26. I've lost the motivation to be my very best.	❏	❏	❏
27. I'm distrustful of others.	❏	❏	❏
28. I feel as if I were pretending or putting on an act.	❏	❏	❏
29. I have negative reactions to events or encounters.	❏	❏	❏
30. Even when I have a strong opinion or point of view, I'm afraid to speak out.	❏	❏	❏

(continued)

ID Your Energy Blockers—Continued

	Often	Sometimes	Never
31. I feel distance between myself and others.	❑	❑	❑
32. I feel that I can't keep my priorities straight.	❑	❑	❑
33. I don't feel committed to anything that I really love doing.	❑	❑	❑
34. I want to do more things that are unique or unusual and make a difference in the world.	❑	❑	❑

Here's a quick guide to whether you're most in need of calm, active, sensory, or heartfelt energy.

Look at statements 1 through 8. How many did you answer "often" or "sometimes"?

All the statements in this section are related to *calm energy*. Turn to page 21 to find the calm-energy switches.

Look at statements 9 through 17. How many did you answer "often" or "sometimes"?

All the statements in this section are related to *active energy*. Turn to page 147 to find the active-energy switches.

Look at statements 18 through 25. How many did you answer "often" or "sometimes"?

All the statements in this section are related to *sensory energy*. Turn to page 247 to find the sensory-energy switches.

Look at statements 26 through 34. How many did you answer "often" or "sometimes"?

All the statements in this section are related to *heartfelt energy*. Turn to page 351 to find the heartfelt-energy switches.

In each part, you'll find specific suggestions and guidelines to turn on the energy switches and discover immediately whether they work for you.

Part 2

Calm
Energy

S he made it look so easy!"

"He set a new record—and didn't even break a sweat!"

How often and in how many different ways have we expressed this sentiment when watching someone excelling at an important task, whether in life, work, the performing arts, or sports?

And when we express admiration this way, it's usually with considerable curiosity or even envy. Wouldn't it be wonderful to feel so comfortable, graceful, and relaxed when facing difficult challenges and overcoming them?

But for most of us, a different kind of energy takes hold when we're trying our best to act skillfully, efficiently, or quickly. In everyday life, many tasks—large and small alike—seem *hard*. Too often, they make us strain and struggle. And at the end of what seems like a trial, we don't feel like elegant, accomplished performers. We feel like we've crossed a tightrope over a 20-foot chasm with nothing to hold on to except ourselves.

The truth is, we need calm energy more than ever because pressures keep going up, with no end in sight. This doesn't happen to only a select few; it happens to every one of us. The difference between those who are at the top and those who are not is in how we handle these pressures.

Dealing with Frenzy

In the everyday business of getting on with our lives, how can we generate more energy and have more fun while making a greater difference in the world, not just a living?

Some people would be happy just to have enough energy to get out of bed in the morning, go to work, look after their homes and finances, make plans for their children and themselves, and handle the emergencies that come up. Beyond this, we all face particular situations that make us more tense than usual or drain our energy more than they should.

Perhaps, for you, the most horrendous source of personal anxiety is preparing for a difficult conversation or meeting—*that's* the event that you'd like to get through with an enviable display of calm energy rather than with nerves, jitters, and anxiety. Or maybe it's the holidays that sap your energy—working out arrangements, preparing meals, making sure that people are attended to, dealing with the emotional roller coasters of life and the shadows of all holidays past.

Or, if you're the kind of person who rises to those challenges and glides through with calmness and equanimity, maybe it's the humdrum evening at home that seems most challenging. These days, many of us seem to scarcely enjoy or relate to the people with whom we live. That situation can be exhausting. It's easy for the first few minutes at home to turn into a championship duel of conflicting needs and emotions that quickly dispels any hope of coolness, calmness, and relaxation.

Making It Feel Easy

The truth is, when you see someone who makes a job, a conversation, a crisis, a meeting, a performance, or managing a household look easy, that person may well be a master of the calm energy that I'm talking about. The star performers whom I've met in sports, business, education, health care, government, the performing arts, service groups, and academia—and those whom I've encountered on a personal basis—do have a special kind of ability. They've found ways to streamline their efforts, to dispense with the unessential burdens and tension, and to make great things happen, not once in a while but day after day.

We can't keep pushing harder and doing more. I could cite extensive statistical figures that would tell you the price that we pay for doing just that. Longer work hours. Higher stress levels. An epidemic of neck and back pain. Rising numbers of people who experience tiredness and grouchiness. Soaring depression. Increased violence in homes and communities.

But you don't need astounding statistics to tell you that. If you're like most of the people I meet every day in my work and travels, you can tell me all about being overstressed, overworked, and overtired. You know what it feels like. And you can tell me the cost in terms of your health, your nerves, your family relationships, your work, and your friendships.

The intriguing thing about this rising tendency toward stress and fatigue is that it's intrinsic. In fact, it's one of the most ancient instincts in the human brain to meet rising stress by taking emergency measures that produce even more stress. If you fall behind in your work, for instance, don't you tell yourself that you have to work harder? If you miss appointments or fall behind in your schedule, don't you try to convince yourself that you need to go faster to catch up?

In the meantime, another voice inside you may be whispering, "I have to do something about this. I have to figure out a way to cut back." That's a good, intuitive message, but it can easily be drowned out by the roar of shifting gears as you go even faster. Maybe you know that you should take a break, slow down, and have more fun. But the ancient, instinctive part of your brain is revving up the stress hormones. You become more tense and more reactive, not because you want to be that way but because you feel as if your very existence is threatened by all the stressful events that are going on.

But what if you could cut through the numbness and listen to the voice that tells you to move ahead with less strain, more fun, and smarter choices? If you recognize and respect that voice, you can increase your calm energy and position yourself for more happiness and success.

From Tense to Calm

Calm energy is a state of low tension and high energy. If that sounds contradictory—and un-familiar—it's because few of us experience calm energy often enough.

Reaping the Benefits

Calm energy will give you:
- Increased effectiveness under pressure
- Reduced tension, distress, and strain
- Greater creativity and inge-nuity in daily life
- Heightened immune function and better health
- Better sleep and rest
- Deepened sense of humor, playfulness, and resilience—even during difficult times
- Increased longevity
- Expanded sense of content-ment and happiness

Calm energy feels remarkably serene and under control. It endows you with an alert, optimistic presence of mind, a peaceful and plea-surable physical feeling, and a deep sense of stamina and well-being. Your mental and physical reserves are high. When you feel calm en-ergy, you have the best combination of healthy vitality and increased creative intelligence.

With calm energy, you can take minor irritations in stride and handle them more easily and efficiently. They don't loom up and be-come major frustrations. Small setbacks stay small—they don't take on the guise of big obstacles. Challenges appear manageable; and you see steady progress in making more of the right things happen throughout the day.

Calm energy produces another benefit as well: It's easier not to get consumed by details and somehow forget the things that are most important to you.

"When an individual feels highly energetic and at the same time is relatively calm, his or her perception of both self and the world is distinctly different from when that person is tired and at the same time tense," says Robert E. Thayer, Ph.D., professor of biological psychology at California State University, Long Beach. "Not only are memories of past successes and failures likely to be different but the perceived likelihood of future successes and failures is also different."

Finding the Flow State

There is convincing scientific evidence that across the full range of life's situations—in work, sports, school, and relationships—the highest level of thinking, feeling, and action comes as a natural expression of the "flow" state.

Does that sound like something unreal or mystical? It isn't. Extensive research conducted by scientists at such prestigious institutions as the University of Chicago and Stanford University confirms the power and value of this state for those who want to excel at virtually any endeavor in life or work.

In today's uptight, hurry-up world, many people simply don't realize that calmness is an integral part of peak vitality and best performance—and that calmness does *not* mean depleted energy or dulled senses. By developing your ability to quickly enter a state of profound, revitalizing relaxation and restful alertness, you can distance yourself from life's noise and distractions and promote clear-mindedness and awareness. When you feel alert and strong, you are also more likely to feel happy.

The opposite of calm energy is tense energy, which creates an illusion of vigor. I describe tense energy as an illusion—and a costly one, at that—because it's often triggered by the buzz of caffeine, by anger, by rushing, or by stress. Hour after hour, this fake energy level interferes with your healthy neurotransmitter (brain-messenger chemical) function. You eventually collapse in a heap, tense and tired, with your mind and senses numb. Along the way, tense energy breaks down health and impedes healing.

It's a tragedy that so few Americans ever experience calm energy anymore, according to Dr. Thayer. Instead, we're trapped by tense energy and its inevitable aftermath, tense tiredness, which have become so common that they seem normal. Therein lies a major risk to health and well-being, both on and off the job.

Getting There

Achieving a state of calm energy won't change your daily schedule very much. But once you learn to turn on the switches that create calm energy, you'll start to flow more readily with life and have much more fun along the way.

On most days, many of us sense deep down that we could be something more than we are right now—leaders or teachers; climbers or explorers; inventors or poets; musicians or independent scholars; scientists, artists, or collectors. I can't guarantee that turning on the calm-energy switches will fully turn you into the person you'd like to be. But I know that it will move you closer to being that person, because we all need calm energy to more fully enjoy the most significant and meaningful activities and pursuits.

If you feel too tense and tired, you sense that you can't handle the constant challenges of life or work. You find yourself settling for something more accessible or doable but far less enriching or rewarding.

With calm energy, you'll be far more effective at turning obstacles into opportunities. You'll be able to call forth more of your untapped capacity, hour after hour and day after day. Instead of feeling beleaguered by pressures or pummeled by adversities, you'll begin to better use them as springboards for new learning and for doing what no one else has done before. In short, calm energy will help you close the gap between where you are right now and where you most want to be.

Launch the Day with High Energy and Low Tension

Considering that this is a book about high energy, you may be surprised to learn that I don't advise anyone to start the day with a bang.

The first few minutes right after you wake up can influence your entire day. So it's worthwhile to take a close look at what happens in those minutes. Turn on this calm-energy switch the right way, and you'll increase your energy level from the moment that you open your eyes. Not only that but you'll also change your metabolism—that is, the way that your body generates and utilizes energy. Turn on Calm-Energy Switch #1, and you'll actually boost the way that you burn excess fat in your body. That change will establish a pattern for the rest of the day.

Lots of people have gotten into the habit of setting their alarms as late as possible to get as much sleep as they can. In the morning, I know, many people prefer to keep the lights dim to ease some of the jolt of waking up. The day begins at the last possible moment with a begrudging jump out of bed—but after that, they're almost sleepwalking through the morning ritual.

When you wake to a last-minute alarm and then stagger through the launch zone of the day, you suffer a tension-producing shock to your system. Your blood pressure skyrockets. Stress hormones pour into your bloodstream. Yes, you may feel awake, but it's a survival signal, not a sign of true vigor, and it won't last long. Add a blast of caffeine on an empty stomach, a dose of negative news on the TV or radio, and then some rush hour anger or time frustration, and you have all the ingredients for the proverbial cannon shot that begins the rat race each day for millions of people. And it's killing us.

Signal Failure

There's another kind of danger if you drag your way through the morning. If your morning ritual takes place in low light and slow motion, your brain has little incentive to push your metabolism much higher than near-hibernation rate. And if you stifle your metabolism even more by skipping breakfast, you unwittingly fail to turn on the first calm-energy switch. As I described in a previous book, *Low-Fat Living*, you may even stimulate fat-preserving and fat-storing processes instead.

These morning wake-up habits are almost sure to backfire. First of all, if you begin the day without any activity or exercise, you slow down your fat-burning metabolism, which has an obvious effect on your weight. When you look at the energy side of this equation, the effects are similar. If you jump out of bed, rush around, and gulp down some caffeine, you actually begin to deplete your calm energy. You throw yourself into a state that will produce increased tension and tiredness all day long.

LIFE BEGETS ENERGY. ENERGY CREATES ENERGY.
IT IS ONLY BY SPENDING ONESELF WISELY
THAT ONE BECOMES RICH IN LIFE.

—Eleanor Roosevelt (1884–1962), former U.S. first lady

Here's how it happens: From the moment that you get out of bed, your brain cues your body's metabolism to match your current and anticipated physical demands. If your mind and body experience a rude or slow-motion awakening without any signals to suggest it's going to be a calm, invigorating, and productive day, you put yourself on a kind of red alert. You start producing all the hormones associated with tense energy, and that production doesn't quit. Ironically, you also diminish your true energy level by trying to conserve energy for some vague yet impending emergency that you may be required to face later on. This is an ancient biological instinct, and it's counterproductive to high-energy living in today's world.

Energy Settings

Amazingly, researchers can predict how much energy someone will likely have in late afternoon and evening by measuring that person's behavior patterns in the morning. You essentially make a choice for your entire day by the way you get up in the morning and by what you do—or don't do—in the first hour or so after rising. In a sense, your metabolism adjusts itself for the day, trying to anticipate how much energy and what kinds of energy will be needed.

With Calm-Energy Switch #1, you can get out of that early-morning sleepwalking mode and start your day in an entirely different way. Here are the five key elements of an effective wake-up call to your metabolism that will prime your day for calm energy.

1. Awaken with a positive response to the upcoming day.

2. Rise slowly and get up on the right side of bed.

3. Get some extra light.

4. Ease your way into at least 5 minutes of relaxed physical activity.

5. Enjoy a convenient, great-tasting breakfast.

According to scientists, by starting your morning this way you move your natural biological rhythms toward faster metabolism and better health. You'll tend to sleep better at night and have even more energy the next day.

These five steps are also fat-burning tactics. Research suggests that there's a significant link between the creation of calm energy and the fat burning that is associated with weight loss. When you take these steps to achieve calm energy, you're not only setting your energy switch for the entire day but also taking steps that will reap benefits for your health and self-esteem. I begin here, with these simple steps, because they truly set the stage for beginning to feel 100 percent alive.

1. Awaken with a Positive Response to the Upcoming Day

Few people realize that they may lose many of the benefits of deep sleep whenever they try to wake up at the last possible moment and dive into their day in a tense rush, with their minds immersed in anticipating problems and pressures. This abrupt awakening takes a toll on their bodies, emotions, and minds—and the effect can last most of the morning.

If you wake up to an alarm, it's important to realize that pleasing music can get the job done yet is much more invigorating and relaxing than the traditional alarm, say researchers. Jarring noises shock your system, and most popular alarm clocks are equipped with beepers or buzzers that are meant to awaken even the most stubbornly resistant sleeper. Remember, even when you awake to music, keep the volume no higher than needed.

The first few minutes after awakening are the start of your warmup for an active day. Think of things that you're looking forward to, not dreading. Imagine yourself at your best, having fun and getting many of the right things accomplished. This initial impression of what's ahead really matters to your energy level. Your metabolism is waiting for these signals. And by easing out of sleep, you retain more of the invigorating power of that sleep. You awaken more rested and resilient as well as calm and resourceful, not rushed and anxious.

2. Rise Slowly and Get Up on the Right Side of Bed

Take a few moments to enjoy not moving and not rushing. Blink your eyes. Take several deep, relaxing breaths. Notice every spot of tension in your body and release it before getting up. Otherwise, you're adding tension on top of tension and blocking calm energy. Open and close your hands. Loosen your shoulders and release any tension in your jaw and shoulders. Slowly stretch your neck and arch your back.

Then, use these wake-up movements to start your day with calm energy.

- Breathe in energy, breathe out tension.
- Move slowly, and let every muscle awaken without strain.
- Imagine the day brightening as you slowly get out of bed.
- Step to a window that is filled with light and the best view that you can find. Soak it in.
- Look forward to some easy, enjoyable activity, such as a brief walk in

(continued on page 37)

TRY THIS NOW!

When we awaken first thing in the morning, most of us fail to notice that we're tense. Your muscles may be sending your brain the message that you're tense, but it's hard to believe. "How can I feel tense," your brain argues, "when I've just had a full night's sleep?"

During the night, you experience various levels of sleep. During deep sleep, called REM sleep, you may be completely relaxed. But toward morning, your sleep becomes lighter. Thoughts and worries about the day begin to intrude, creating tension even before you're fully awake.

Even if you try to wish away your tension, that doesn't help to relieve it. If you just leap out of bed, your first action of the day produces even more tension. Subsequent activities may leave you increasingly tired. Eventually, since you're not doing anything to relieve tension, your muscles stop conveying the tension alarm to your brain. The tension stays, but you scarcely notice it.

To increase calm energy, it's vital to tune your senses to become much more aware of tension—and then to release it on the spot, whenever it appears. And your first chance to do that is first thing in the morning.

A method called one-touch relaxation is one of the simplest ways to defuse tense energy and increase calm energy, anywhere, anytime. Relaxation is elicited through key muscles that, under gentle fingertip pressure, trigger a cascade effect that quickly dissolves tension throughout the body. This concept has been explored by Vernon H. Mark, M.D., a neurosurgeon at Massachusetts General Hospital in Boston and coauthor of *Brain Power: A Neurosurgeon's Complete Program to Maintain and Enhance Brain Fitness throughout Your Life*.

Here's How

I recommend doing one-touch relaxation first thing in the morning, while you're still lying in bed. But you can also use it any time during the day. Here are the steps.

1. Press your fingertips on your jaw joints, just in front of your ears.
2. Inhale. As you inhale, tense your jaw muscles, bringing your upper and lower jaws together, which will feel like you're clenching your teeth. Hold this clench for several seconds.
3. Exhale. As you exhale, let your jaw muscles go totally loose, releasing all tension. Let your lower jaw drop, and relax your tongue.

As you do this exercise, focus on what it feels like. Feel the contrast between the sensation of tension and the sensation of relaxation.

Repeat the exercise, but this time, tighten your jaw muscles half as much. Hold for several seconds, then release. Do two more repetitions, reducing the tension each time—one-fourth the original tension, then one-eighth. With each repetition, hold the tension for the same amount of time. You'll find that when you're using only one-eighth as much tension, you can hardly discern the difference between clenching and unclenching.

Then, try it one final time, without any tension at all.

1. Take a deep breath. As you do, press your fingertips against your jaw just once.
2. Exhale, relaxing your jaw muscles completely so you feel your jaw slacken.
3. Let your tongue release tension. Let it settle into the bottom of your mouth, with the tip lightly touching your lower front teeth.

(continued)

4. As you do this, imagine that you're breathing out all of the tightness in your body. Put aside all of your duties and emotional burdens, completely eliminating all of the *shoulds* in your life.

What you're doing is using touch to set a sensory cue for relaxation. As soon as you feel your fingertips pressing on your jaw muscles, you have the highly desirable sensation of releasing tension. The process is triggered by your touch and the accompanying mental command to relax.

Once you've practiced this technique with your jaw muscles, you'll find that you can elicit a similar response anywhere on your body. If your shoulders are often tense, for instance, here's how to get a similar relaxation response.

1. Inhale, lifting your shoulders toward your ears. Touch one shoulder with your fingertips.
2. Exhale, relaxing all of the muscles in your neck, down your shoulders, and across your chest and upper back.
3. As your upper body relaxes, breathe away stiffness and inner pressures.
4. Repeat, reducing the tension each time, until you get an instant release as soon as you touch a shoulder with your fingertips.

Once you've practiced using these exercises for your jaw and shoulder muscles, you can apply the same techniques to any other areas of your body that tend to stiffen up when you're sleeping or when you feel stress mounting during the day. For instance, you may want to apply this quick release to your lower back or abdomen. With some practice, you'll be able to use a single touch to trigger an immediate wave of relaxation through the area that needs release. You get such an instantaneous payoff because you elicit a powerful calming and energizing response from your brain.

the morning air or some relaxed stairclimbing or simply a 5-minute tour of your favorite spots in the house.

- Think of a light meal that would taste great this morning—and prepare to enjoy it.
- Feel yourself gathering your best energy to meet the day ahead.

Think some invigorating thoughts about the great things that could happen today. Remind yourself of the reasons that you're getting out of bed, such as to provide for your loved ones, to keep learning, and to make more of a difference in the world, not just to make a living. This is something that we all too often forget about in our rush to get moving.

When you get out of bed, do it slowly and smoothly, giving your muscles a chance to ease into action. They'll stay loose and limber.

Done together, these early-morning actions generate calm energy.

3. Get Some Extra Light

On sunny mornings, do you step outside for a breath of fresh air? Do you take a moment to soak in the brightness?

This may seem like a luxury that you can't afford. But if you don't get light, you're missing a wake-up call that can be far more effective than a morning cup of coffee.

There is a neurological link between the retina of the eye and a small area of the brain known as the suprachiasmatic nucleus, according to professors Richard Kronauer, Ph.D., and Charles Czeisler, M.D. The suprachiasmatic nucleus, they believe, plays a key role in helping us to focus our attention. In a 3-year study conducted at Harvard University, Dr. Kronauer and Dr. Czeisler were able to link the impact of light on the retina to better attention focus and energy production in the brain. The study used light with an intensity between 7,000 and 12,000 lux, which is comparable to daylight just after dawn.

Other studies have shown that the body has hundreds of biochemical and hormonal rhythms, all keyed to light and dark, and that the human brain is powerfully affected when the body is exposed to bright light.

Even if you wake before dawn, you can send a wake-up call to your brain just by switching on more lights. When you get out of bed tomorrow morning, switch on every available light—from your nightstand lamp and overhead bedroom light to lights in the hall, bathroom, and kitchen. Leave these lights on for at least the first 15 minutes after you get up.

If the sun is up, step outside for a minute or so to flood your eyes with daylight. Feel the difference in energy, which can readily grow and last. For many people, the added light boosts mood and triggers an instantaneous alertness signal in their brains. This is the phenomenon that Dr. Kronauer and Dr. Czeisler noted in their study. Bright morning daylight is far more intense than indoor lighting, and with exposure to it, your whole physiology changes. You turn away from sleep. Your body prepares for a new day filled with more calm energy and higher metabolism.

4. Ease Your Way Into at Least 5 Minutes of Relaxed Physical Activity

Morning exercise may not appear to be much fun. According to national surveys, many of us prefer to remain sedentary during the morning hours. We are much more likely to exercise in the afternoon or evening, if we exercise at all. And we pay a price for this, energy-wise, all day long.

The truth is that morning activity primes your metabolism and has a fat-fighting effect. Moderate exercise in the morning, before you eat breakfast, may give you an extra boost in burning off excess body fat. After a full night's sleep, there is little glycogen—stored carbohydrate—in your muscles to supply energy. If you exercise before you eat anything, your body needs to draw on more body fat to find the fuel that it needs.

In addition, there is increasing scientific evidence that moderate exercise, even just a few minutes of it, increases calm energy and reduces tension. Whether it's before or after breakfast, light physical activity within an hour or two after awakening also helps to increase your metabolism throughout the day. Without doing something—even a limited amount of light activity such as walking around your home or yard—your metabolism stays sluggish, and you're primed for tension and tiredness, not calm energy.

Here are a few ways to ensure that regular physical activity becomes part of your morning.

Make it routine. One of the pluses of morning exercise is the way that it can easily become a habit. A study by the Southwestern Health Institute in Phoenix found that three out of four people who did some light morning exercise continued the exercise habit 1 year later. In comparison, only half of those who waited until midday to exercise were able to keep up the habit. And among those who said, "I'll do it in the evening," only one out of every four were still exercising a year after the study began.

That makes intuitive sense, doesn't it? If you don't rev up your metabolism and increase calm energy early in the day, it's probably easier to make excuses as your busy day sails forward and your tension levels rise. Not surprisingly, one excuse is likely to be "I'm too tired."

But even if the will is there, what's the way? How can you fit 5 minutes of morning exercise into your schedule? If, like so many people, you feel like you're a slow riser, how can you get enthused about doing exercise early in the morning?

Well, for one thing, that feeling of morning sluggishness may be directly related to tense energy. As you get used to morning exercise, you'll

TRY THIS NOW!

As little as a minute or so of light physical activity sends an immediate and powerful signal to your brain to reduce tension and increase alertness and calm energy, according to researcher Martin Moore-Ede, M.D., Ph.D., associate professor of physiology and director of the Institute for Circadian Physiology at Harvard Medical School. "Taking a walk or stretching can stimulate your level of alertness," says Dr. Moore-Ede.

Here's How

You don't have to travel far to verify Dr. Moore-Ede's observations. In fact, you can demonstrate the principles of exercise-induced alertness right now. Wherever you are, you can generate some very light physical movements.

1. Stretch your arms and back.
2. Extend your legs, then relax them.
3. Shake your arms, letting your wrists hang loosely so that your hands feel nerveless and floppy.
4. Do the same with your feet, shaking your legs one at a time so that your ankles wobble freely and your feet feel loose.

find that it's easier to do because you'll notice immediate rewards of more calm energy. Once you start to release tension and increase your level of calm energy, you'll feel very different in the morning.

But don't start off with unrealistic expectations that you'll leap out of bed and eagerly begin morning exercise. You're probably going to do it a lot more comfortably if you *slowly* get out of bed, get dressed, and then *gradually* increase your activity level.

5. Gently rotate your neck and shoulders.

6. Take several relaxed breaths.

As simple as they are, these exercises teach a quick lesson about movement, if you just become aware of your body's responses. Every half-hour or so throughout the day, your brain and senses expect you to shift position and release tension by becoming more physically active without straining or becoming tense. In other words, this is easy, natural motion, not formal exercise. You satisfy that expectation—and set the right pattern for the rest of the day—if you do some simple, enjoyable, light activity as soon as you get out of bed.

It's important to try these techniques. Millions of us have unwittingly taught ourselves to work in fixed positions, almost statuelike and immobile. Yet we pay a huge price for immobility. It leads to lower metabolism—that is, less energy burning—which in turn contributes to weight gain and its many associated health problems. Your brain and senses await your signals. In a sense, you're the conductor of an orchestra. If you want your body to play, you have to raise the baton and give the signal.

Get your togs ready. You can make morning exercise easier if you plan ahead. Lay out some comfortable physical-activity clothes the night before. Simply seeing them beside your bed in the morning may help remind you—and inspire you—to get up and get moving. That's especially important if you plan to go out for a morning stroll. Having the clothes right there at your bedside will eliminate the getting-dressed issue.

In comfortable clothes, before or after eating breakfast, go through a gentle warmup routine. Then, do a few minutes of light physical activity such as taking an easy stroll or slowly climbing and descending a few flights of stairs. If you have home exercise equipment, you can listen to music or the morning news as you pedal a stationary bike at a relaxed, moderate pace; take some smooth, balanced steps on your stairclimber; or do some strokes on a rowing machine.

For variety, you can do some moderate strengthening or abdominal-toning exercises. I think that you may soon enjoy this active time so much that on some days it will stretch into 10 or even 20 minutes.

5. Enjoy a Convenient, Great-Tasting Breakfast

Don't skip breakfast. Of all the foods that you'll eat throughout day, these first bites are the ones that matter most.

In a surprising number of ways, your breakfast is a turning point. What happens to your energy in the hours that follow breakfast will depend on what you eat before you head off to work or get started on the day's chores. When you eat a low-fat, high-fiber breakfast—even a small serving—you switch on and turn up your calm energy.

Even if you are in a hurry, you can grab a good-tasting morning meal on the run. It really doesn't take much—say, a bowl of old-fashioned oatmeal with 1%, 2%, or fat-free milk and a piece of fruit. Or try a slice of whole-grain bread with low-fat cream cheese and all-fruit preserves.

When that food reaches your stomach, it triggers responses in your brain and senses. With the extra supply of energy, a transformation takes place. There's a shift in messenger chemicals known as neurotransmitters that influence your brain and are essential to alertness and energy.

According to research, breakfast eaters are usually leaner than those who skip breakfast. They have an easier time maintaining their ideal

IT IS ENERGY THAT PRODUCES

THE MIRACLE OF ENTHUSIASM AND WILL DO ANYTHING

THAT CAN BE DONE IN THIS WORLD.

—Johann von Goethe (1749–1832), German poet and philosopher

weights and sticking to healthful, balanced diets. In addition, they have lower blood pressures, show less irritability and fatigue, and demonstrate a more positive attitude during difficult times. If you eat breakfast, studies show, you're more alert and you perform better at work. (The same goes for kids: Those who eat breakfast tend to be alert, high performers at school.) You're also better able to maintain balanced blood sugar and have a greater sense of energy and strength.

Food First

"We can't overstress the importance of the morning meal," say Peter D. Vash, M.D., an endocrinologist and internist at the University of California, Los Angeles, Medical Center who specializes in obesity and eating disorders; and dietitians Cris Carlin and Victoria Zak. "When you wake up and get started on a new day, you must have breakfast to turn on your thermic switch, moving your body's rhythm from low ebb to high tide." According to these researchers, the thermic switch is what turns on your crucial ability to burn fat and produce energy, two of the body processes that are essential for lasting calm energy.

When you eat a breakfast that is rich in carbohydrate, protein, and fiber, you stimulate your sympathetic nervous system, that is, the neurons that cause important energy functions to happen automatically. That stimulation revs up hormones and neurotransmitters in your brain. In fact, the right kind of low-fat breakfast may help boost your calm energy for your entire day. As we'll see in part 3, low-fat, high-protein food also sets the rates for another kind of energy, active energy.

To get the most from your breakfast, the key is to choose carefully. A high-fat breakfast won't do the job. If you have scrambled eggs with sausage, instant oatmeal with whole milk, or buttered white toast with jelly, you invite a very different kind of body response. Instead of stimulating the sympathetic nervous system, you trigger the processes that generate fat and produce fatigue and tension.

No More Skipping

Your early-morning need for quality, low-fat protein can be fulfilled by pouring low-fat or fat-free milk on cereal or drinking a glass of it. Or you can eat some low-fat cottage cheese, nonfat yogurt, or nonfat cream cheese. For dietary fiber, the optimum sources are whole-grain bread and cereal.

And if you skip breakfast? It's an insidious way to cheat yourself of calm energy—insidious because the damage may not register until late afternoon or evening. Those are the times when people who skip breakfast are most likely to gorge on high-fat or high-sugar foods, according to research by Sarah F. Leibowitz, Ph.D., of the Rockefeller University in New York City. The reason, Dr. Leibowitz says, is that your body experiences an exaggerated increase in neuropeptide Y, a brain chemical associated with tension and cravings. Those cravings may be delayed, but by the end of the day, you're likely to turn to high-fat or high-sugar foods in response to neuropeptide Y.

Another compelling argument for the low-fat, high-fiber, high-protein breakfast comes from Lawrence E. Lamb, M.D., a national medical

The Weight-Loss Benefit

While the right kind of breakfast is an important first step toward calm energy, it will also provide weight-loss benefits. When your breakfast is low in fat and contains a moderate amount of metabolism-boosting protein and plenty of fiber-rich complex carbohydrates, studies suggest, you're less likely to overeat or eat high-fat foods at lunch. You're also less likely to reach for impulsive, high-fat snacks. "Skipping a meal leads to hunger-related tension and binging," observes Kathy Stone, R.D., president of Strictly Nutrition, a dietetic consulting firm.

"Eating breakfast is also essential to help control eating after dinner. Surprising, but true," says Stone. What you eat in the morning affects how full you feel at the end of the day, she says. Many people, she notes, skip breakfast almost as a way to test their willpower. They figure that if they go as long as possible without eating, they'll be better off.

But people who skip breakfast often overeat later on, Stone points out. "If you think you are actually better off on the days when you go as long as possible without eating, think again," she says. "What happens when you finally start eating? Most times, you lose control."

columnist. In the morning, notes Dr. Lamb, your liver is about 75 percent depleted of glycogen, the energy fuel that is derived from blood sugar and that you need for any kind of sustained energy. When there's a shortfall of glycogen, your liver begins making glucose to help sustain your energy. It uses your body protein to manufacture that much needed glucose. But you need that body protein, especially muscle tissue. To make sure that it isn't sacrificed during your morning activities, you had better eat some carbohydrate food for breakfast to replace that glucose. "Your brain will function better, too," notes Dr. Lamb. "It needs that glucose to maintain its ability to do all the complex tasks required of it."

A New Routine for Breakfast Skippers

If you routinely skip breakfast, changing that habit can prove to be a challenge. But there are a number of easy ways to meet that challenge. Here are some tactics.

Answer to hunger. Do you wake up with no morning appetite? Maybe it's because you've learned to override your morning body clock.

Whole-Grain English Muffin Cheese Melt

1   whole-wheat or multi-grain English muffin, halved

1   slice low-fat cheese (such as Swiss, Cheddar, or mozzarella), halved

Place ½ slice cheese on each half of the English muffin. Microwave on high for 30 seconds or until melted.

Fruit Smoothy

¾   cup unsweetened frozen fruit, such as bananas or peaches

¼   cup unsweetened frozen berries

½   cup plain nonfat or low-fat yogurt or soy yogurt

½   cup fat-free milk or low-fat soy milk

Dash of cinnamon

In a blender or food processor, combine the fruit, berries, yogurt, milk, and cinnamon. Blend until smooth.

However, once you reestablish your normal, healthy metabolic routine and a higher level of calm energy, you'll begin to feel some natural hunger pangs when you climb out of bed. That's a good thing.

If you've long avoided a morning meal, begin simply. You might have a piece of ripe fruit—an apple, banana, orange, or half a grapefruit, for example. Have some whole-grain toast or a whole-grain bagel with nonfat cream cheese on top, and a cup of tea or coffee. On some mornings, you may enjoy mixing whole-grain cereal with a 4-ounce serving of nonfat or low-fat yogurt.

Sit with the family. Can you make breakfast a time for family connection? Most of us crave added time and attention from loved ones, but we keep rushing through those moments that we could be spending with them. Here's the antidote: Begin a breakfast partnership. Share your healthy breakfast with your spouse or children, with a few minutes in the morning to talk about the day ahead. With friends or coworkers, you can meet to eat. Stop on the way to work or school; meet in a park; or visit each other's houses first thing in the morning. Make the first meal of the day more fun and interesting—and get closer to the people about whom you care most.

Munch as you cruise. Many breakfast foods are easy to take along with you. Stock up on those, and your breakfast can be part of your morning commute. If you add some frozen berries and a handful of nonfat whole-oat granola to a cup of nonfat plain yogurt, you have a complete combination of fiber and protein. Take advantage of red lights or traffic jams to dip into that morning meal.

Of course, if you have a long drive with few stops, it's easier to eat bread or bagels than a carton of yogurt. Spread some nonfat or low-fat cream cheese on a slice of fresh whole-grain wheat or rye bread. Or have a pumpernickel bagel with or without the cream cheese. Other options include a container of fresh orange juice, hot tea with fat-free milk, or a nonfat, whole-oat granola bar.

Savor the ultimate energy breakfast. One of the world's best-known natural-healing medical facilities is the Bircher-Benner Clinic in Zurich, Switzerland. The atmosphere there is invigorating, and so are the meals. One of the pillars of the Bircher-Benner energy-building regimen is a cereal adapted from a morning meal that has long been favored by European mountain people. This cereal, called muesli, is easy to make and very satisfying. Old-fashioned oats are soaked overnight, instead of being cooked, and are served with just-ripe fruit and nonfat or low-fat yogurt.

The night before, put ½ cup of old-fashioned slow-cooking oats in a bowl and pour on just enough water to cover them. Cover the bowl, place it in the refrigerator, and let the oats soak overnight. When you're ready for your high-energy breakfast in the morning, take the bowl out of the fridge and stir in 1 cup of nonfat or low-fat plain or vanilla yogurt, 1 to 2 teaspoons of brown sugar, and pieces of just-ripe fruit such as apples, bananas, oranges, or berries. Add cinnamon, vanilla, or other flavorings to taste, depending on your preferences.

You can make all sorts of variations on the muesli recipe. It's up to you. You can use canned, unsweetened fruit instead of fresh fruit. You can also add fresh strawberries, fresh kiwifruit, or lemon-flavored yogurt. Sometimes, my family likes to add a teaspoon of ground almonds, cashews, or hazelnuts; sunflower seeds; dried tart cherries; raisins; or currants. For sweetness, try a teaspoon of honey or maple syrup.

Find Instant Calmness

Most of us are accustomed to viewing tension as inevitable. It is not. With few exceptions, tension and tiredness don't come upon us by accident or seizure; instead, they build slowly and insidiously in response to what we do and don't do throughout the day. By evening, millions of us feel depleted and exhausted by life's demands.

After days, weeks, or months of feeling this way, you may begin to believe that there's no alternative. But there is.

The early-morning habits that turn on Calm-Energy Switch #1 will start your day off right. But how do you sustain calm energy as the day *really* begins and you face one tension-creating situation after another?

The key is to become aware of tension, distraction, and fatigue the moment that they appear. Then, you learn to release them on the spot, using some of the techniques that you'll find in this chapter. Don't tell yourself that you can wait until later, when you will have time to "relax." You may have to wait for hours, which will likely be too late. By then, all those stress-causing forces could be too monstrous to deal with, or you'll be too uptight or numb to be effective.

Often, the day's tension spots come in very small doses that can sneak up on you. Even worse, when you feel tense and tired, there's a natural tendency for the constant flurry of daily challenges and small problems to appear magnified. Disappointments loom as disasters; helpful advice stings like criticism; and daily hassles feel like a personal curse from the Almighty.

When the Little Things Get You

When you're tense and tired, there's a greater chance that you'll get upset and distracted over trivialities that, when at your best, you could readily take in stride. It may seem like such things are too small to drive you over the edge. They are not. More people than ever before are feeling numb and rushed.

I have long appreciated the truth in this poem by Charles Bukowski called "The Shoelace":

> It's not the large things that
> Send a man to the madhouse . . .
> Not the loss of prized possessions
> But a shoelace that snaps
> With no time left . . .

We are faced with a mounting wave of stimuli, not just in our rushing everyday world of responsibilities and work but also in the withering barrage of messages and distractions. With answering machines, cell phones, and pagers, along with incoming messages that many of us get from regular mail and e-mail, it may seem impossible to escape the constant reminders of commitments and obligations. With the distractions of TV and the Internet, it all adds up to overload.

In frustration, people sometimes exclaim, "That's it!" and pursue elab-

MOST PEOPLE PURSUE SUCCESS AND
HAPPINESS **WITH SUCH BREATHLESS HASTE**
THAT THEY HURRY RIGHT PAST THEM.

—Søren Kierkegaard (1813–1855), Danish philosopher and theologian

orate and time-consuming "cures" to release all the tense energy that's pent up inside them. But, as we all know, heavy drinking, overeating, and vegging out in front of the TV are not really cures. And even quick getaway vacations are not a lasting solution for tense energy if we come back to find that our messages and missed appointments have accumulated to gigantic proportions while we were away. If we want to tame tense tiredness, we have to do it daily, even hourly, using preventive measures that stop it from building rather than relying on day-after reactions that add up to too little, too late.

Recognizing Tense Tiredness

Tense tiredness has many manifestations. It may express itself in the form of a headache, a stomachache, or a tight neck and shoulders. Some people wear tense tiredness on their faces or in their voices: You can see it in their expressions or hear it in their words. Or you find that they express their tense tiredness in brief, unpredictable bursts of irritability.

No matter what situation you face, you're less able to cope with it and put it in perspective when you're consumed with tense tiredness. One troublesome symptom of excessive mental stress and tension is a distortion of your sense of time. This distortion can result in extraordinary pressures—the feeling that time is running out or that there's no time to lose or similar feelings of extreme urgency.

Larry Dossey, M.D., an internist and the author of *Meaning and Medicine: A Doctor's Tales of Breakthrough and Healing,* has treated many executives who experience mental stress—what is sometimes called hurry sickness. His diagnosis begins with asking the patient to rest quietly in a chair and say when he or she thinks a minute is up. It's a simple but telling way to understand the person's concept of time. Some of these executives think the minute is up when only 30 to 40 seconds have passed. For many, the "minute" is much less. According to Dr. Dossey, the record was set by a manager of Electronic Data Systems, the famously hard-driving organization founded by H. Ross Perot. The manager said, "Now," after only 9 seconds.

Costs of Frustration

The truth is, many of us waste enormous amounts of energy reacting automatically and unconsciously to even the most minor delays, with thoughts such as "There's never enough time" and "What else can go wrong today?" If you notice that you have these feelings of time frustration day after day, it may be an early warning sign that your burden of stress and tension has reached an intense and potentially harmful level.

That sort of time distortion can easily express itself by hurting your health. Numerous studies show that prolonged or increased stress may raise your risk of physical problems such as high blood pressure and heart disease as well as emotional conditions including anxiety and depression. At the very least, stress may cause aches and pains or induce ongoing fatigue. All of these are also signs of tense tiredness.

Of course, there are many stopgap measures that you can use to mask tense tiredness or temporarily relieve it. If you tend to get tension headaches, perhaps you take over-the-counter painkillers for relief. If you

The Foundation of Quick Relief

Recent medical discoveries have shown that minor, daily mood fluctuations are associated with immune functioning.

Tense, anxious moments essentially pile up, creating a long-term impact on our health as well as our attitudes. Without a way to neutralize the pressures that accumulate, both health and performance suffer. When mishandled, the chronic, unavoidable small stresses of everyday life may accelerate aging, according to research done by experts at Wake Forest University School of Medicine in Winston-Salem, North Carolina.

One of the principal dilemmas with many of the popular calmness-oriented programs, including biofeedback, relaxation training, and passive meditation, is not only that they are time-consuming but also that they have a lack of transference. That is, techniques that may work well when you're alone in a quiet meditation room or doctor's office are extremely difficult to apply to situations in the real world. It seems all but impossible to calm down when you're hit with problem after problem all day and you just can't take time out to go relax or meditate.

According to neuroscientists, one of the most effective ways to master pressure-filled situations is to learn how to respond immediately to signals that you're getting tense or tired. Chemical and hormonal changes in your brain and body can tighten muscles and unleash negative emotions so quickly that it's much more difficult and time-consuming to reverse tension or tiredness once they've occurred. You're far better off, say neuroscientists, if you can catch the first stimuli or signals of mounting tension and trigger an immediate control response.

like to exercise, you may try to push tension away with an extensive exercise program. Or maybe you wait until you're at home and you can crawl into your bed or put your feet up in a comfortable chair and turn on some music. All of these measures may help. But they don't get to the *source* of tense tiredness, which is rooted in the buildup of dozens of stressful moments all day long.

So what's the alternative?

The Instant-Calming Sequence

More than 15 years ago, I began some pioneering research on a calm-energy strategy that I called the instant-calming sequence, or ICS for short. It received praise from a number of scientists and performance psychologists and was immediately popular with individuals and groups around the world. Over the years, I have made further revisions as I have continued to explore its effectiveness and application.

Small frustrations can take a big toll, and recent scientific research has shown us just how great that toll really is. At first glance, the irritations of everyday life may seem fairly minor. We all encounter little annoyances; we all have our moments of tension or anger.

During the typical day, we're faced with delays, interruptions, disappointments, and feelings of frustration. People break appointments. The phone rings insistently when we're least inclined to answer it. Financial worries crowd into our thoughts. Not to mention the myriad other annoyances we encounter, ranging from bad weather and traffic jams to the deadlines set by spouses, family members, employers, or ourselves.

How we handle these challenges, researchers have found, is often a far better predictor of psychological and physical health than is our reaction to major life crises. That may seem counterintuitive because we often think of the big pressures as the real test of our mettle.

Facing the Music

What about the challenges of facing final exams, getting married, getting divorced, or changing jobs? What about the birth of children or the numerous crises that they—and we, with them—encounter when they're clambering up the rungs of adolescence toward adulthood? Or what about the illnesses and deaths of friends and relatives? Aren't those the really big challenges that overload us with stress?

Almost miraculously, we almost always find the inner resources to face these challenges—and we develop confidence in our ability to do so. But daily life poses another challenge, exacts another toll. We need a different set of inner resources—essentially, a modified tool kit—to handle the quiet frustrations that creep into everyday life.

In day-to-day living, the smallest delays and interruptions can be the most annoying. What exacts the greatest toll? That varies from one individual to another. But one thing we know for sure is that daily hassles can't be ignored. And while we can't change the nature of those hassles very much, we can alter the way in which we respond to them.

The ICS is a way to instantly deal with stressful moments before they mount to their natural, debilitating conclusion, tense tiredness. The ICS stops negative effects of stress and helps you stay in control of your thoughts, feelings, and actions whenever you're under pressure. This simple five-step technique can produce exceptional inner calmness over your mind, emotions, and body whenever peak stress situations occur. The ICS can help you take a higher vantage point and avoid anguishing over life's many hassles and unexpected challenges. It can provide a buffer against worry and guilt while preserving more of your best physical and mental capabilities in the present moment.

The Step-by-Step Approach

Research supports the benefits of each of the ICS steps. The instant and automatic stress-management concept has been verified through successful results in behavioral workshops with thousands of participants, and it is endorsed by experts in the United States and Europe.

The beauty of the ICS is that you don't wait for tension to grow to the point where it's a monstrous force. Instead, you use a simple sequence, a clear, brief series of well-defined actions, to release tension as soon as you sense it and before it builds momentum.

What's the best way to test the instant-calming sequence? I encourage you to simply try it. When I've taught it to business leaders and members of their families as well, they've been able to use it immediately in their jobs and homes. These are people who are dealing every day with events and schedules and impending crises that would be insurmountable without an effective coping mechanism. In fact, my own family members and I use it every day. We've found that it can nip tension in the bud.

Clearing the Air

The ICS is effective whenever you don't want frustrations or distractions to cloud your thinking, lower your mood, or interfere with your actions. No matter what pressures you face, whether they're major out-in-the-open crises and performance challenges or quiet, nagging self-doubts that worsen each time something or someone reminds you of past mistakes or present weaknesses, the ICS is a direct and simple skill that you can start using right away.

Unlike the relaxation tapes or exercise machines that are so often used to release tense energy, the ICS "removes" you from the scene for just an instant. You don't do anything that can be observed by others. Instead, you use one of the most important triggers in your brain to create a split-second response that results in calm energy.

Here are the five steps.

1. Continue breathing.
2. Lighten your eyes.
3. Release tension.
4. Notice uniqueness.
5. Call upon your best self.

At first, these five steps have to be practiced consciously, but they soon become automatic. You perform ICS while you are fully alert, with your eyes open, therefore you may use the technique unobtrusively in a wide range of circumstances. The ICS is successful whether you're standing, sitting, or moving. You can call upon this response at the first sign of irritation, tension, or anxiety.

ICS Step 1: Continue Breathing

When you are tense and tired, your breathing tends to become shallow and intermittent. Each time stress levels rise, most people tend to halt their breathing, if only for a few seconds. This creates a ripple effect of tension and anxiety. Small problems loom up as insurmountable and distressing obstacles. Slight delays can feel interminable.

When most of us think of breathing, we think of our lungs filling with air. But there's more to it than that. Breathing can be difficult or easy.

There's a rhythm to it, and that rhythm, as we know, can be fast or slow. Breathe easily, with a steady, natural rhythm, and the result is a steady consumption of oxygen. It's a critical process because that oxygen feeds the 100 trillion cells in your body and enables you to produce biological energy. And the *way* in which you breathe will enable to you to produce calm energy instead of tense energy.

Using the transference of oxygen from air to blood—the process that takes place in your lungs—your body produces a substance called adenosine triphosphate, or ATP. This is, quite simply, the currency of life. ATP is an enzyme that acts as a catalyst in your body's energy-production process. Think of it as a match that lights a campfire. Your body has plenty of fuel in the form of blood sugar, or glucose, but you need ATP to turn that fuel into energy that stirs your blood, moves your muscles, and helps you use your senses and brainpower. Without ATP, there is no physiological energy. It is ATP that you utilize to act, think, and feel.

Your body and brain are extremely sensitive to even very small reductions in ATP production. When there's a shortage of ATP, your body's reaction is expressed in terms of aches, pains, confusion, intermittent fatigue, and greater susceptibility to infection.

All of these sensitive reactions are initiated by the fundamental act of breathing. Breathing well is one of the most important things that you can do to improve your life. That's why the first step of the ICS is simply *continue breathing*. That means breathing without interruption, smoothly, deeply, and evenly.

Activating Step 1

If breathing without interruption sounds easy, perhaps you haven't paid close attention to what happens to you when you're suddenly frightened, alarmed, or under a lot of stress. The next time you hit a snag in your

TRY THIS NOW!

Research indicates that smooth, steady breathing is one of the simplest ways to activate calm energy, enabling you to experience life more fully and vigorously. It can break the grip of tension and tiredness and provide a refreshing release in the rush and roar of everyday life. Good breathing plays a vital part in expanding your capillary network and producing increased feelings of alertness and well-being.

Here's How

Right now, you can experience the calm energy that arises when you take a full, relaxed breath. Here are the guidelines.

Don't force it. As you breathe in, simply be aware of the air coming in. Feel the sensation. Does the air feel warm or cool?

Open up. On the inhalation, relax your shoulders, straighten your back, and let the air "open" your chest.

Use images. As you inhale, vividly imagine yourself drawing in vitality and strength from the air. Imagine drawing the air into every cell of your body, and imagine new light filling every corner of your mind.

Let it go. As you exhale, release every bit of tension from your thoughts and muscles.

schedule—or traffic—take a moment to notice your respiration patterns. Most of us unknowingly halt our breathing for several seconds or more during the first moments of each stressful situation. This propels us in a split-second, so fast that we scarcely notice it happening, toward feelings of anxiety, panic, anger, and frustration. The breathing interruption creates a serious domino effect. We lose our perspective and then overreact.

We feel a general sense of victimization and loss of control. And this all happens so fast that we're often not aware of where it came from.

ICS Step 2: Lighten Your Eyes

It's all but impossible to maintain a state of calm energy with a scowl on your face. Yet that's the expression that many of us wear. If we're tense, tired, rushed, and distracted, we show these feelings on our faces.

Yet when tension is visible in a person's expression, it's more than a one-way street. Ironically, the muscles of your face not only react to your mood, they help *set* it. If you tried the one-touch relaxation in Calm-Energy Switch #1 to relax your jaw, you may have noticed that your whole body became more relaxed along with your jaw muscles. Conversely, when your face or jaw is tense, within moments you feel increasing tension throughout your body. You rush ahead, numb with hurrying, with tense energy transcribed from your face to your whole being.

Often, you're not aware of your expression. Why should you be? After all, an expressive face is truly a mirror of your emotions, and you can't force yourself to adapt an impassive expression. Nor would you want to.

Activating Step 2

What you can do is use your facial expression as a means of influencing how you react. This is the key to step 2 of the ICS. A relaxed and positive, or at least neutral, expression produces a positive response of calm energy within your own body—and in others too.

One reason for the speed and power of this response is that positive reactions in your facial muscles increase bloodflow to your brain. Nerve impulses are transmitted from your face and eyes to your limbic system, a key emotional center of your brain. That's where your core perceptions of life and your immediate reactions to it are guided.

The Eyes Have It

What does it mean to "lighten your eyes"?

Just imagine the clear, attentive, and focused gaze of someone who is totally awake, relaxed, and aware. You may see that expression in the faces of people enjoying quiet music or playing a game that they enjoy.

It's easy to practice. Just look in the mirror and let your expression change. As you lighten your eyes and smile, there's actually a change in your neurochemistry. You have more favorable emotions. Research shows that these changes are powerful and swift. You can learn to flash a slight smile the moment that pressures rise or a challenge appears.

Although new science supports this interpretation of the process, the evidence that it works can be traced back thousands of years. In the martial arts and in traditional practices of meditation, practitioners wear genuinely positive or benign expressions that are a sign of attentiveness, curiosity, and concentration. It's no coincidence that the expression of contemplative wisdom is so easily recognized in many cultures.

Characterized by a slight smile and positive brightness in the eyes, that expression infuses the wearer with attentiveness and curiosity. You don't need to bubble over with happiness, joy, or even enthusiasm, for that matter. It's attentiveness that counts; and if you maintain that, along with curiosity, you can reset your entire nervous system so that you're less reactive to frustrations, pressures, tension, and fatigue. "Smile inwardly with your mouth and eyes, and say to yourself, 'Alert mind, calm body,'" advises Charles F. Stroebel, M.D., Ph.D., professor of psychiatry at the University of Connecticut School of Medicine in Farmington and author of *QR: The Quieting Reflex.*

TRY THIS NOW!

The more deeply you learn to relax, the more effective is the calming wave of the instant-calming sequence. One way to help yourself feel this wave is by using a one-word vacation. This technique will help you create an island of mental and emotional calmness that alleviates excess physical tension on the spot.

There is evidence suggesting that this brief, vivid escape will help keep you feeling younger. Even more startling, "the chemistry of billions of cells throughout your body—especially in your central nervous system—will immediately change in response to what you vividly visualize," says performance psychologist James E. Loehr, Ed.D.

Here's How

The objective of a one-word vacation is to anchor a sense of calmness in a single word cue. The word can be any one of your choosing, as long as it has pleasant associations. It might reflect an idyllic setting such as *beach, lake, meadow, garden,* or *forest.* It might describe something visual such as *moonlight* or *starlight.* Or the word might represent a specific location with pleasant associations—*Caribbean, Hawaii,* or *my own backyard.* Whether it's a favorite getaway scene, a location that you enjoy thinking about, or some-

Lightening your expression goes along with controlling your breathing response. As you ease off the intensity in your eyes and maintain a slightly positive facial expression, the expression combined with the breathing creates calm energy. Then, you're ready for the third step in the ICS response.

thing that you've experienced in person, the word should evoke warm, positive feelings of calmness, relaxation, or support.

Once you've selected the appealing word, spend a few minutes making it more vivid. It's important to use all of your senses—to see the place in your mind's eye, hear the sounds, enjoy the pleasant smells, and experience the tastes if you can.

At first, this evocation may take real concentration. You'll have to close your eyes and visualize it intensely so that all of your senses are engaged. But as you repeat this exercise at different times and in different places, you'll find that the word itself begins to switch on all of those associations. You'll need much less time and effort to create the sensation that you're actually there, totally engaged in the experience. Before long, whenever you simply think or say the word, the feeling of being there will come over you in a moment.

The symbolic word-image is then something that you can use whenever you begin feeling signs of stress. It immediately releases the pressure grip of a tense situation. It takes only a moment to evoke the mood and sensations that give you instant release; and after that, you're free to move forward, invigorated with a refreshed emotional and mental attitude.

ICS Step 3: Release Tension

Frequently, we react to sudden rises in everyday pressure with a posture that's known as somatic retraction. In this posture, your chest is collapsed, with your shoulders rolled forward and down. Your abdomen, back, and neck are tensed.

In some people, the somatic retraction is obvious. These people almost double over toward the floor. In others, the reaction may be subtle—slight shoulder movements and tensing of their necks, jaws, backs, or chests.

But whether it's obvious or subtle, somatic retraction comes with a cost. When you react this way, your breathing becomes restricted, so step 1 of the ICS is impossible. Bloodflow is reduced by as much as 30 percent, depriving your brain and senses of much-needed oxygen. Muscle tension increases, reaction time is slowed, and the somatic retraction magnifies feelings of panic and helplessness.

Step 3 of the ICS helps to prevent or counteract that response to stress.

Activating Step 3

First, you need to balance your posture. The key is to keep your posture buoyant and upright; don't let it become tense or collapse even slightly. You should feel as if an imaginary hook were gently lifting your whole spinal column upward from a central point on top of your head. Keep your head up, with your neck long, your chin slightly tucked in, and your jaw and tongue relaxed. Lift your chest so it feels open, as if it were floating upward. Extend your shoulders to their full expanse so they feel broad and loose. Keep your pelvis and hips level and your back comfortably straight, with your abdomen free of tension.

With balanced posture, you have an exhilarating sense that movement takes no effort at all. You should feel as if you were moving buoyantly and comfortably in space.

Next, perform a split-second tension check. To locate tension, scan all your muscles, from your scalp, jaw, tongue, and face to your fingertips and toes, in one fast sweep of your mind.

Finally, flash a mental wave of relaxation throughout your entire body.

WE MUST NOT JUST PATCH AND TINKER WITH LIFE.
WE MUST KEEP RENEWING IT.
EMBRACE NOVELTY AND UNIQUENESS.

—William James, *Pragmatism*, 1907

You should feel as if you were standing under a waterfall that washes away all unnecessary physical tension. Keep your mind fully alert, your senses engaged, and your body calm while the tension evaporates.

ICS Step 4: Notice Uniqueness

Imagine what it would be like to find a devilish knot in your shoelaces every morning. The first morning, you might muster the patience to calmly untie the knot. You'd surely think to yourself, "I'm going to make sure this doesn't happen again." But what if the knot reappeared the next morning? And the morning after that?

It would surely replace calm energy with tension and frustration. And unless you were truly blessed with the patience of Job, your frustration would increase every morning, until you were ready to trash those annoying shoes and tangle-prone laces.

Needless to say, a lot of us face the same old tangled shoelaces of life time and again. Patterns start to feel old. Didn't we solve that problem yesterday? Didn't this person have the same issue last week? Not surprisingly, when the tangle appears again, frustration can flash to the boiling point. We're likely to overreact, lash out at others, or feel victimized.

"Not again," we think. Or, "He's *always* doing that!" The pattern seems familiar—and so does the outcome.

Of course, we know that we can't throw people or problems on the trash heap, which means that, in order to bypass frustration, we need to come up with a different way of thinking about these seemingly repetitive problems. That method is what John L. Horn and Raymond Cattell, professors at the University of Southern California in Los Angeles, have called fluid intelligence.

According to Horn and Cattell, there's a clear and distinct difference between fluid intelligence and its opposite, which they call crystallized intelligence. Someone with fluid intelligence, they note, is capable of highly adaptable, loose, and ingenious thinking. To someone with fluid intelligence, each person is a unique individual. Each problem is an opportunity to use fresh and often innovative solutions.

Crystallized intelligence, on the other hand, is much more likely to be "frozen." To someone with crystallized intelligence, each problem seems like the same problem. Every individual is seen as being cut from the same cloth: Their uniqueness is missing, and without that, we quickly lose interest in the novelty and distinctiveness of each encounter.

Of course, we all have a tendency toward crystallized thinking because it often seems like the easiest, fastest, and most familiar way to solve problems. But there's a way to head off this natural tendency.

Activating Step 4

When I introduce people to ICS step 4 and ask them to *notice uniqueness*, they sometimes look at me in complete wonderment. Why this? They ask. Yet in practice, the process is far from abstract. The key is to focus on specific items or details that are absolutely unique to each situation, person, or challenge.

For example, wherever you are, notice precisely *where* you are. Clearly observe your environment, what's happening inside and around your space right now, how it feels. Notice the lighting, the sounds, the movement, your posture, other people. Then, within that sharpened scene, pay closer attention to exactly *what* you are thinking, feeling, saying, seeing, or hearing, and exactly *how* you are doing those things. Simply by increasing your awareness in this manner, studies indicate, you'll likely be more efficient, more directed in your actions, and less prone to tension and common mindless errors.

Take a conscious moment to identify the unique features of each challenge. No situation can be exactly the same as another, because time passes, the scene changes, and people (believe it or not) also change. Notice the differences between the present situation and whatever happened in the past, and you'll be clearer about the uniqueness of this event. Even if you're dealing with the same person or group of people, you can find out what's different today, right now, in these individuals, their lives, and the world you share with them.

The ability to recognize uniqueness can make an immediate difference in your home life as well as in your working life, according to Gerald Nadler, Ph.D., IBM chair emeritus in engineering management at the University of Southern California, and Shozo Hibino, Ph.D., professor at Chukyo University in Japan. Your brain has a lightning-fast tendency to categorize situations and render snap judgments. Essentially, you're always trying to put your problems into neat "boxes," a convenient way of attempting to solve new challenges with old solutions.

But the packaged solution is rarely, if ever, the best solution. When you face a unique situation and try to apply crystallized thinking ("It *must* be done this way!"), you're sure to be uptight when the tangle gets worse instead of better. Solving the same old problems in the same old ways gets to be immensely frustrating.

ICS Step 5: Call Upon Your Best Self

In large part, what you do with your mind and heart in the initial moment of a challenge determines the outcome. In the first split second of

Keeping Your Cool the ICS Way

The instant-calming sequence (ICS) can be a lifesaver. Not only can using the ICS to gather calm energy help you out of predicaments, it can also help prevent an escalating, high-tension reaction that might get you in serious trouble.

Let's consider a real-life situation for using the ICS. You're rushing to get to an urgent meeting and running short on time when your car breaks down on a badly lit road a few miles from your home.

It's easy to fume and curse. That's what you'd usually do, especially since you're pressed for time and your adrenaline is racing. But what if, by using the ICS, you arrived at another sequence of actions?

In the time that it would take you to swear furiously and jump out of the car, you could, instead, carry out all five steps of the ICS.

And where would that get you?

With more calmness and forethought, you might lock the car doors and turn on the emergency flashers. What if, by doing this, you were to catch the attention of an approaching car driven by a neighbor?

Without the ICS, you would have likely gotten more tense and angry by the moment, and you could have still been pounding the steering wheel in frustration, muttering, "If only. . . ." You wouldn't have turned the flashers on; the neighbor wouldn't have noticed your predicament.

Or suppose that no one were to come and you were to end up walking

a crisis, your nervous system reacts and can choose a panic-paralysis or positive-action response.

Far too many of us get caught up in bemoaning every challenge that we face. "Not another problem! Why does this always happen to me?" Or "Well, that blows the day! It's just been one disaster after another."

a mile to a nearby house to make a call for help. If you use the ICS, that walk could be brisk and easy rather than an exercise in high tension and frustration.

Or suppose that you were to have children with you. Wouldn't you set a better example if you could handle the pressure by taking the circumstances in stride? Looking back later, minor disasters can become positive and, often, humorous memories. Children learn from the way that you behave when things go wrong. Wouldn't you rather have them observe your calm actions than listen to you curse?

The ICS helps you to plan for the future as well as deal with the current "crisis" in a calm, reasoning manner. So following the experience, you would likely have the calm energy and clear-mindedness to sign up for the American Automobile Association or to get a cellular phone or both. Or you might take more care about preventive maintenance on your car.

Without the ICS, many of us end up feeling that we're the victims of circumstance. We end up blaming the whole world because we have problems, and we do little to improve our attitudes or lives.

When in doubt, ask, "Will tension and anger help me here?" The answer is almost always no. Using the ICS, you have a far better chance of staying on top of life and making the best of things during crunch times.

Or "Please, not now! I need more time or money or energy or rest or experience to prepare for this." Or "Oh, no! Why couldn't I be somewhere—anywhere—else right now?"

By wishing that the situation weren't happening, regretting that you didn't have more time to prepare, wanting to be somewhere else, or anguishing over life's unfairness, you set off a biochemical avalanche of victimizing thoughts and feelings. Without realizing it, you actually help yourself lose control and get loaded up with anxiety and frustration. When mishandled, a single stressful moment can disrupt your entire day.

If you look back at a time in your life when you reacted poorly to situations, it's usually easy to see that you could have chosen a better response during the crisis. But you would have had to remain calm and think more clearly.

Often, if you can just *call upon your best self*, the fifth step in the ICS, you can emerge from a situation with more calm energy and also with a lot more clear-mindedness. But if you want to emerge with flying colors, you need to establish that calm energy in precisely the right place: at the beginning of each high-pressure challenge or situation.

With practice, you can train your focus to put things in perspective. In the split second when your mind makes its choices, you can instantly recall what it feels like to be at your best and seek solutions instead of getting locked up with tension or worrying about problems.

One of the simple keys here is to train yourself to shift your view of time. In this way, you pay attention to what you *can* control rather than to what you *can't*. Yes, hurry when you must, but do it while recognizing why you're doing it, and remember that when you're at your best, you can move rapidly but calmly. When you do this, you'll hurry through your tasks and obligations with a lot less tension.

If you find that, as you rush ahead, your mind is making lists and compelling you to accomplish every last thing on them, remind yourself that some of it can probably wait. Move forward on the most essential points.

With this fifth and final ICS step, you make a commitment to recalling what it feels like to be at your best, and you remain open to learning new patterns rather than rely on habits that you've acquired by reacting in predictable ways. Shift your view of time, and you'll be able to pause for a moment and listen with an open mind instead of blindly responding. This step gives you a tool to resolve conflict rather than create it.

Activating Step 5

The idea in this step is to develop powerful radar that instantly scans each new situation, magnetically seeking and drawing out all your options for most effectively dealing with it. When your imagination, dread, and tense energy have already made a mountain out of a molehill, this step restores the molehill to mole size again.

Here's how to activate the fifth step.

Acknowledge reality. Sometimes, it's tempting to ignore problems, hoping that they'll simply disappear. Call it wishful thinking. It rarely works.

Instead, practice this key thought again and again: "What's happening is real, and I'm finding the best possible solution right now." This is crucial to what performance psychologists call the flow state, in which you think, feel, and respond exceptionally well, with a high level of calm energy, by avoiding the paralysis of analysis.

Recall what it feels like to be at your best. "Recall" doesn't simply mean to remember; it means to "call forward into the present" your best state of mental, emotional, and physical vigor. This helps you face pressures with the greatest calmness and effectiveness.

You can learn to instantly elicit surges of your best energy and reduce or eliminate many common anxiety reactions using a technique called anchoring. Anchoring calls forth positive physical, emotional, and mental states by linking sensory cues to feelings of competence.

"We all have within us the key to feeling stronger, more confident, more resourceful, and more successful," observe psychologists Bernie

Human beings loathe criticism.

   Did you take that as a criticism? Then you know what I mean.

   But why do we react this way? Research shows that it's because an area of the brain called the reticular activating system seems to magnify negative incoming messages and minimize positive ones. Criticisms are shouted to the higher brain centers, while compliments are merely whispered.

   Critical remarks trigger a huge number of misunderstandings and arguments and can be a major cause of tension and tiredness. But you can use the instant-calming sequence (ICS) to help you handle criticism in positive ways, turning that criticism into a benefit rather than an energy-depleting cause of anger and resentment.

Here's How

Imagine that you were being criticized right now. If you were to internalize those harsh words, they could zap your calm energy and interfere with your life.

Zilbergeld, Ph.D., and Arnold A. Lazarus, Ph.D. "By recalling and focusing on times when you were successful, you recreate the feelings of confidence, power, and accomplishment that are associated with these successes, and that helps to ensure good feelings and positive results in the present and future. Recollection of past achievements is one of the most powerful kinds of imagery available to anyone. . . . All of us have been successful and effective at something, but it's amazing how quickly we forget or minimize these experiences."

When you assemble a set of anchors that help you recall what it feels

Instead of letting that happen, pause at the first moment to use the ICS. Continue breathing, lighten your eyes, release tension, notice uniqueness, and call upon your best self. From there, ask yourself, "Is this comment coming from someone who genuinely cares about my well-being?" If the answer is yes, it's worth thinking about or talking about. If not—if this person appears to be filled with jealousy, envy, anger, tiredness, or tension, or if he just plain doesn't know you very well—express empathy instead.

"I hear what you're saying," you might respond. "It sounds like it's been a tough day for you too."

With the calm energy produced by the ICS, you can help the other person calm down. You can also better deflect barbed words aimed directly at you. Pick the moment when you want to disengage or wrap up the interaction, and end the exchange gracefully and with kindness. That gives the other person a better memory of who you are at your best and how hard it is to knock you off-balance with angry words.

like to be at your best, you can gain calm energy in a split second whenever you need a boost of confidence or strength.

Think of the strong feelings that you immediately get from vividly recalling any of your great moments. Those memories might be of experiences that you had in sports, public speaking, art, music, dating, parenting, working, traveling, or pursuing a hobby. Any peak experience is an anchor. You can choose to take greater charge of your own life by forming positive anchors.

Experts say that the most effective anchors are multisensory; that is, they involve several senses unified into a single nervous system cue that recaptures the sensation of being your best.

To create an anchor:

1. Sit in a comfortable, quiet place and take some time to relax deeply.
2. Vividly imagine yourself thinking, feeling, looking, sounding, and performing with excellence in a specific past circumstance. (Real-life experiences are best, but imaginary moments are also effective.)
3. Keep the mental picture moving in slow motion. "Summon an image of yourself at your best, a time when you were able to respond effortlessly no matter how demanding or intricate the challenge," advises one scientific report. "Recall your finest moment in every detail, using every sense. . . . Etch it into your consciousness so that you can summon it in an instant when facing a crisis."
4. Develop every aspect of the image: Were you indoors or out, in sunlight or shade, with clear skies or rain or snow? What was the temperature? Did you notice air currents? What were you wearing, and how did it feel on your skin? What could you see in all directions from the surface (hard, soft, cold, or warm) where you sat, stood, or lay? What did it smell like there? How did the muscles in your body feel? What were the sounds around you and off in the distance?
5. At the peak moment of the imagined experience, make a unique sensory signal. Choose a touch (such as your thumb against the second knuckle of your index finger with a specific amount of pressure), a mental picture (of yourself in a fluid state of confidence and control, performing at your best), and a sound (a personally meaningful word or phrase: *calm, confident, clear-minded, joyful, creative, I can handle this,* or any other choice). This combined sensory signal becomes your anchor.
6. Wait a half-hour or so and repeat the process.

TRY THIS NOW!

Some participants in one of my seminars came up with a reminder system that helps them with the instant-calming sequence (ICS). They decided to use visual symbols to remind them about using it. Since they're often on the telephone or in a work area, the best location, they decided, was somewhere right next to them.

Here's How

At any office-supply store, buy some stickers in the shape of brightly colored dots. Put one on your telephone or desktop. Whenever the phone rings, the dot should remind you to go through the ICS in the next moment before you pick up the receiver. It will help you be more calm and confident in conversations. Here are some other good locations for the dots.

• Watchband
• Computer monitor
• Television screen and remote control
• Bathroom mirror
• Car dashboard
• Wallet or checkbook cover
• Alarm clock
• Appointment calendar

In addition to placing the ICS reminders in these strategic locations, you might begin practicing the ICS before you get out of bed each morning and whenever you have to wait in line or stop for a red light. You'll find dozens of situations for using the ICS in response to daily stress cues—every single time you start to feel annoyed, anxious, tense, guilty, worried, or angry.

7. Later in the day, test your anchor. As you imagine the first sign of a stressful situation in which you'd like to recapture the "best-moment" state, initiate your anchor by firing the sensory signals—a touch, a visual image, and a cue word. When the anchor works, you will feel a quick surge of energy, inner peace, and confidence. With practice, you can make the anchor stronger.

If your anchor doesn't seem to be effective at first, you probably haven't used a vivid-enough image. Rehearse it several more times. Go back through the process of forming the anchor, increasing the richness and brilliance of the scene.

How *exactly* did your best moment look, feel, sound, smell? Sense the lighting, colors, shapes, temperatures, textures, movements, tastes, physical sensations, and feelings. Be certain that your sensory cues are unique—try modifying your anchor touch or gesture to see how that works.

For example, if you want to improve your ability to speak effectively to certain people to advance in your career, you may wish to form an anchor to help you. Sit quietly at a table, relaxing thoroughly. Place your hands on the table and use touch to re-create the sense of command that you felt when you were speaking confidently to a group. Close your eyes and imagine the faces of the people who listened closely as you communicated clearly and from the heart. Hear the sound of applause that greeted the end of your presentation. All of these sensory and imaginary cues form your anchor.

But, you may be wondering, how do you form an anchor for situations where it seems that you have no related experience? Authorities confirm that you can create anchors that build on your past best performances by creatively imagining a new personal strength and then anchoring that image.

Begin using positive anchors whenever you are faced with difficult situations. You'll be surprised at how helpful anchors can be in boosting your resourcefulness and responsiveness.

Extend your time horizon. Most of us feel a compelling sense of urgency when we're facing a crisis. It's a kind of panicked reaction. Our minds get dramatic and tell us that if we don't solve this crisis in the next few seconds or the next 5 minutes, dire things could happen.

But ask yourself how important the problem is going to be in an hour, a day, a month, or a year. If you can take the longer view, scientists have found, you are more likely to show adaptability in the face of change. And the long view also bolsters your ingenuity. Imagine, for instance, that you were facing a financial crisis. Your immediate, panicked reaction might be to sell stocks at a loss or quickly borrow money, either of which could be a mistake. With a more deliberate, ingenious, long-term view, you are more likely to come up with a long-term plan that would prevent the crisis from happening again in the future.

Here are some of the questions to ask yourself.

- What is the real problem that I'm trying to solve?
- What new learning will I get from this situation?
- How, specifically, does this fit into the greater picture of my priorities or vision?
- If I get angry or impatient, what will the consequences be in the long term?

The ICS is a simple, logical, scientifically founded skill that enhances every aspect of high-energy living. But it's not automatic. Most of us who are in the habit of overreacting to daily hassles find it challenging to break those habits. If you've had many years of practice at reacting unproductively, using the ICS may seem like a novelty. You may have to rehearse it in your own mind and then practice it a number of times before it starts to become second nature. But once you've grasped it, you'll have a much larger repertoire of responses that you can use in any situation.

Developing the ICS as an Automatic Response

How do you learn to use the ICS? You rehearse it here and there throughout the day, in slow motion, gradually increasing the speed. You can use simple cues, such as each time the telephone rings or whenever you walk to a chair to sit down or any time you answer a question. You choose to use it every day. Notice that I didn't say "try" or "hope" to use it. "Choose" means bring the skill to life right now. Here's how.

First, think back to a particularly stressful situation. Sit down, take some time to relax, and vividly imagine, in extra-slow motion, that this particular tension-producing or pressure-filled situation were just beginning to happen. Stall the stress signal right there. Then, picture yourself effortlessly, successfully going through the ICS: (1) Continue breathing, (2) lighten your eyes, (3) release tension, (4) notice uniqueness, and (5) call upon your best self.

Next, repeat the process, a little faster. Remember, the ICS is a natural, flowing sequence. You unleash it; you don't force it. Practice a number of times a day, using different stress cues and increasing the vividness of the mental images and the speed of your ICS response.

If at first you have difficulty with any of the steps, practice them one at a time until they become comfortable. If you get partway into the ICS and feel yourself starting to lose control, back the sequence up and slow things down. Be absolutely certain that you freeze the image of the stress cue at the first instant—don't let the stressful image keep rolling to the point at which you become tense or anxious.

Ongoing Training

When you can automatically apply the ICS at the first signal of pressure or tension, it makes all the difference in the world in the outcome. When rehearsing for especially intense situations, you might try lightening the image of the pressure cue (by seeing yourself move farther away from it in your mind or by dulling the vividness of the scene) until you are at ease with using the ICS to handle it.

You can begin applying the ICS to many everyday situations. How long does it take until you don't have to think about it anymore? In some cases, only a few weeks, but on average, 4 to 6 months. At that point, the ICS should become a truly automatic part of your response to stress—and then it should last for a lifetime.

Be patient with yourself, especially during the first weeks. The really tough stress challenges often require quite a bit of rehearsing before you can handle them with ease. Remember that most of us have had years of practice at strengthening the bad habits that the ICS is going to replace.

If you try the ICS for a particularly difficult challenge and happen to get impatient and revert to an old victimizing response, don't worry about it. Simply take some time later in the day to sit in a quiet place, relax deeply, and replay the beginning of the scene in slow motion in your mind, clearly seeing the ICS succeeding this time. Each time you use it, the sequence will flow more easily and become more automatic.

Flow Show: Using Fluid Intelligence

You may be wondering: If the instant-calming sequence is a five-step process, how can all of those steps occur in a fraction of second?

To demonstrate how it's possible, here's a quick, simple exercise: Blink your eyes.

Done?

If you take just a moment to try to analyze that simple exercise, I think you'll find that it's actually a multi-step process. Step 1: Read the words. Step 2: Interpret them, understanding that you're supposed to blink. Step

3: Send a message from your brain to your eyelids to make them shut quickly. Step 4: Send another message to your eyelids, telling them to open rapidly.

Of course, the blink of an eye is never as complicated as that, because you do it all in a single fluid action. That action uses a combined response that seems to happen all at once.

Messages travel fast along the fluid intelligence pathways. The speed of those signals is measured in thousandths and ten-thousandths of a second. During a single hiccup or eye blink of neurological activity, there are complex interactions and sequences in perception, attention, neuromuscular activation, and responsiveness.

Your brain can recognize the meaning of more than 100,000 words or images in less than 1 second. It takes only $\frac{1}{100}$ of a second for your eye to blink completely. At least 600 individual muscular actions can occur in a single second, and the number may be much higher, say researchers.

Of course, you've had many years and many occasions to practice blinking, and you can do it without thinking twice. The interesting thing is that some scientists believe that other skilled actions can be stored in similar ways. Essentially, you can load up with chunks of instructions instead of with single steps. These chunks "can be called up and executed by a single command," according to one scientific report. This may account for the deep relaxation and control—the flow state—felt by top musicians and athletes.

With practice, your nervous system can enact the entire ICS in a fraction of a second. Like a musician learning a symphony for the first time, you may have to go through repetitions of each of the steps, slowly at first, then gathering speed as the steps become more familiar. With repetition, you'll find that the steps aren't really steps anymore: One flows into the next, and they happen in such rapid sequence that the ICS comes to you as naturally as blinking your eyes.

You'll discover just how useful this is at the first instant that tension strikes or pressures rise. In place of an unconscious, habitual response that gets you tied up in knots of tension, anger, or anxiety, you'll be able to substitute a powerful, positive self-command that is activated instantaneously. If you notice yourself getting anxious or hurrying so much that you're snapping at others, pause and use the ICS—several times, if needed.

Here are just a few of the daily situations where you can use the ICS.

- You try to do more than you can in a limited time—and you fall behind.
- You feel frustrated because other people seem to be moving too slowly.
- You turn to answer the phone or reach for your notebook or purse and spill something on your clothes.
- You make a mistake or mispronounce a word in front of other people.
- Your boss is mad about something, and you begin to panic because you haven't been listening and you can't remember what your boss just said.
- The person ahead of you in the express lane of the grocery checkout decides to write a check instead of paying cash.
- Your computer locks up while searching the Internet for a key fact or while you're rushing to finish a report.
- You drive at the speed limit on the highway and notice a tailgater in your rear-view mirror.
- You get some bad news.
- You notice yourself making a careless error.
- You have an emotional downturn without knowing why, and you begin to feel pessimistic.
- You're angry at another person and are about to curse at them or wish them harm.

In short, your can use the ICS in any of life's various stressful moments.

Keeping Step

All five ICS steps are critical. Unlike some pep-talk motivators and psychologists, I don't believe that positive thinking or "mental self-talk" is sufficient to help most people master stressful situations. Positive thinking can be valuable, but it won't do the job all by itself. You need to have your heart involved as well as your head (see part 5 of this book).

Also, the key physiological steps, such as continued breathing, lightening your eyes, and immediately releasing tension, can be every bit as vital as the mental elements of the ICS. Positive affirmations may be helpful, but they can't create calm energy by themselves. Your physical, emotional, and mental actions need to be in alignment. If you halt your breathing, frown, collapse your posture, tense your muscles, and open the floodgates to negative emotions, calm energy is almost impossible to achieve.

One final note: Keep practicing. It may be the best investment in boosting calm energy and health that you have ever made.

Hold Your Head High

Hunched shoulders. Bowed head. Shuffling gait. These images immediately suggest advanced age and, with the burden of gravity and years, the depletion of energy.

But which comes first, the depletion of energy or the hunched–over posture? Surprisingly, they may seem to be closely interrelated.

We rarely think of the cause-and-effect relationship between posture and outlook or posture and vigor, but these connectors exist, according to intriguing research from the University of Southern California in Los Angeles.

When you're stooped over, you not only look old and out of touch with life but you also tend to feel that way, according to René Cailliet, M.D., chairman of the department of physical medicine at the Santa Monica Hospital Center in California and former chairman of the department of physical medicine and rehabilitation at the University of Southern California School of Medicine.

My own grandfather battled this after each of his four heart attacks.

The Balancing Act

In the continued exploration of mind-body interactions, scientists have discovered that posture can affect mental attitude just as mental attitude affects posture. It's not surprising, then, that calm energy is raised and sustained by great posture.

"Posture is not solely the manifestation of physical balance," writes occupational-medicine specialist David Imrie, M.D., who has spent many years investigating the links between posture and energy levels. "It's also an expression of mental balance. Think about the way you stand when you are depressed or tired: You stand with your shoulders rounded and drooping. Your body represents your emotions by giving up the fight against gravity, sagging just as low as you feel."

The language of physical balance has also become the language of mental and emotional balance, says Dr. Imrie. "It's also notable that the term *well-balanced* is used to describe someone who 'won't go over the edge' and whose emotions are 'on an even keel,'" he says.

As the heart attacks took their toll, he began using canes to walk. He might have steadily collapsed into the image of Father Time: slow, bowed, hesitant, and shuffling. But that wasn't the grandfather that I knew. Instead, he found every way possible to develop a new, more careful posture and infused it with his inner strength and calm energy. The cane was included in his walk—and he needed it for standing, too, when he was tired—but his posture told me that he still supported himself, comfortably and completely.

I have since come to understand that he accomplished what I call *balanced posture.*

My grandfather knew instinctively, as experts now know from studies, that tension builds on top of tension. Essentially, tension is the "web" that so many of us sense and feel as we get older. What drags us down and can change our very posture and way of moving is not gravity but what our tendons, nerves, and muscles are doing to themselves. And this tension, the clear and visible appearance of tense energy in all of our limbs, actually brings us down in body and spirit.

When you instead uplift and relax your body alignment you can actually help prevent or reverse the aging process, says Dr. Cailliet.

An Uplifting Experience

It's easy to change your posture. If you doubt that statement, just take a moment, right now, to change the way that you're sitting. Adjust your position in the seat of your chair. Lean a little more to the left or the right. Take a deep breath and pull yourself upright, relaxing your shoulders.

If you're aware of what you're doing, you can feel the subtle changes move through your hips, your lower back, your shoulder blades, your neck, and your arms. One small movement, and your entire attitude or energy level can change.

With that small sample exercise, you've just caught a glimpse of what changes in posture can do for your calm-energy level. How much real effort does it take to shift position in your seat? What powers of concentration do you have to muster to stretch your shoulders back a fraction of an inch? I think you'll agree that the effort is simple and direct. But the rewards of these small changes are vitally important to the calm energy in your life.

Research suggests that how you sit and stand may exert a powerful influence not only on how rapidly you age but also on your mind and mood. It makes scientific sense when you realize that slouching or hunching over in your chair creates 10 to 15 times as much pressure on your lower back as sitting up straight does.

When you're slumped in your seat, that posture also restricts your breathing and impedes your circulation. Even the simple act of rounding your shoulders forward may cut by up to 30 percent the amount of oxygen that's headed to your brain.

The Costs of Slouching

Intuitively, you may already be aware of what happens when you are tensely hunched over. I'm sure that you have gone to special occasions where you reminded yourself to stand tall. The wedding you attended. The speech you gave. An induction, graduation, or awards ceremony.

Your mind acknowledges, instinctively, that these are important events when you welcome the present and face the future with pride, energy, attentiveness, and optimism. Your body automatically acknowledges these moments with a posture that expresses your willingness to be present and your eagerness to meet the occasion with energy and pride.

Day to day, good posture is not automatic. If and when you remind yourself to sit up straight, you may feel like the effort is forced. And the repeated admonition to stand up straight may actually have negative associations, reminding you of anxious, authoritarian, or frustrated parents or teachers.

Needless to say, you can accomplish a upright posture on command. It takes just a second to broaden your shoulders, tuck in your butt, suck in your stomach, and straighten your back. And if you've been in the military, that single action sends a surge of adrenaline through your whole system. The trouble is that this well-intended position of combat readiness doesn't work very well in day-to-day life.

WE OUR BOUND TO OUR POSTURE

LIKE AN OYSTER TO ITS SHELL.

LIFT IT. CARE FOR IT.

—Plato (ca. 427–347 B.C.), Greek philosopher

The reason is simple. If you tighten your muscles, you end up stiff and well-braced. But you can't maintain this tiring, unnatural position for long.

Good posture can't be forced. But it's not automatic, either. "We're not born knowing how to do it right," says posture expert Wilfred Barlow, M.D., medical director of the Alexander Institute in London. "No reflex system sets up good posture. We have to learn it."

The Energy-Posture Connection

Fortunately, you don't have to train many muscles to get in the habit of sitting and standing in ways that maximize your calm energy. Of the nearly 700 muscles in your body, excellent, natural posture relies on only 5. Those key muscles hold your chest, shoulders, neck, and head upright. If you keep those muscles reasonably well-tuned using a few methods that I'll discuss in this chapter, your posture will become buoyant and comfortable.

In addition to having more calm energy when you train these muscles, you will have better health. Research shows that poor posture creates some of the obvious damage that you'd expect: It distorts the alignment of your bones and makes your muscles chronically tense. With poor posture, you're likely to have stiff joints and pain symptoms such as headaches, jaw pain, and muscular aches. It has been estimated that 80 percent of all cases of back pain are related to poor posture.

But in addition to these problems that are clearly related to your muscular and skeletal systems, researchers report some health effects that you would hardly suspect. For instance, a hunched-over posture can reduce vital lung capacity by 30 percent or more. That means you have to work harder for each breath, and even when you try to capture more air, your lungs probably don't fill all the way. With diminished air intake, less oxygen reaches your brain and senses. Inevitably, you feel increased fatigue. You're also less alert, which can affect productivity.

A series of studies reports that, compared with people who have good postural positions, those with slumped postures were more likely to experience feelings of helplessness and frustration during work tasks. They also perceived themselves to be under greater stress. Other researchers have reported that poor posture decreases mental alertness and increases work errors.

Other side effects of poor posture include premature aging of body tissues, faulty digestion, and constipation. In addition, it can impair creative thinking and emotional control and slow your reaction time.

Even mood is affected. People with poor posture tend toward cynicism, pessimism, drowsiness, and poor concentration. They also have magnified feelings of panic and helplessness. And some studies have shown that, in some people, poor posture may be one of the contributing causes of depression.

In a Slump?

"It's extremely difficult to work in a technological society and not develop a forward head," says Dr. Cailliet.

"Forward head" is a curious expression, but you've seen people with that posture—and you probably recognize it in your own profile. If you sit in front of a computer or work behind a counter or on an assembly line, chances are that you have a forward head. Even cooking, cleaning, reading, and desk work can produce that posture.

Forward head is a constant postural stress that contributes to tension headaches, vision problems, and jaw and neck pain. In a way, it's natural to adopt this posture when you're working at a desk job or peering at a computer screen. To an outside observer, it may appear as if you were intent on your task or trying to concentrate better. But inside you, that posture is having quite a different effect. Combine a forward head and a slumped seating position, and you have all the elements of a stress-filled, discouraging, numbing, and ultimately mind-dulling work experience.

Can so much be inferred just from the way you sit?

Danger for Desk Jockeys

If you have a desk job or any kind of job that requires sustained concentration, your posture is one of the most influential components of your work environment. Sitting and standing with upright, relaxed posture is a choice that you make—or fail to make—every minute of your life. Whether or not you consciously control it, your sitting position creates its own momentum. If gravity gets a grip on your tilted head or drooping shoulders, your body starts to feel as though it were being overtaken by a slow, heavy wave. Slouching gradually become slumping, and ease turns into effort.

Even if you don't sit at a desk for the greater part of the day, you always have the element of choice about posture. Whether you spend time sitting in the car, standing in line at the store, doing housework, or answering phone calls, you will be more aware of your posture if you take a mental snapshot of your body's profile.

Fortunately, at any point in your life—and what better time than now?—you can break the habit of forward head.

Breathe Right and Think Taller

In Calm–Energy Switch #2, I described how you can release tension by moving into a position of balanced posture. That's a good technique for instant calming. But something more is required if you want to *always* have the kind of uplift in your posture that helps you maintain calm energy.

The best posture isn't forced. Rather, think of it as being unlocked. Your body creates a balanced platform where good posture can occur, and with a few minor adjustments good posture happens.

To understand this a bit better, just think about the weight of your head. Your head weighs between 10 and 15 pounds. It may have more gray matter than a bowling ball, but the plain fact is that it's just as heavy. If you wanted to hold up a 10- to 15-pound bowling ball, you would center yourself exactly underneath it, where it would be perfectly supported by the upright structure of your whole body. Your head needs the same kind of precise support.

If your head is tilted to one side or the other, the effort of holding it in that position is significantly magnified. But if you're right underneath all of that weight, it's a simple and effortless task to keep your head aligned and centered over your body, because your body happens to be a magnificently well-balanced supporting structure.

A New Alignment

To avoid placing undue stress on your neck, shoulders, and spine, your head must be poised in a comfortable, centered position. But perhaps you've paid little attention to that ideal placement. If so, here's one way to make yourself more aware of the most comfortable position possible.

1. Sit comfortably in an armless chair or on a bench, with your feet flat on the floor. You can keep your eyes open while you read these in-

structions, but after you get used to this exercise, try it with your eyes closed. Breath naturally and comfortably.

2. Lengthen your neck and let your head move upward. As you raise your head, bring your chin slightly in, broaden your shoulders, and flatten your lower back.

3. Gently lean your head to the left, then to the right. Finally, return your head to the most central, balanced position—that is, the place directly over your body where you can balance it without feeling any muscle strain.

4. Move your head slightly forward and then back. Then, find the precise center once again.

5. While you do this, work with the following image. Think of yourself as carrying a weight on top of your head. Your task is to push up against that weight, holding it in position so it won't fall off. If you keep in mind this image of a weight, you'll give your senses instant, valuable signals that will help balance and stabilize your head and neck.

I suggest using this awareness exercise whenever you sit down, when you're waiting in line, and when you're about to start some chore. Using these movements and this imagery enables you to relax your neck. You'll quickly and consciously choose where to hold your head with the least strain.

But beyond this exercise, there's something that you can do automatically. I call it thinking taller. Encourage your head to rise upward as easily as a float that's buoyed by water. You don't have to push or strain your neck. Simply think tall until you bring your head over your shoulders, with your chin slightly in. After you have felt the difference, you may want to try this in front of a mirror, where you will be able to see the difference as well.

Take It Easy

Whenever you sit down, it pays to briefly pause to choose the most balanced, comfortable sitting position. Here's how.

Sit squarely. Make sure you don't slump. Center your buttocks on the seat. If you lean to one side or sit off-center, you throw off the alignment of your body—and gravity does the rest. When you're in that unbalanced position, your muscles have to do more work defying gravity, which creates excess tension. Also, your bloodflow is reduced in key areas whenever your posture is out of alignment. If you've ever stayed in an uncomfortable or restrictive position for very long, you know that your limbs can feel tense, stiff, or numb because of restricted circulation. This can negatively affect tissues, nerves, and muscles in that part of your body.

Adjust your armrests. If you work in a chair, I recommend choosing one that has armrests that can be adjusted to a comfortable height. By resting your lower arms, even lightly, on the armrests, you can relieve up to 25 percent of the load on your lower back, according to rehabilitative-medicine authority Janet G. Travell. The armrests also help provide stability and support when you're changing positions.

Empty your pocket. If you're used to carrying your wallet, car keys, pen, comb, or checkbook in a back pocket, find some other place for such items. This is particularly important if you're a man who is used to carrying a fat wallet in your back pocket. According to a study published in the *New England Journal of Medicine*, some men with back pain experienced complete relief of their symptoms when they simply stopped sitting on their wallets. Insignificant though it may seem, that small bump under one buttock can be enough to throw the entire spine out of alignment.

Bend at your hips, not at your spine. When you first take your seat, your lower back should be straight, centered, and far back in the chair. Smoothly

TRY THIS NOW!

You don't need to be standing up to improve your posture. Here's a simple posture exercise that can be done lying down—and because it involves deep breathing, it's a superb way to get in touch with your calm energy. This exercise also helps increase the elasticity of your rib cage.

Here's How!

Once you start this exercise, you'll find that gravity does at least half of the work for you.

1. Lie face up on a rug or exercise mat.
2. Relax your body and gently press your lower back toward the floor. At the same time, keep your head aligned with your spine, with your neck long and your chin slightly in.
3. Place your hands lightly on either side of your rib cage.
4. Inhale slowly and deeply. Lift and expand your chest fully as you maximize the inhalation.
5. Exhale slowly.
6. Breathe normally, allowing your whole body to rest.
7. Repeat the exercise. This time, as you expand your chest, lift your ribs a little higher as you apply some light hand pressure.

As a variation on this exercise, try inhaling with a number of short breaths rather than with one deep breath. Continue the breaths until your chest is completely expanded. Then, exhale slowly with a number of short breaths until all of the air is released.

OVER 99 PERCENT OF US **PULL THE BACK OF THE SKULL** DOWN INTO THE BACK OF THE NECK AS WE SIT DOWN AND STAND UP. IT'S A MIRACLE THAT WE SURVIVE THIS POOR POSTURE.

—Wilfred Barlow, M.D., medical director, Alexander Institute, London

put your upper body against the back of the seat. Breathe. Release all excess tension. Hold your head high, relaxed, and centered over your shoulders. Your upper body will be suspended squarely over your hips.

Watch what you cross. If you want to shift position and cross your legs, try just crossing your ankles instead. Even if you feel like crossing your legs at the knees, avoid it. By hoisting one leg over the other, you misalign your pelvis, which can lead to back tension and pain if you hold that position for too long.

Have flat feet. Keep your feet flat on the floor as much as possible. If you get restless in that position or just need a change, lift one foot onto the rung of a chair. Or pull over a small stool and place one foot on it.

Do the head nod. When you're comfortably seated, do the head-nod exercise in "Try This Now!" on the opposite page to make sure that your head is centered over your neck.

Trim your torso. You can align your torso using a technique that's similar to the head-nod exercise. With your eyes closed, shift your torso right, then left, and finally to the center, moving from your hips. Repeat with a similar movement forward, then back, then to the center.

Bring up those pages. When you read at the office, bring your reading material up to your field of vision to avoid the strain of dropping your head. At home, use a reading chair with high arms to help support

TRY THIS NOW!

Calm energy is often won or lost from the neck up. Neck position strongly affects the placement and comfort of your shoulders, chest, and back.

At the crest of your spine is a small muscle called the rectus capitis anterior. It positions your head atop your neck and shoulders. Toning this muscle is one of the keys to maintaining good neck posture.

Here's How!

To tone the rectus capitis anterior muscle, try a gentle head-nod exercise. You can either sit or stand when you do it.

1. Bring in your chin just slightly, which will create the feeling that the crown of your head is rising. Your head should feel as if it were gently extending upward, as though it were being lifted by an imaginary skyhook or cord attached to the top of your skull.

2. With your neck in this slightly elevated position, bring your head forward and nod just slightly, as if in agreement. (*Note*: Don't nod so sharply that you bow your head.)

Repeat this simple, relaxed nodding action 10 times during the course of the day.

---

your elbows, bringing the book up to eye level. If you're traveling on a plane or train, you can pull out the tray table from the seat in front of you, then use a pillow or folded coat to support your elbows or forearms.

Avoid the shoulder jam. When you're talking on the phone, keep your uplifted posture and bring the phone up to your ear. Don't cradle the phone between your ear and shoulder, or you'll force your neck to the side, which can create the worst kind of neck tension.

Take time to align. Especially for prolonged hours of work, choose an adjustable chair. Take time to adjust it properly before you begin working. And if you don't have exclusive use of that chair—if someone else in your family or your place of business has access to it—be sure to readjust it each time you get it back. This should become as automatic as adjusting your car seat, steering wheel, and mirrors after someone else has driven your car.

Even if you love it, leave it. No matter how comfortable you are in your chair or how caught up you are in your work, you need to take breaks. To remain seated all day is stressful, no matter how ideal the chair and work-surface design. Make it a priority to get up from your desk at least once every half-hour. The breaks don't need to be long, just a minute or two, but you definitely need them.

Call on the ICS when needed. Whether you're seated or standing with the right posture, don't accept tension as a normal consequence. It's important to respond to the first sign of tension with the instant-calming sequence (ICS) from Calm-Energy Switch #2. The longer a muscle area stays tense, the more your awareness of it will dim and the greater your tendency to lock in that tension will be. So whenever you notice a stiffening or tightening in your body due to stress or slumping, immediately release it with the instant-calming sequence. That may be all you need.

A Walk on the Tall Side

Most of us think of walking as pure action, and it's definitely one of the key strategies for active energy. But posture is an essential part of walking, as you can see if you witness any group of people traveling on foot.

Often, you see people walking stiffly. They look tense and retracted. Their eyes are down as they move along, and every step seems to be an effort.

What goes through your mind when you walk? Do you view it as an exercise, at best? Or is it merely an inconvenience? So many people seem to choose walking only when they've run out of other alternatives such as driving, taking a cab or bus, or getting a ride from someone.

In my opinion, relaxed walking is one of the simplest and most useful ways to keep generating and sustaining calm energy. There's a rhythm, ease, and grace to walking that surpasses most other activities. And no wonder, since we know that humans have been practicing this expert balance-and-motion act ever since the first humans clambered to their feet.

But just because we know, genetically and behaviorally, how to walk, that doesn't mean we get all the calm energy that we can from it.

As you walk, hold your head high, with your neck and shoulders relaxed and your lower back flat. For the sake of your posture, here are five things to be conscious of while you walk.

1. Keep your feet pointed straight ahead.
2. Don't hyperextend your leg. If it locks at the knee as you swing it forward, it is extended too far.
3. When your leading heel comes down, make sure it touches the ground lightly.
4. Roll your weight forward across the sole of your foot, then push off gently with your toes.
5. Swing your arms easily and naturally, using a heterolateral pattern:

Your left arm should move forward as your right leg advances, with your right arm swinging forward as your left leg advances.

Slow-Mo Moves

If you practice the relaxed-walking step in slow motion, you'll find that your body naturally assumes good posture. The easy motion of your legs, with a balance between the heel of one foot landing and the toes of the other pushing off, assures that your body is well-balanced at the midway point. And the heterolateral pattern of your swinging arms maintains that balance.

You can also be aware of posture when you're working. In fact, good posture not only boosts calm energy but also saves a lot of people from back pain that's initiated when they lift, drag, or pull in the wrong way. Here are what I consider the two cardinal rules for everyday movements.

1. Whenever you turn to reach for something, take a step toward the object that you're going to pick up. This step helps coordinate and focus your power and integrates your body as it moves. By better using your legs and trunk, you take strain off your back muscles.
2. When you reach, bend, or turn, lead the movement with your head. Let your head "float" upward, followed by your whole body.

Do Less
to Get Ahead

Today, many of us find ourselves with an inner state of tense energy caused by what is commonly called the rat race. Tense energy is the antithesis of calm energy.

The more we try to get ahead by rushing and competing, the more tension we feel. We have less ease in our lives, and we're probably not having as much fun as we'd like. Instead of getting ahead, we find ourselves in a state of near–constant emergency. It's like inner gridlock.

When there's an urgent need to move in many directions at once, you may feel as if you couldn't move at all. You come to a standstill, with all lights red and all lanes blocked. But even then, you can feel the mounting stress created by tense energy.

That's when you need streamlining.

When you streamline, you get to the essence of living and working. You find every way that you can to dispense with what doesn't matter. You lighten your load and mute the roar of duties that clamor for attention and the doubts that warn you of failure and disaster. You stop wasting calm energy and focus it, instead, on aligning your talents and strengths with your truest aims. This is the "high level of energy" that ranks number one on the *Harvard Business Review*'s list of essential qualities for success at work.

Getting on Target

Essentially, streamlining means that you commit, absolutely, to what you can do. All the rest—the mountain of details that grows ever-higher—you delegate, delete, or minimize. When you effectively streamline, you devote the least possible time and attention to the things that *deserve* less time and attention.

There are two primary aspects of streamlining. First, you need to stop competing with others. When you streamline, competition becomes irrelevant and an impediment. Your focus shifts to excelling instead. Though at first this may seem like a small distinction, as you'll see, it makes all the difference in creating calm energy rather than tense energy.

The second aspect of streamlining is doing less to get ahead. I know that this sounds contradictory. The idea of doing less is certainly contrary to what most of us have been taught. That's why it can be such a breakthrough.

Here are the approaches that I recommend to accomplish these two steps.

Streamlining Step 1: Stop Competing and Start Excelling

In a world where competitiveness is almost worshiped, many people are surprised to learn that an intensive focus on competing is, in fact, one of the primary barriers to calm energy and exceptional performance. Not only that, but competition can stand in the way of a happy, healthy life.

When it comes to your own life and work, where do you put your energy and attention, on competing or excelling? You cannot do both.

WHEN **WE ARE UNABLE TO FIND TRANQUILLITY**
WITHIN OURSELVES, IT IS USELESS
TO SEEK IT ELSEWHERE.

—François La Rochefoucauld (1613–1680), French author

Competitors rely far too much on tense energy and on wanting others to lose so they can win. They repeatedly, and sometimes almost constantly, compare themselves to others—to family members, friends, coworkers, cover models, Hollywood stars, and TV personalities. What do they look like? What are they thinking, saying, doing?

Whenever it appears that anyone else may be catching us or surpassing us, it's easy to feel defensive, anxious, envious, or jealous. This promotes tense energy and blocks us from being our best.

Even when competitive people compare their own children to other children, they use the same mind-set. No matter what, competitors want to look successful and keep up with the Joneses.

Competitors lose a huge piece of their lives to this. It has become so common that many people assume that's just the way life is. It isn't.

In contrast, those who excel flow well with pressures and give every ounce of their attention and ingenuity to giving their best individual effort. No one else has to lose for them to win.

Consider the story of Mika Häkkinen, who won the 1998 world championship in Formula One auto racing. His calmness is perplexing to sports writers, who are used to interviewing braggarts with flamboyant personalities. Before winning the Formula One championship at age 30, Häkkinen nearly died in a crash in the 1995 Australian Grand Prix. Though he survived, he was in a coma for a week and was hospitalized for 3 weeks.

"I learned to walk a little bit slower," Häkkinen recalls of his recovery. "I learned that you don't have to rush. People tend to forget that in their lives. They keep panicking, panicking, until one day they realize, 'Finished. I'm not going to do this anymore.' "

That's the approach that he invested in his racing. Of all the top drivers, Häkkinen is known as the one who makes the fewest mistakes at top speed. That's the power of calm energy.

To compete means to run in the same race. That's fine, of course, if we are actually *in* the same race, if we're doing what everyone else is doing and we actually want to beat them at playing the same game.

But that's not quite how it is in most life situations. For instance, consider a very typical office situation in which you and a coworker are both in line for promotion. Aren't you in the same race? Shouldn't you be competing? It may seem like you have no choice, especially if only one of you can get the promotion. But if you focus solely on that competition, you may be hurting yourself.

For you, a promotion might be the right step. But you also have to consider the possibility that you might want to spend less time working or focus on an avocation or launch a new business. And you don't know what's really going on with the other person, either. Yes, that person may have their eye on a promotion, but they might also be thinking about leaving for a new company, going to school, or starting a family.

If all you do is compete with that other person, there's a good chance that you'll lose sight of what's best for *you*. You might become so preoccupied with "winning" that you miss other opportunities that pop up. Or you might undermine all your chances for a more satisfying job by competing so intensely that you fail to support or cooperate with the person whom you perceive as a competitor.

Our pursuits are as diversified as our lives. I know that I'm not in the same race as my next-door neighbor—or, for that matter, as anyone who's working in a nearby office. And if we're not in the same race, it's certainly the wrong use of energy and a sure path to frustration if I try to compete with them.

Besides, whenever you don't know if someone else out there wants your glory, credit, fame, or advancement, when faced with vagueness about the motives or intentions of others, your brain's ancient instinct is to assume the worst. There's a voice that tells you, "Yes, people want you to fail." And when you listen to that voice, you react accordingly, treating life and work as battlegrounds rife with tense, not calm, energy.

Double-Check Your Attitude

There's another aspect to competition that's destructive. Many people believe they can win by tearing down their competitors. Today, this mind-set seems to be infiltrating our personal lives as well as our professional relationships.

In far too many families, groups, and organizations, competition has become an immense distraction. Without realizing it, we compete against siblings, peers, friends, bosses, employees, and nearly everyone else in our neighborhoods, communities, and industries.

One problem with constant competitiveness is the way in which it can infect everything that we do. Sometimes, of course, competition sparks action. But it goes too far when you begin to feel as if everyone, including family or team members, were a real or potential competitor and as if there were no safe retreat from the race. Calm energy vanishes, and one thing that's guaranteed is that you're no longer at your best.

In an atmosphere of constant competition, people in organizations as well as in families and communities vie for position, promotion, or profits. And competitiveness can transfer into our personal lives as well. It can get to the point where we feel that we must be vigilant and mistrusting. Wherever it dominates, competition keeps us ever on the alert for people who will attempt to move past us. How can we trust others when we're looking at them that way?

Competition has become so ubiquitous that many of us don't even recognize what a toll it takes. It destroys commitment and loyalty. It thwarts creativity.

If we sense that we're losing or that someone is gaining on us, we get anxious and preoccupied. It's likely that we'll criticize or try to sabotage our rivals, if only as a self-defense measure. Even if we don't know these people personally, the competitive outlook can make us so wary that we feel compelled to do whatever we can, openly or covertly, to derail people's progress or tear them down.

With anger or false smiles, they reciprocate—in the spirit of competition, of course. There's no room for calm energy here.

The Excel Factor

What's the alternative to competing? I ask people to think in terms of excelling.

To excel means to reach beyond, to make a difference, or to stand out from the crowd. It means to run your own race.

For you as an individual, it means that you don't compare your success to the successes of your classmates, coworkers, colleagues, or neighbors. For your family, it means that each member values and celebrates the unique talents and capabilities of every other member, without comparing the achievements of one sibling or relative to the success of another. Among members of a team, the emphasis on excelling rather than competing means that each individual focuses on performing to the best of their ability, complementing the best efforts of others, demonstrating the full range and extent of personal capabilities, and setting goals that truly represent a personal best.

In the many organizations with which I've worked—even in those that have a fiercely competitive culture—I've discovered that placing the emphasis on excelling over competing creates new standards in the levels of performance and interpersonal interactions. People in those organizations discover that they can set and achieve goals in terms of absolute maximum-performance capabilities. When the old goals of winning and beating are set aside, there's new room for creative achievement that transcends rivalries and one-upmanship.

In the Passing Lane

To excel means to fluidly and ingeniously work at the upper edge of your capabilities, not once in a while or in certain circumstances but all the time. Those who excel, rather than compete, can perform well consistently and with collected, calm energy in the midst of stress, uncertainty, and wrenching changes. They may have sky-high expectations, but those are expectations of fulfillment rather than of continued frustration.

There are sound reasons why those who excel can consistently outperform those who compete. Beneath its bluster, the ongoing battle to be competitive rarely produces anything more than lost time and costly mediocrity.

While competitors struggle for a few inches of gain on a traditional field of battle, those who excel are more likely to streamline their efforts and marshal all their ingenuity to redefine the field. Often, star performers demonstrate abilities that are a dimension beyond the vision of those who focus on competition. They give every ounce of their best effort to reaching the upper edge of their capabilities. For those who capitalize on

TRY THIS NOW!

In 5 quiet minutes, you can become much more aware of what you can do to streamline your efforts. You can focus more clearly on connecting your efforts with your deepest values and beliefs. Almost at once, you'll likely feel tense energy replaced by calm energy.

Here's How

Look at the next few items on your to-do list. Ask yourself, "How much does each item actually move me toward what really matters most to my life? If I commit to these items, will I be reaching for my own best efforts and learning?"

Our days are busy, and some are so busy that they seem frenetic. You may think that all of this busy-ness is productive. But is it really?

You can be maximally efficient—in motion every moment of the day, accomplishing long lists of tasks—but get nowhere in terms of your long-term goals or purpose in life. Sometimes, you need to say no,

calm energy to live and work at the peak of their possibilities, there's not a moment to be wasted with the distraction of tearing anyone else down.

When faced with change, those who excel ask, "How can I turn this into new opportunities—or, at least, new learning?" Competitors worry, "How can I defend my position and bring others down or block them from making progress?"

Consider the amazing contributions and accomplishments of such people as Helen Keller, Nelson Mandela, John Glenn, Oprah Winfrey, or Michael Jordan. Consider the remarkable accomplishments of Michael Dell, the visionary founder of Dell Computers; Lance Armstrong, who won the Tour kindly but firmly, to demands on unnecessary or unpleasant uses of your time and energy.

To say no is difficult. But it doesn't imply rudeness or rejection. It simply says that you have other plans for the use of your time.

When faced with the prospect of a new task, ask yourself, "Would anything terrible happen if I didn't do this?" If the answer is no, consider not doing it.

Look again at your list of tasks. Are there any that could just as well remain undone? If so, cross them off. Maybe you'll have to call someone, express your regrets, and let that person know that you have to say no.

You may be surprised at the results. Your "no" is a simple statement that you need time to do what's important to you. It may not be important to anyone else, but keep in mind that you're not competing with anyone else. If you're not competing for attention, affection, popularity, acceptance, or promotion, then your time is yours alone. You can use it for your own purposes—to excel at the things that you most want and like to do.

de France after recovering from cancer; or the entire 1999 U.S. women's national soccer team, who defied all expectations to win the Women's World Cup. At their best moments, their efforts and actions weren't predicated on tearing anyone else down. By excelling, by reaching into themselves to give the world the best that they had, they have each made history.

In many different and sometimes small yet always significant ways, this is the opportunity that we are each given in our life and work. Unfortunately, we tend to make things harder on ourselves by getting caught up in the tense energy that comes from getting mired in competition. You can choose another way.

Streamlining Step 2: Doing Less to Get Ahead— And Getting Ahead Faster

Calm energy promotes happiness and ease. At the same time, it enables a wide variety of your best-ever actions in life and at work. Streamlining is a way of using calm energy to move through challenging times more elegantly and efficiently.

According to researchers, people are usually happiest when they're flowing with life, very aware of whatever experience they're in but not struggling rigidly or feeling desperate in trying to control the outcome. Such attempts at perfectionism or end gaining rarely work anyway.

Because of this, streamlining begins with letting go. Stop overanalyzing things. Get more integrally involved with each process or experience of life that will shape its own results according to how much of your best you put into it. Think of a conversation with a friend or associate at work during which you are distracted by details of the task at hand or by other obligations. What happens when the other person doesn't get your undivided attention? He or she fidgets, tenses up, and feels increasingly impatient, invisible, disrespected, or devalued. Then what are the results you achieve?

Compare that with giving your full energy and concentration to the person and moment at hand, and receiving the other person's complete attention in return. The richness of what happens increases dramatically. Attitudes loosen. Perspectives broaden. Humor surfaces. Learning happens. In short, the conversation amounts to something valuable. You can get to the point sooner. There is reduced chance of misunderstanding. You can listen as well as talk, and when you listen, you're not miles away thinking about something else or worrying about what you're going to say next. Instead, you absorb what's happening. It's easier to be open and honest, instead of tense and controlling. In most cases, you struggle less and accomplish more.

WITHIN US THERE ARE WELLS

OF VISION AND **DYNAMOS OF ENERGY**

WHICH ARE NOT SUSPECTED. . . .

—Thomas J. Watson (1874–1956), U.S. executive

Stop Struggling and Start Flowing

In something as common as everyday conversations or as rare as record–breaking efforts in sports, the arts, invention, or service, calm energy is the foundation of success.

When you are streamlining and relaxing in the moment, you are priming the most creative parts of your nervous system, including the visualization center in the posterior part of your brain. Scientists believe that this frees up your mind, senses, and emotions by turning off the parts of your brain that drain energy into anxious or neurotic thinking. As NBC medical correspondent Bob Arnot, M.D., author of *The Biology of Success*, explains, "When you see a great movie, opera, ballet, or sports event, you become totally absorbed in the moment, flowing with it, and the visual centers in your brain glow brightly as the anxious concerns of the day take a rest. It is one of life's great ironies: We believe we accomplish so much by constantly worrying, when in reality we prevent ourselves from opening the most magnificent parts of the brain."

Streamlining depends on stripping away the tensions and distractions that keep pulling you off in other directions. It requires you to focus more fully on the possibilities right in front of you and creatively make the most of them.

TRY THIS NOW!

Streamlining is a technique perfected by athletes, but all of us can use it just as well in our everyday lives.

Before beginning an important activity or task, allow yourself some brief, focused mental- and emotional-preparation time. Take this opportunity to streamline your focus, that is, to prepare in a streamlined way for what's ahead. Doing that can make a major difference in the outcome, according to researchers.

In these moments, you gain extra calm energy by extending your time frame and planning ahead. You figure out how to accomplish your task more by choice and less by chance.

These brief times can be tied to other breaks during your day. Or you can choose a moment in the shower or a few minutes after lunch. Some people with whom I've worked prefer to do it when walking or jogging, or even when taking a commuter train or bus. If you're in a situation where you can close your eyes, all the better. All you need is a little time when you can achieve a relatively deep state of focus without disruption, at least for a few minutes.

Here's How

Here are several simple yet practical ways to maximize the positive outcome of streamlining.

When possible, add music. Instrumental movie soundtracks without lyrics are less distracting and can be excellent because they are specifically composed to set a background mood. Events take place in front of the music, not within it. Similarly, I find that a soundtrack lets my focus go its own way. The background music, whether relaxing, uplifting, or contemplative, helps to generate feelings of confidence, calm energy, and hope. That's the setting that you need in order to let your thoughts focus. Specific soundtracks that can help include those from the films *Everest*, *The Last of the Mohicans*, *Crimson Tide*, *Dances with Wolves*, and *Lonesome Dove*, according to performance psychologist James E. Loehr, Ed.D.

Shift to a present focus. You'll be able to concentrate more clearly and with less strain if you use the instant-calming sequence described in Calm-Energy Switch #2. It will help you quickly establish a peaceful sense of calm energy.

Streamline your time and commitments. As you think ahead to what's coming up, contemplate specific ways that you can streamline the process. Is there any way that you can take work out of your efforts? In what precise times and ways can you best apply your talents, strengths, or passions to move things forward? If parts of this project are likely to be tiring or irritating, how can you minimize or delegate these aspects of the work?

Ask, "Is this worth giving a piece of my life to?" Life is enriched through questions. If you ask yourself this question at the beginning of each project or endeavor, you'll never have to wonder, "Why did I do that?" or "Why did I waste my time?" after spending time on something that was not important.

In my own family, "Is this worth giving a piece of your life to?" was a question that my grandfather would ask me at the start and end of each effort or initiative. Perhaps it is my memory of that question that always makes me pause. I wonder what I'm doing each day to shape my own

(continued)

"footprints across the sands of time," to borrow a phrase from the poet William Wordsworth.

Consider a realignment. Think about what you've done recently. If you can't honestly say, "This was worth giving a piece of my life to," then it makes sense to reconsider your course. Will you be doing something tomorrow that leaves you feeling the same way, or can you make a change now instead of later?

When I come home from work projects or business trips, my two young daughters always tell me about what has happened in their lives, and then we talk about my travels. Because I have had to leave them to do my work, I feel that it's imperative to answer the question behind their words: "Was it worth it?" If my answer is no, I challenge myself to make changes in my work approach and to realign my efforts and commitments.

It's easy to put off the tough questions that you need to ask yourself about what you'd like to *stop* doing, *keep* doing, and *start* doing. These are the questions that shouldn't be deferred. But how frequently should you ask yourself for answers?

I have used this approach once a month over the past 10 years, and it has kept me in far closer touch with what matters most to me. It has helped me say no to dozens of things that I was doing—and was efficient at doing—but that I would never have been doing had the conditions of this check-in been true. Even if you can't make instant changes, if you consistently use this check-in, you'll automatically begin streamlining.

Step Forward into Life

Streamlining is making the choice to engage more fully in what's happening at each moment and to flow with it. If you're frequently distracted by tension or stress, keep applying the instant-calming sequence (ICS) described in Calm-Energy Switch #2. Pick several practice times during the day—such as when you're in conversation with people you care about, taking a brief walk, or running a routine errand—and challenge yourself to flow with them.

Once you choose an experience to practice streamlining, consciously set aside your distractions. Skip dabbling and, instead, immerse yourself as completely as you can in the activity. Absorb yourself in it. Engage your senses. Soak in every aspect of what's going on.

Still hearing background chatter in your mind? No problem. Dive into the present moment more deeply. Each time you do this, you activate the visual-imaging capacities in the posterior part of your brain, where creativity and enjoyment are fueled. Many of the great scientists, poets, inventors, leaders, and musicians were highly skilled at accessing these parts of their brains. Jump into the deep end of each experience. Notice what's unique, humorous, and most valuable. Remind yourself that you'll have plenty of time later to worry about other things, if you really want to.

Use Small Rituals to Be Your Best

Simple daily rituals are the foundation of consistently generating and sustaining calm energy. The ICS is one example. Surgeons have exact preoperative routines. Mountain climbers never ascend without a specific preparation ritual. Pilots count on preflight sequences. Race car drivers use precise start-up rituals before the green flag. Through simple, specific sequences of actions, these men and women are able to increase and sustain their reserves of calm energy and their great senses of inner confidence and initiative. They rarely get sidetracked by irrelevant details, needless tension, or petty frustrations.

These rituals save you time; they are automatic and can be used whenever needed. They're also crucial to creating brain energy. This is because they synchronize your biological clock and enable you to approach life's challenges with greater creativity and ingenuity.

During crazy times, simple rituals are akin to landing pads and launching sites to provide breathing space and reestablish your bearings. They give you something focused and familiar to count on. Performance psychologist James E. Loehr, Ed.D., says that the most accomplished performers have defined specific rituals in daily life, whereas those who are less successful have not.

Examples of rituals include brief, specific preparation sequences before working, creating, planning, or making decisions; a set time each day for interacting with your family; and specific times for rest, reflection, hobbies, eating, sleeping, playing, exercising, and working. Rituals depend on setting clear, specific times for all of your routine activities. Plan a week ahead. The best rituals boost your energy and reduce tension levels.

Get More Kicks

Here's a final though on streamlining: Play harder. In the pell-mell rush of working and meeting our obligations, we often forget about the essence of life: fun. What activities do you pursue purely because you get a kick out of them? Yes, your work is demanding. But it's my guess that your play is too often dull, limited to activities like reading on a beach, watching your kids play sports, running errands, and standing in line for museums, theme parks, and movies. Play should invigorate your brain and get you flowing better with challenges and opportunities.

When you play hard, many chemical messenger molecules called neurotransmitters are activated. These include serotonin, opioid peptides, gamma amino butyric acid, and catecholamines (dopamine and norepinephrine). Each finely tuned cascade of these neurotransmitters targets your brain's principal "reward site," the nucleus accumbens, which results in your feeling good.

So don't just sit there. Now and then, step out for a deep breath and a burst of daylight. Kick up your heels and (okay, when no one's looking) dance a bit in the hallway when you're headed from point A to point B. Call a family member, colleague, or friend about something that has you excited. And never miss a single chance to laugh out loud or spend a lounging minute with your feet up on the coffee table. Even when you're extremely busy, finding moments like these to play hard in the middle of working hard puts more of the zest of life within your reach.

Every day, you can make better choices that determine the level and quality of your calm energy. You can choose to excel rather than compete. And you can streamline, eliminating needless tension and self-imposed resistance so you can move faster and further ahead with less effort. Few investments of your time and attention pay greater dividends throughout your life.

Find Breathing Space

I f only I could get a little breathing space."

When we say that, we're usually not begging for extra days of free time. Just a little break to—well, you imagine it. For some people, breathing space is a few well-protected moments when the phone doesn't ring. For others, it's enough time for a long walk or hot bath. Even the literal meaning of breathing space holds for some of us—an empty room or open space where they can take a deep breath, release tension, get going again.

How often have you wished for that lately? Nearly all of us have a deep craving for more chances to step back from life and loosen up, to let go and have more fun. And that's breathing space. It's one of the quickest and most often overlooked igniters and sustainers of calm energy.

Doing Too Much and Living Too Little?

Years ago, I went to a research seminar that was attended by more than 150 doctoral-degree candidates. All of us were conducting studies at major universities.

THE GOAL IN LIFE
IS TO **DIE YOUNG**—
AS LATE AS POSSIBLE.

—Ashley Montagu, Ph.D., Rutgers University, New Brunswick, New Jersey

The leader of the session, a professor who was an authority on advanced research methodologies, began by saying, "Some of us in this room don't know how to lime."

"Not only do I not know how to do it," I thought to myself, "but I don't even know what it means."

The professor explained. Years before, while coordinating research programs for a number of universities, he and his colleagues had worked in Trinidad and the West Indies. To their delight, they had found that people who had grown up on these islands were willing, alert, and energetic workers. Every morning, the men and women showed up full of enthusiasm. They were quick to understand assignments, very focused on expectations for the day, and enthusiastic about their jobs. The professor and his colleagues remarked separately on this phenomenon, but only when they observed the Trinidadians *after* work did they begin to understand what was behind their remarkable energy and enthusiasm.

Making the most of Caribbean pleasures, the professors customarily took their lounge chairs down to the beach every evening, and by 7 o'clock, they were enjoying the beverages of their choice while watching the sunset. But the local people, they observed, had quite another evening regimen. They didn't come to the beach alone. Their families were with them. Far from tucking themselves into beach chairs, they would dance on the beach, play games, sing songs, tell stories, and laugh with enjoyment at the smallest things. The holiday-style celebrations, repeated nightly, continued far past sunset.

Random Energy

At first, the professors thought that the nightly celebrations must be special occasions. Or perhaps, they thought, the merriment was the result of hyperactivity or, worse, some form of drug addiction. "This can't be normal," they agreed. "No normal person can have this much energy and this much fun every evening and show up the next morning enthusiastic and focused. How can it continue day after day?"

But after the professors had been there several weeks and had observed no letup in the festivities, they decided to do what professors instinctively do. "We should study them," they declared. And they did.

Though hardly self-conscious about their customary activities, the Trinidadians did have a name for it, the name that the professor sprang on our lecture group. In the islands, the nightly and weekend celebrations are called liming.

Liming means doing what you want to do—whatever healthy things you most enjoy doing—guilt-free. For these people, it was partying, playing games, singing, dancing, whatever happened to be fun and invigorating. As the professors observed, these men and women weren't just good at liming, they were great at it.

And the word itself? Apparently, it had been in their language for more than 300 years, originating at just about the time that the first Europeans arrived on the islands. Some of the ships, the islanders observed, brought Europeans who were dead or dying, sickened by scurvy during the long ocean voyage. On other ships, however, the Europeans were alive and well. These were the ships that had limes on board. The crews, called limeys in their own country because of their dependence on the fruit, had eaten the citrus fruit during the voyage. From the limes, they got enough vitamin C in their diets to stave off the ravages of scurvy. Overjoyed at reaching the island, they came happily ashore. From the celebrations of sailors deboarding lime-bearing ships, the word *liming* came into island currency.

As I listened to this story, which has been confirmed many times in recent years by people in my seminars who grew up in Trinidad or the West Indies, I found myself recalling the essayist Alfred Kazin's description of an ideal enthusiasm for living as "a lifetime burning in every moment." The people who had taken up liming seemed the perfect embodiment of such a quality. Their health, their focused energy, was directly linked to a sense of fun and lightheartedness.

Liming is one of the cornerstones of calm energy. The lightheartedness may pass, of course, but it feeds a human need and gives us what we need to face difficult challenges with greater commitment and ingenuity.

How to Do Nothing, Guilt-Free

Doing nothing can be harder than you think. A lot harder.

I'll be the first to admit that I can always use some remedial help in this area. There may have been a time in preschool when I could do nothing without feeling guilty, but by the time I heard the word *liming* in that seminar, I'd completely lost the knack. Sure, I could relax, but I had to plan ahead to find the time. And if the relaxation time lasted too long, I got anxious. I thought that there must be things that I was forgetting to do. Was this downtime really well-spent?

The sight of a hammock alarmed me. If I got into one, I might never want to get out! Then what would happen?

Goals are essential, aren't they? You don't want to lose your edge. So, I was driven. But the problem with being driven is that you may be driven away, inadvertently, from the life that you most want to lead.

As the research professor brought up the concept of liming in that room full of goal-oriented, achievement-oriented, time-cramped doctoral candidates, I'm sure that he sensed our unease. "I want to challenge every one of you," he said. "You are bright men and women. You are doing research that can have an influence on the world. But what I promise you is this: The heights of your intellectual brilliance will be enhanced by the extent to which you can let go and lime."

Was he exaggerating? Hardly, though when we think of brilliant people with great talent or intellectual stature, their ability to have lots of fun may not be the first thing to come to mind. But ever since that seminar, I have paid more attention to the liming that exceptional people instinctively do and the healthy, energizing impact that it has on their lives.

Merrier Go-Round

There's a famous picture of Albert Einstein in his fifties, riding a bicycle in a circle with a huge smile on his face. No place to go, just gliding around having fun. Getting breathing space. That's one of the images that comes to my mind when I think of liming.

I doubt that Einstein was dreaming up the theory of relativity at that moment, but the man on the bicycle with that boyish grin is the same human being who imagined a beam of light pedaling along through the universe.

The concept of liming also makes me think of the movie *Amadeus* and the insanely joyous, abandoned antics of Wolfgang Amadeus Mozart—a dramatic characterization, but nonetheless based on the real musician's reputation for sheer, exuberant musical celebration.

No, we don't turn ourselves into Einsteins or Mozarts by whooping it up. But there is increasing scientific evidence that, to be healthy and fully alive throughout our lives, we need to play often and with abandon. We need the release and relief of liming. Research also shows that repetitive patterns can be deadening.

We've all observed in our own lives what happens if we don't get breathing space. If we just keep working harder, longer, and faster, sooner or later we severely limit our capacities and thwart our own genius.

Breathing space is a necessity. We can't afford to skip it. We can't make everything serious. In our time away from work, our time with friends and loved ones, we need liming for calm energy as surely as those European sailors needed their storehouse of limes for survival.

Lessons from the Young

Five-year-olds are pretty good at liming. As I write, two of my top liming instructors are my elder daughter, Chelsea, and my younger daughter, Shanna.

Actually, Shanna was just 4 when she taught me one of her liming lessons. I had gone to pick her up from a summer preschool class. She and her friend Audrey were playing outside, running and laughing.

Naturally oblivious to the timepiece on my wrist and my wound-tight schedule, they continued to play after I arrived. I walked up and pointed to my watch, saying, "We only have 1 minute. Then we have to go." As I turned toward my car, with my cell phone ringing, I thought, "What are you doing, Robert? They don't really know what *1 minute* is."

But one thing that Shanna knew was that if she and Audrey could slip to the back of the school, they could play longer because I would have to walk back to get them. That is what happened. I turned around after my phone call and they were gone. "Great!" I thought, as I marched around the school, knowing that I was falling farther behind, time-wise.

When I found the girls at the back of the school yard, they were teasing each other, howling with laughter. Everything was fun and funny, the bugs, bushes, flowers, everything. As they dashed around the playground equipment, I felt myself getting even more impatient and frustrated. Didn't they know that adults have to be on time in life?

I was tense and tired, not feeling much calm energy at the end of that long day of work. Plus, I'd hoped to finish up a difficult project before the end of the day, and the prospects of succeeding at that grew fainter with each passing moment. Was I going to abandon my entire late-day schedule just to give them a few more minutes on the slide and swings?

"Come on, Shanna, we have to go . . . right now," I said, pointing to my watch.

No response. They waved to me and dashed off, laughing, in the opposite direction.

"Now!" I shouted.

"I have to get Shanna a watch—soon," I thought to myself. She might as well learn to be aware of time. After all, we all have to learn sometime.

I jogged across the playground to where the girls were playing.

"Shanna, we have to go now! There's no time to play!" I shouted.

Either the intensity of my voice or my words gave her pause. She stopped and looked up into my face with intense curiosity. In her sweet 4-year-old voice, she said simply, "But, Daddy, if there's no time to play, what's time for?"

I suddenly felt about an inch tall. What could I say? Oh, time is for getting in a car with a tense, anxious adult and driving too fast?

No, Shanna, you don't need a watch, not yet. You don't need to check things off your list and rush breathlessly from one errand to the next. As I walked her back to the car, I thought, "I'd better learn when to take my watch *off*."

Timeless Liming

At its purest, liming is a break from the stress of clock watching. Surprisingly, this kind of daytime rest, which is as much mental and emotional as physical, is also vital to your memory power. It gives your brain a much-needed opportunity to sort out the load of information that has reached it during the previous several hours.

As little as a few moments of breathing space can really pay off. Be

(continued on page 128)

TRY THIS NOW!

Take a break.

Sounds easy, doesn't it? Ironically, many of the obstacles to doing it well are internal rather than external.

Just think about how most of us react when friends, family, or coworkers advise us to relax or slow down a bit. Don't you feel a little insulted to be given that advice? First of all, if there were *time* to relax, you'd do it, wouldn't you? Second, if you didn't get things done, who would? If everyone just kicked back and relaxed, we'd have a pretty big mess on our hands.

Not surprisingly, that is how most of us react to this well-meant advice. "I'd love to take a break," we say. "There's no time."

We dedicate our lives to doing. And we have plenty to do. So it makes sense that we always feel as though we were falling farther behind.

We have to figure out a way to become great at the one thing that we can't let ourselves do, which is nothing, of course. Could 10 golden minutes of blissful procrastination be worth not getting something done? In its own way, yes. In fact, it may be even more valuable for some of us.

But grabbing that time means that we have to get over the trap of conditional happiness. That trap is setting up breathing space as a reward for accomplishment. "Once I finish this project, I'll take a nice break," we say to ourselves. We set up criteria that will "allow" us to take a break: "After I finish cleaning the house . . ." or "After I finish that task . . ." or "After the quarterly report is done. . . ."

But when breathing space is a reward on the other side of accomplishment or completion, like the little pot of gold at the end of a big rainbow, we rarely, if ever, give ourselves the time-out that we promised ourselves.

Why? According to one survey, each of us constantly has at least 35 hours of unfinished work waiting for us. That's right, we'll never finish. We'll never be completely caught up with all the tasks that we think we have to do.

That being the case, we have to fight the impulse to put off pulling back. If we're going to let go once in a while, we have to learn to do it by choice, on the spot, anytime and anywhere.

Here's How

If you think that you don't have time for a break, think again.

There's time, and then there's time.

Here's how to prove it to yourself. Take off your watch and hold it in your hand. Check the time, then close your eyes. Breathe steadily as you wait for 2 minutes to pass. When you think it has, open your eyes and check your watch.

When most people do this, they say that it's the longest 2 minutes they've had recently. That's a lot different from the stressed-out 2 minutes that fly by when you're trying to get out the door on time or get to the store before it closes or get to a meeting before your name becomes mud.

It's a timewarp—and a delicious one. It means that the time that you spend doing nothing is long, rich, and full. It may be only 2 minutes, but if you're truly doing nothing, it's as satisfying to your time-sensitive nature as a much longer spell of rest and relaxation.

So when you find yourself saying, "I don't have the time to take a breather," don't believe it. I know that you can find 1 to 2 minutes here and there. Seize them; use them. Do nothing during those minutes, and you may boost calm energy in one of the simplest ways of all.

sure to experiment with one of the simplest actions of all: Take a break to do absolutely nothing. That's one of the fastest ways to generate or renew calm energy.

Instead of speeding up and losing perspective, you can slow down and take a good look. This is what Ellen J. Langer, Ph.D., professor of psychology at Harvard University, has described as "shaking free of the mind-set of exhaustion."

Your mind and body have an innate conception of time that can fluctuate wildly, depending on who you are, what you're doing, and what pressure you're under. For someone who's on a tight schedule and under constant stress, the minutes get shorter. In fact, it may be revealing for you to try a time check on yourself. Check the time on your watch, then close your eyes. Wait until you think a minute has passed, then look.

Was it a minute? Or was it much less?

You may recall a similar test that I mentioned in Calm-Energy Switch #2, in which Larry Dossey, M.D., an internist and the author of *Meaning and Medicine: A Doctor's Tales of Breakthrough and Healing*, tested a group of high-powered managers. One of them thought a minute had passed in 9 seconds.

If *your* minutes are passing by in a matter of seconds, it's no wonder that you feel as if time were flying by. I believe that many people end up in this time crunch now and then.

The Big Slowdown

Time doesn't fly. *We* fly through time. Yes, we pack more in. We get more done. But we feel like the minutes were zooming by. If we actually perceive a full minute as a minute even with our eyes closed, we stand apart from the crowd.

You can step off the fast track whenever you choose to. You can breathe or listen or watch or wait or savor a momentary pause. In the middle of a traffic jam or when running for a plane. When you are up against a deadline or in the course of a meal.

With some practice, you can get the hang of what I call the liming minute. It doesn't require a course in meditation, but for some people, a well-timed liming minute can create as much calm energy as a lengthy relaxation session. Here's how you do it.

1. Let go of time.
2. Think of something funny.
3. Imagine something fun.

1. Let Go of Time

How do you let go of time? Hide your watch. Ignore the clock. Do the instant-calming sequence that I described in Calm-Energy Switch #2 to become focused in the present. When you let go of time, you simply release your concerns about what has just happened or what is coming up later.

2. Think of Something Funny

A sudden smile or pulse of laughter is one of the fastest igniters of creativity. Studies show that people who are quick to laugh, especially at themselves, are generally more active, more energetic, healthier, and better able to bounce back from stressful situations. But it's sometimes hard to get an instant chuckle, especially in a high-stress situation.

Here's a clue: In order to laugh at yourself, you have to forgive yourself for not being perfect. All right, so you should have seen the banana peel before you slipped on it. So what?

A forgiving attitude allows you to step back from your humanity and laugh at yourself. In truth, humor has very little to do with telling jokes.

It's about perceiving and chuckling at the absurdities of everyday life, from hassles to heartaches to hard times, and taking yourself more lightly even when you're doing serious work. As the editor of a very successful magazine said about his energetic, creative group of editors, "We take our work seriously, but we don't take ourselves seriously."

The fact is, you goof up. We all do. The bottom of the paper grocery bag gets wet, and all of the groceries fall out in the middle of the parking lot. Did you space out or was this just bad luck? Or both? Could you have avoided it? Could you have gotten plastic bags or noticed that the paper bag was wet on the bottom? Sure. But you didn't. So what? Seeing all of those loose apples rolling across the parking lot could be a sign that your whole day is going wrong and, furthermore, that you're incompetent.

Or it could just be pretty ridiculous and even hilarious. The most important thing to remember, with a smile, is to avoid oncoming cars as you run around retrieving the apples. Keep your balance and focus on what you *can* control, not on what you can't.

That's the concept of finding something that's funny. It's all about light-heartedness and laughing a lot harder and more often than most of us usually do. Humorous thoughts and, in particular, mirthful laughter work their wonders by initially arousing and distracting you mind, then by leaving you feeling more relaxed. We're all nut cases in our own little ways. So why not enjoy it? You're allowed to: It's for your own health.

Scientists have found that laughter stimulates the production of brain chemicals called catecholamines and endorphins. These chemicals affect hormonal levels in the body that are related to feelings of joy, the easing of pain, and strengthened immune response. Laugh at those runaway apples, and you stand a better chance of fighting off the next cold virus. How's that for a reward?

Admittedly, when you're under pressure, your humor button gets rusty. It sticks or freezes up. You try to push on it as if it were a badly wired doorbell, and what do you get? Nothing.

Here are several ways to get that button rewired, unfrozen, and working again.

Cultivate cosmic humor. If you're in the biggest hurry to get to the airport, you will get stuck in a traffic jam. If you're going to a meeting where it's absolutely essential to look your best, you can be sure that a spot will appear, as if by magic, on your suit. If it's of the utmost importance to be polite, be assured that some nondeliberate inept remark will slip out. In other words, the cosmos will play tricks on you. It comes with the territory. All you can do is your best in this comedy. The rest is dictated by that pair of rolling dice that we call destiny.

As for exercising absolute control over that destiny, well, forget it.

Multiply your mirth. Start looking for more of the ridiculous, incongruous events that go on around you all of the time. When you have the radio on in your car, notice the people on the sidewalk who stride in time to the music. Not that they realize it. But look for it, and you'll see it.

Watch a kid eat an ice cream cone. How can he get so much ice cream on his face or on the puppy that's sharing the cone? See how the little boy seems to enjoy the ice cream even more when that happens.

Look for coincidental names that are incredibly appropriate: the candy-store owner named Jellybean, the bank manager named Cash, the undertaker named Grim, the podiatrist named Corn.

What is the funniest thing that happened today? Is that the number one story that you take home to share with others? Any great conversations that you overhear are entertainment for the whole family. Rehearse them if you have to, but make sure that they get retold. You never know when a story may take on a life of its own.

TRY THIS NOW!

We all know that the daily newspaper has more than its share of grim or worrisome news. But the oddball, hilarious stories are there too.

As I write, I'm reminded of a news story reported to me by a friend. Timothy Boomer, a 25-year-old factory worker from Pittsburgh, fell out of his canoe when it hit a rock in the Big Rapids River on a bright summer day in 1998. Unfortunately, when he got his dunking, he let loose with a stream of expletives, well within earshot of a number of families.

Unbeknownst to Boomer, his expletives violated a Pennsylvania law drafted in 1802 that prohibits men from cursing in front of women and children. Among the bystanders, however, there was someone who knew about the law. One year later, Boomer stood convicted of—well, what do you call it? Assault with a dirty word?

However heinous his crime, Boomer was convicted of the charges, according to the news article. The second paragraph of the story contains this zinger: "Boomer did not show any reaction when the verdict was read." This raises the question, what was he supposed to show, deep remorse? What if he'd broken down and cried and begged the judge for mercy for all those expletives overheard by children?

Needless to say, that's a story that I'll add to my humor library. I may not read it often, but when I do, there will always a new twist to con-

Start a humor library. What makes you laugh? Whether it's news clippings, cartoons, letters from friends, posters, biographies, old or new comedy movies, joke encyclopedias, or humorous stories, expand your collection. Pay attention to whatever harmless humor tickles your funny bone and make it a point to keep it close by at all times.

sider. Like, what if Boomer had started swearing in the courtroom? Would the judge have arraigned him a second time for violation of the cursing law? Would the charge of courtroom swearing be added to his conviction for river swearing?

The mind, as they say, boggles.

Here's How

Find a manila folder or an envelope and label it "cosmic humor." Then, check your local paper to find at least one item to go in that newly created file. It shouldn't be hard. Find the headline that says something that it doesn't mean to say ("Driver Says He Lost His Head"). Look for the story of someone getting away with something amazing (the first grader who ordered a house, a Jaguar, and a Rolex watch on the Internet for $900,000). Or discover the absurdities that hover around normal events (the couple who lost their rental car in a 6-acre parking lot or the bank manager who had to show his ID at his own bank). This is, after all, the era when information that moves at the speed of light can be stopped by a single hacker and when cars that can go from 0 to 60 miles per hour in 6 seconds are forced to move at the speed of snails in traffic. Absurdities abound.

When you need a break, just open your cosmic-humor folder and enjoy at your leisure. This is one of the candy stores of calm energy.

3. Imagine Something Fun

Think of a beach. A beautiful view of nature during a hike. A sunrise. A favorite friend. Looking up at the stars on a crystal-clear night. Breakfast in bed at your favorite getaway place. Give your mind a rest in the most pleasant place you can find. Picture anything that reminds you of what you've enjoyed in the past and look forward to in the future. Have you ever found a patch of sweet grass warmed by the sunshine? Go there anytime—there's nothing to stop your mind from wandering there.

Basic Deprogramming

In some ways, we're pretty well programmed *not* to lime. We almost have to deprogram ourselves to escape some of the seriousness and intensity that closes in on every side.

Am I kidding? Not by a long shot. Think of all the years of training that went into making you a time-conscious, schedule-conscious, responsibility-conscious individual. Now, all I'm asking you to do is spend a few minutes deprogramming, getting the opposite kind of training.

Here's a little deprogramming exercise. Stand beside a big pile of unopened mail. Don't open any of it. Don't even look at the envelopes. There might be a check in there. More likely, bills. Perhaps a personal letter or two. Ignore all of it. Walk away and sit down, going through the liming minute: Let go of time. Think of something funny. Imagine something fun.

Can you feel the tension? Something tugging inside you that's telling you to go ahead and at least flip through the envelopes? When you feel that, you're dancing with one of the most powerful pulls of all: the doing instinct.

Here are some other challenges that are not for the rigid or rule-anchored.

• Spend some time watching a cat. Cats know almost everything there is to know about calm energy and liming.

THE DAYS AND MOMENTS
THAT MAKE US HAPPY **MAKE US WISE**.

—Witold Rybczynski, professor, McGill University, Montreal

- Practice lounging. When you're with others, whether at home, out in a restaurant, or on vacation, don't think or talk about goals and deadlines, urgencies or mistakes. Put your feet up on the coffee table.
- Listen to what's going on outdoors, in the street, or in a crowded room. Let the sounds wash over you.
- Eat for pleasure. Savor every single sip of tea and bite of food.
- Sink deep into an easy chair. You're not allowed to move suddenly. You can't leap up when the doorbell or phone rings. Your requirement is to lounge with as little tension as you can.
- Let the phone ring without answering it.
- Tune out workplace gossip.
- Turn off the radio or television just before the evening news.

A Balancing Act

What happens when there are demands on your time? When a child, for instance, approaches you with a problem?

You can't underestimate the ability of other people to spark your doing instinct. When a child, especially, voices frustrations, you're likely to feel a strong urge to fix whatever is wrong. You probably want to get all the details and guide your kid in what you see as the right direction.

But all of that doing could rob you of the very breathing space that could do the most good. Ironically, despite your good intentions, you could be robbing your child of something as well. Listen, by all means.

But just because you listen, that doesn't mean that you have to go out and fix things for your child. If a child can begin to self-manage emotional upsets, it's a good sign of emotional intelligence—the ability to sense and apply the feeling side of highest intelligence, which helps predict success later in life.

Be a Walden Walker

Here's one more exercise in liming training: Try taking a walk without your watch and without a map or goal. That's what Henry David Thoreau did. Thoreau called it sauntering.

"When I go out of the house for a walk," he said, "uncertain as yet whither I will bend my steps, I submit myself to my instinct to decide for me."

The point of all this is to try to see small things that you've never noticed before. Enjoy living, not just doing. The goal of not doing is to experience this feeling so fully that you will instantly realize when you begin to get tense and trapped in the rat race. No more numbness.

The better you get at not doing, the better you also get at doing things well in less time.

Head Home without the Headaches

If you work outside of the home, you need to develop a liming routine that will help you escape the work environment and free your mind and body so you can come safely and comfortably home again. You need a method of escape.

The word escape comes from the Latin and Old Northern French and originally meant "take off one's cloak." Today, as never before, we each need to be able to take off the cloak of work at the end of the day and on weekends. But just as most of us don't know how to lime, neither do we have the skills to downshift from work activities to nonwork activities.

Even if you've been at home all day, either in and out of a home office or consumed by daily chores, it's just as hard to free yourself from the mind-set of work.

By the time you walk in the door at home or finish all of the appointments, chores, and housework for the day, you are probably still firmly seized by the mind-set of work. You know the feeling: loose ends, items left undone, mistakes made.

If you get no break, the tension mounts. You can feel your knotted muscles. As you head home, the headaches on the home front begin to intrude on your consciousness. True, work is left behind, but what about those recurring concerns about your children and their future, or your parents and their problems? What about today's world news?

Compounding all of these concerns, you probably have an extensive list of the things that you have to get done—yard work, errands, meals, bills, cleaning, home repairs, laundry. There's always something.

Back at Home

Up to half of the most damaging arguments in a family relationship are started or magnified within 15 minutes of people greeting each other at the end of the day, according to a researcher at the University of California, Los Angeles, Medical School. Despite all the talk about how important it is to create some kind of work-home balance, most people aren't sure how to make this a reality. Here are a few practical approaches that you can use.

Make a brief transition away from work at the end of the day. Devote the final minutes of your working day to low-pressure tasks. Still have some phone calls to make? Talk only to people who are likely to be supportive and positive. You can call the complainers and the monsters in the morning.

Straighten up your work area. This is a simple thing, but it can finalize the day for you.

Look at your schedule for the next day. You won't be caught off-guard.

Put pen to paper. There's a certain finality and a sense of completeness when you make a list. When you find your thoughts ablaze with uncompleted business, make a note of whatever projects are pending or likely to nag you overnight. And list any calls you have to make the next day, including the difficult ones that you've just postponed. Sure, you'll have to face that list and make those calls in the morning, but it's better to do it when you're fresh. In the meantime, you can put that list out of your mind.

Sketch out the evening. If you're planning to tackle some after-hours work, ask yourself, "What's the best use of my time tonight, for myself and my loved ones? Can this task be postponed or delegated? Can I realistically complete it, or will I be distracted and frustrated because I can't finish what needs to be done?"

By making a clear separation in your mind between your work life and your home life before you reconnect with loved ones, you're already taking greater control of your work-family balance.

Let go of tensions all the way home. In interviewing leaders and professionals, I'm amazed at how many of them curse and fume at traffic delays, make risky driving maneuvers, and generally treat the trip home like a combat mission. Research suggests that we're far better off if we take a few minutes longer to arrive home and shed excess tension and work intensity every mile of our commutes. Consider taking off your watch, breathing more slowly, relaxing tense muscles, and thinking not of working but of your own nonwork passions. Think of the people whom you love and whose lives you are working to benefit.

If you feel that you're losing out because someone is cutting in front of you or getting in the faster lane, measure the risk against the gain. The gain is probably a minute, maybe two. The risk is quite possibly your life. Aggressive driving just isn't worth it.

Building a Buffer Zone

I believe that it's essential to create a 1- to 15-minute buffer zone for yourself that starts at the moment that you walk in the door of your house.

Often, partners are primed for a mutual rendition of "Here's what happened today" as soon as they see each other at the end of the day. Little do we realize that this is a danger zone for relationships, a prime time for dumping complaints on each other and triggering fatigue-driven arguments.

Consider an alternative: Negotiate in advance, with your spouse or other family members, a different kind of greeting. Let your first comment be 25 words or less: "What a hectic day! It's great to be home"; or "Things were really crazy at work, but I'm really glad to see you!" Hug each other.

Is that enough? For the moment, yes. You're glad to be home. The day was eventful. But leave it at that. Without ignoring your partner or other family members, delay talking about your day. In return, others have to acknowledge that you're not ready to listen, either. Later on, you can hear about your partner's day or what the children experienced or argued about, which household appliances broke or who needs money.

But before all that, take some buffer-zone minutes. This is an opportunity to climb to a higher vantage point and take better care of yourself and your relationships. You might use this brief interlude to exercise, take a shower or hot bath, or change clothes. Or enjoy a small pre-meal snack. There's evidence that simple hunger-related tensions trigger many needless arguments, so that little snack may help prevent an argument as well as protect your buffer zone.

A Sitter Situation

For some families with young children, the end of the workday is one of the best times to have a babysitter come in. Often, we act as though it were legitimate to take time for ourselves, even just a few minutes, only when we have satisfied all of the demands of others. In other words, never. But such an interlude is time that we both need and deserve.

In any relationship that involves caring and intimacy, you and your partner need time to relate to each other. What makes people get along in a relationship is "the ability to feel relaxed together," says William Nagler, M.D., psychiatrist at the University of California, Los Angeles, School of Medicine, who specializes in effective relationships communication. "Do you want a relationship that is satisfying, makes you happy, and will last? The truth is that happy couples don't try to entertain each other, they relax and enjoy each other's company. . . . Tension reduction is the most important thing you can do to make your relationship last and to make it better."

Given a respite, you and your partner can go for a walk, sit for a while outdoors, or give each other a back rub. Enjoy some relaxing music, or sip your favorite glass of wine or cup of tea.

This is also a good time to share the absurdities and funniest pratfalls that you observed during the day. In one study of married couples, psychologists found that humor was a key component of happiness. Seventy percent of the couples who ranked high in happiness also displayed significant amounts of humor in their relationships. In particular, the researchers found that happiness was often tied to having an amusing, energetic partner who finds simple ways to make you laugh.

Cut Up a Bit

Using humor to defuse tension and anger can work in all kinds of situations. What if your spouse comes home after a rough day at work and takes out frustrations by yelling at you or the kids? Instead of becoming angry and emotionally off-balance, try a dose of humor or fun.

For example, you might imagine your spouse as a grouchy, irritable-yet-cuddly teddy bear in dire need of a hug or a kiss or a kind word. He or she is asking for your help because of a difficult day at work. You can take the grumpiness less seriously because what your spouse really needs is your support and care, rather than more yelling, or a confrontation and a ruined evening or weekend.

In response to grumbling complaints and grouchy comments, you might take a deep breath and say, in as warm a tone as you can muster, "I can tell that you've had a really rough day." Reach out to give a reassuring pat on the back or squeeze on the arm. "I'm happy you're home now, here with us," you might add. Contrast that to the probable outcome—and the mood of your entire evening—if you snap back with something like, "If you think that *you* had a rough day. . . ."

If the grouchiness is a chronic behavior, it may call for other strategies. But if it happens only occasionally, your willingness to be compassionate and have fun can be contagious. Humor and good jokes that are well-timed, that are backed with kind words, and that provide a chance for your spouse to cool off can lighten almost anyone's burden.

Try the "What a . . ." Response

Whenever you find yourself feeling a surge of anger or hostility, shift your attention. Ask yourself whether the action that has provoked your anger is really a deliberate affront. Try to reframe the provocation and see things from the other person's point of view. Tell yourself, "There's no need to get upset about this. Maybe he's actually angry about something else and is letting off steam."

Then, be sure to relax your tense muscles. Slow your breathing. Whenever possible, use humor.

Again, you may be better off if you have a well-developed ability to detect silliness or at least imagine it. If you're driving and someone else has failed to signal and cuts into the lane ahead of you during rush hour, it's appropriate to think, "What a clown!"

But your anger may still be surging. Take the next step, which will bring you calm energy. Envision a huge clown face, red lips and nose pressed to the wheel, fumbling to steer down the road.

Or follow the suggestion of psychologist Martin E. P. Seligman, Ph.D. In his work, Dr. Seligman has one particular tactic to deal with the growing phenomenon of road rage. When that driver cuts in front of you, he suggests that you say, "What an ass!" Then, go ahead and visualize a pair of buttocks steering the car ahead. When you're vividly imagining that absurd image, it's almost impossible to get mad. How can you be enraged at an ass behind a steering wheel?

Master the Simple Daily Pleasures

One of the ways to deepen and expand your experience of liming and, at the same time, gain a variety of well-documented health benefits is to reclaim some of the small daily pleasures that have probably fallen by the wayside in your busy life.

A Japanese study comparing workers in New York, Los Angeles, and Tokyo found that each group had differing amounts of time for relaxation at home. Those working in New York or Los Angeles had 4 to 5 hours of free time after work. In Tokyo, where there are even longer commuting hours, the average time for relaxation at home was only 3 hours. Yet in all three cities, the hours at home were usually filled with one primary, voracious activity: watching television. Three hours a day means 15 hours during every work week. Five hours a day adds up to 25 hours—and that's not counting weekend TV watching.

Whichever modern city you choose to observe, you'll find that working people are spending an unprecedented chunk of time devoted to one after-work pastime: They're staring at a glowing cathode-ray tube. It's an activity that requires little energy and virtually no imagination. And it can virtually eliminate calm energy.

In fact, the energy-draining effects of TV watching have been studied with objective tests. Evidence suggests that you may burn 10 to 15 percent fewer calories while watching television than you do when sitting still with the television off.

Get Your Active Relaxation

In his research on stress-resistant people, Raymond B. Flannery Jr., Ph.D., professor of psychology at Harvard Medical School, discovered that the healthiest people, those who had the lowest levels of distress and the lowest rates of illness, were those who enjoyed some daily forms of active relaxation that lasted at least 15 minutes. In Dr. Flannery's research, this ranged from more formal pursuits such as meditation or relaxation exercises to such informal activities as knitting or playing solitaire. When asked about relaxation, the people who were more vulnerable to stress were likely to reply, "I don't have time to relax."

As you ease away from television, it's the small, simple pleasures that usually pay the greatest dividends. As with any other change of habit, a gradual switch is best. You might start by cutting out one television show on a certain weeknight and substituting some other enjoyable activity. But whatever you do, you'll reap the benefits of calm energy. Here are some options.

- Listen to your favorite music.
- Study stars against the night sky.
- Watch a sunset from beginning to end.

- Play a musical instrument.
- Write poetry or a short story.
- Paint a landscape.
- Relish a novel.
- Play cards or tackle a crossword puzzle.
- Go for a relaxed run or a pleasant walk.
- Sip tea, reflecting on life or snuggling with your romantic partner.
- Play hide-and-seek with your children or grandchildren.
- Swing in a hammock.
- Throw a Frisbee.
- Shoot some baskets.
- Watch home movies, look through family photo albums, or tell your favorite stories.
- Sit down with your parents or elderly neighbors and ask them some questions that you've never asked before.
- Write down your thoughts and dreams in a journal.
- Play a rousing, laughter-filled board game.

The only requirement is that the activity must give your heart and spirit a boost. This is what, most of all, ignites and sustains the calm energy that you require to be fully alive.

Part 3

Active
Energy

All of us know people who look or act half their ages. Of course, such a gift is partly a reflection of genetics. But there's more at work here. To a great extent, extraordinary youthfulness at any chronological age is due to active energy. It is produced by movement. It rejuvenates us and makes us feel vibrantly alive.

Some of the most memorable notes that I have ever received are from Charles Eastwood, a mentor of mine many years ago. I worked with him for more than 3 years, and he kept reminding me that life is short. He challenged my capacity to make a difference in the lives of others and to contribute to the world. He signed his notes, "Vigorously yours."

This man had survived the Pacific battles of the Second World War. He held two doctorates from Northwestern University in Evanston, Illinois. But what I remember most about him was his exceptional attentiveness and energy in the face of difficult times and daunting circumstances. He had learned to develop and maintain a high level of active energy.

Active energy provides the get-up-and-go that helps you give your best at work and enjoy your life. It enables you to effectively face challenges and to bounce back from life's inevitable difficulties. Without active energy, it's hard—and sometimes scarcely even possible—to stay enthusiastic or vigorous in the rush and roar of everyday living.

Any kind of physical movement is initiated by a set of alertness switches in your brain. And once you're in motion, those switches are stimulated, in turn, by your movements. It's a continuous and self-propelling cycle: The switches stimulate physical activity, and your body movements trigger switch activity. So active energy is a primary source of physical pep and mental drive.

Burning More Body Fat—And Enjoying It More

With a high level of active energy, you increase your ability to lose excess body fat automatically, even while you sleep. When the switches of active energy are turned on at the right times throughout the day, your metabolism—the biochemical processes of making new energy molecules in your brain and body—is naturally higher, and so is your ability to burn off excess fat and stay healthier during stressful times.

The opposite of active energy is reserved energy, or inertia. Examples are driving instead of walking, sitting instead of standing, or watching television instead of participating in active pursuits. This has become the predominant pattern for almost half of Americans.

As parents, we inadvertently take this energy away from our children. "Sit still," we say. "Stop fidgeting. Act like an adult. Stay right where you are. Don't move."

Have you ever observed how difficult it is for children to comply with these restrictions? Even if they want to cooperate, they can't seem to do it. They have to move. They tap their toes. They squirm and giggle. They drum their desks with pencil erasers. Look at a roomful of young children, and you'll see—no, you'll feel—evidence of the active energy that's as strong as a flood tide.

For many of us, the active-energy instinct is evident in subtle ways. We may try to behave like "adults"—that is, "properly" and, in some cases, statuelike—but even when we're sitting still, it's not for very long. Active energy connects us with the world by moving us into it. Sitting motionless is against our inherent biological nature. We were born for motion, for activity.

Gearing Up for Action

Lucky for all of us, the world is full of interesting things to learn and do. But what happens when you suppress your instinct for active energy? Your imagination suffers. Your mental triggers get underused because your body is not activating or being activated by them. That causes a loss of attentiveness and vigor as well as a feeling of tiredness or lethargy.

When active energy is engaged, you have more attentiveness and vigor to fully explore your most compelling interests, talents, needs, and passions. The active-energy connection is evident in people who are doers. But in truth, we are all doers by nature. The poet or musician, writer or explorer, astronomer or gardener, inventor or sports enthusiast, community volunteer, independent scholar or scientist, artist or collector are all actively doing things. What we underestimate, however, is how much the doing generates the increased active energy that is required to do more of the things that matter most.

For instance, imagine that you wish to do something as apparently simple as writing a letter. Start the old-fashioned way, with pen in hand. You only have to think of what you want to say, and you're ready to start writing. You haven't composed the whole letter in advance. You may not even have a clue about how long it's going to be, what will come to mind as you're writing, or when you'll feel that it's finished. Many of those decisions are made in the process of writing, and if it's a great letter or you're writing to someone whom you really care about, the process itself can be energizing.

In a way, the decisions that you make when you're writing are not even conscious decisions. They're the result of a steady flow of signals between your mind and body as your hand moves along, writing steadily, stimulating your brain to think of new ideas, perhaps stirring memories, bringing up word associations, and creating a fresh image of a person or place in your mind. As soon as those ideas are generated, your hand springs into action again, penning the words that describe what's in your mind.

What's to Be Done

In everything that involves doing, this active-energy link is paramount. From hour to hour, your active energy must be switched on again and again.

But there's nothing complicated about these switches. If you are writing a letter, the movement of the pen (or the action of your fingers on a keyboard) is the switch that raises your metabolism, increases your attentiveness, and stimulates your imagination. Other active-energy switches are similarly easy to learn and use. Turn on those switches, and your overall vigor and vitality will noticeably increase.

"A person's alertness is triggered by key internal and external factors that can be considered switches on the control panel of the mind," observes Martin Moore-Ede, M.D., Ph.D., associate professor of physiology and director of the Institute for Circadian Physiology at Harvard Medical School. "Understanding these key switches and how

Reaping the Benefits

Active energy will give you:
• Peak alertness with physical vigor and mental drive throughout the day
• Increased fat-burning power, even while you sleep
• Better self-regulation of moods and motivation
• Greater ability to handle pressure
• Extraordinary attentiveness to people and tasks
• Increased confidence and ingenuity in facing challenges
• Heightened ability to unwind and relax
• Exceptional stamina all day long
• Deeper sleep and rest

to manipulate them is the secret of gaining power over one of the most important attributes of the human brain."

In this part of the book, you'll discover the key energy switches that turn on active energy. How often you use these switches and which ones you use are entirely up to you. But the important thing is to try them out.

The following chapters are designed to help you gain control over some of the most important aspects of the active energy that fuels your life and work. The truth is, with a bit of practice, most of these switches can save you time and produce measurably more energy and attentiveness.

It's essential to begin with systematic self-observation of your active energy, including when you need it most, what causes it to fade, and how to most simply and readily increase it. The following switches are quite simple to turn on anywhere and anytime.

Plan Your Time-Outs

I t's a paradox of modern life: To get ahead, you have to know when—and precisely how—to pull back.

But pulling back is directly at odds with the way that most of us are accustomed to living and working. We get up earlier and earlier in the morning. We drive ourselves and others harder and longer. "I have to keep at it or I'll surely fall behind," we say.

But we're wrong. Many people will endure months and even years of pushing nonstop, making a futile attempt to stay on top of everything. They seem to be in motion at all times. But when they look back, years later, they realize that they were numb from constantly trying to keep moving, and they unwittingly ended up blunting their active energy and accomplishing few of the things that mattered most to them.

For active energy to thrive, you must learn to pace how much you do and how long you do it. Otherwise, the harder you push, the further behind you may actually fall.

To prevail in life, we need what can be called smart pacing. It is based on extensive research with star performers in all fields, the men and women who consistently excel under pressure and make more of the right things happen.

Why Pacing Is Important

The top players in tennis know that they must develop the skill to deeply relax for a few key moments between shots. In the middle of each challenging set, they have to fight the impulse to drive harder. Even if it's just for a moment, they need to relax. If they wait to rest until the end of the game or day, it's too late; they overexert themselves and underperform, losing on all counts.

It turns out that the harder and longer we push ourselves nonstop, the more prone we are to mistakes and errors. That's because the more we're driven by internal and external pressures, the less active energy we have. This can hurt our health as well as our performance.

If we deprive ourselves of conscious, controlled breaks during our waking hours, our bodies' natural instincts take revenge. We get hit with thousands of individual space outs and micro-sleeps. They're caused by never stopping.

Many automobile and airplane accidents are attributed to such brief and preventable oversights. "Impaired alertness is one of the greatest potential dangers of contemporary life," observes William C. Dement, M.D., Ph.D., professor of psychiatry and behavioral sciences at Stanford University School of Medicine.

Of course, even when those moments sneak up on us, when we space out, we continue to rationalize. We say that we have to keep going to catch up. That's an illusion.

WITHOUT ENERGY, LIFE IS MERELY
A LATENT POSSIBILITY. **THE WORLD**
BELONGS TO THE ENERGETIC.

—Ralph Waldo Emerson (1803–1882), U.S. poet and essayist

When we work for longer than 20 to 30 minutes straight on a single task, studies show that the time we need for problem solving increases by up to 500 percent. That is, the task that could take only 5 minutes to complete takes 25 minutes instead. So when we're constantly driving ourselves, there really *aren't* enough hours in the day. But that's not because the days are shorter. It's because we're spending more time than necessary on each individual task.

In short, we're in far worse shape when we try to stay focused and neglect to give ourselves breaks. But so few people around us are stopping for even a moment that we have come to believe that we shouldn't stop either. We're wrong.

Slip Off the Straitjacket

Children instinctively take pauses throughout the day, both at home and at school. We chide them to focus, to sit still, to stop their natural instinct to chat and laugh. We grow tired of hearing them say that they're thirsty or hungry. Yet these are their natural voices of biological energy calling.

Even though nearly all of us adults have silenced those biological voices, it doesn't mean that we're smarter than kids. It simply means that we're following the patterns of many other adults, without ever figuring out whether they've found the best way to make use of their biological energy.

But when you think about it, why should any of us—including our children—be expected to feign attention? It's as if we were at war with our own natures. While we instinctively fidget around, we tell ourselves we should be sitting up straight and paying attention. Why should we force ourselves to conform to this image of statuelike attentiveness?

The Pause That Revitalizes

I recommend a simple and vital technique that requires only a half-minute of your time to produce 30 straight minutes of active-energy boosting. It is a half-minute break that I call the strategic pause.

Over the years, I have learned that strategic pauses create a ripple effect. The ripple builds to a wave of increased energy that has real lasting power. With each brief pause, you do more than refresh your mind and invigorate your senses and stamina. You also send a series of simple yet powerful signals to your brain and senses about how alive you want to feel and how active you want to be. Each of these feedback loops generates increased energy and makes it easier for your senses to notice whenever your level of vitality fades and to respond on the spot to raise it again.

When you take strategic pauses, it's harder to be chronically inactive. It's easier to have the energy and attentiveness to keep abreast of your priorities.

The simplest reminder system is a time cue: Take a 30-second strategic pause once every half-hour.

But there's another way to schedule strategic pauses. You can use body cues. While this may take some practice, you'll find that you can get natural signals from your mind, muscles, or senses that tell you when your active energy is beginning to dip. Those signals tell you instantly that you need to stop pushing so hard or fast.

For most people, the signs of reduced attentiveness or energy appear about every half-hour or so during the day. The very first feelings of increased tension, tiredness, distraction, or anxiety should tell you that it's time to take a strategic pause.

Customize Your Pause

During a strategic pause, you can try a number of different approaches to get the break that you need. This is the time to use any of the calm-energy switches that affect your breathing, posture, and focus, which you read about in part 2. You can use the instant-calming sequence (ICS) from Calm-Energy Switch #2 during the strategic pause, but there are some other very effective approaches as well. Here are some that I recommend.

Shift your gaze. Many people don't realize that accumulated eyestrain can actually cause tension and fatigue or make it worse. Of course, that's especially true late in the day. The tiny muscles in the human eye use more energy than any other muscle fibers in the body. You're constantly working those muscles, and unless you give them a brief break every half-hour or so, they get tired. The exhaustion of those tiny muscles contributes to headache, fatigue, and related tension in your neck and shoulders.

The proliferation of computers has only made things worse. One study of 2,330 people from 15 different regions of the country reported that 77 percent of the users of computer monitors reported problems with eyestrain. Among those who didn't use computers, the reported incidence of eyestrain was 56 percent.

Whenever you're doing close work, you need to take a few moments

Water Works

According to scientific reports, dehydration has a number of negative effects on your metabolism. A decrease in water consumption not only contributes to fatigue but also may cause fat deposits in your body to increase. In contrast, an increase in water intake may actually help *reduce* fat deposits.

"Water may be one of the simplest, most powerful keys to increased energy and the loss of excess body fat," says Ellington Darden, Ph.D., a strength expert and exercise scientist who has been director of research for Nautilus Sports/Medical Industries in Colorado Springs for the past 20 years.

You get even more benefits by drinking ice-cold water, Dr. Darden suggests. "A gallon of ice-cold water requires more than 200 calories of heat energy to warm it to core body temperature," he says. His findings suggest that ice-cold water not only may increase energy but also may actually help to burn excess body fat.

And there's more. People who drink lots of water are more likely to have smoother skin and more regular and softer bowel movements. They also have increased resistance to infections because of the moisturizing effect on the mucous lining of the respiratory tract.

Other benefits of good hydration include a higher volume of urine production, which decreases fatigue, and lessens the risk of elevated blood pressure, kidney stones, and urinary infections. Also, if you drink more water, you're less likely to have that problems with fluid retention that are known as edema.

to blink your eyes and look at more distant objects. Turn away from your area of focus and gaze at a picture or poster on the wall. Take in the scenery that's outside your window. These easy actions help provide a brief and vital rest for the most active eye muscles.

For anyone who wears contact lenses, some added tactics can be helpful. You blink less when you concentrate, so your eyes can get very dry at work. But contacts need constant remoisturizing, or they'll start to irritate your corneas. You'll need to look up from your work more frequently than someone who doesn't wear contacts. When you give your eyes that moment of relief, researchers have observed, your blink rate has a chance to return to normal.

Sip ice water. Consume small amounts of chilled water every 20 to 30 minutes during the day, and you provide a clear, repeated signal to your metabolism to keep your energy and alertness levels higher. In addition, you improve your overall health and resistance to illness.

Active energy depends on fluids. Water provides the medium for nerve-impulse conduction, the transmission of other biochemical processes, immune functioning, and the muscle contractions that stimulate metabolism. When your body is fully hydrated, it enhances the physiological processes that release fat cells' fatty acids into your bloodstream so they can be delivered to your muscles for burning.

Dehydration occurs when you don't take in enough water to replace all that's lost through perspiration, respiration, urination, and other body processes. Dehydration reduces blood volume, leading to thicker, more concentrated blood. That blood is more difficult to pump, which puts more stress on your heart muscle. It is also less capable of providing your muscles with the oxygen and nutrients they need, and it's less efficient in transporting, carrying away, and eliminating accumulated wastes.

Many factors contribute to invisible fluid loss. When you're in a well-

(continued on page 162)

TRY THIS NOW!

Studies show that a very small water loss can lead to significant changes in the way that your body works. "Even a tiny shortage of water disrupts your biochemistry," says Michael Colgan, Ph.D., nutritional researcher and visiting scholar at Rockefeller University in New York City. "Dehydrate a muscle by only 3 percent, and you lose 10 percent of contractile strength and 8 percent of speed. Water balance is the single most important variable in lifelong good health and top performance."

It takes surprisingly little fluid loss—only 1 to 2 percent of your body's water content—for you to become dehydrated. You may think that you would instantly become thirsty when you're dehydrated, but in fact, thirst is an unreliable indicator of mild water loss. That's why physicians have long recommended that we each drink six to eight 8-ounce glasses of water every day for best health.

"Because a deficiency of water can alter the concentration of electrolytes such as sodium, potassium, and chloride, water has a profound effect on brain function and energy level," says Vernon H. Mark, M.D., a neurosurgeon at Massachusetts General Hospital in Boston and coauthor of *Brain Power: A Neurosurgeon's Complete Program to Maintain and Enhance Brain Fitness throughout Your Life.*

"Even a slightly dehydrated body can produce a small but critical shrinkage of the brain, thereby impairing neuromuscular coordination, concentration, and thinking," add sports-medicine researchers Robert Goldman, M.D., president of the National Academy of Sports Medicine, and Robert M. Hackman, Ph.D.

Everyone begins the day with a water deficit. During the night, you lose a normal amount of water that's exhaled with every sleeping breath. When you open your eyes in the morning, your body is already thirsty.

Water loss continues throughout the day. Each day, the average person loses at least 2 cups of water through breathing, another 2 cups through invisible perspiration, and 6 cups through urination and bowel movements. That's 10 cups a day that you lose automatically, even if you don't do any high-intensity exercise or hard physical work.

Many foods contain a large amount of water, and you obtain approximately 3½ cups of water from what you eat over the course of a day. Interestingly, your body's metabolism itself is another source. As your body uses energy, it produces about ½ cup of water as a by-product. Taking into account the approximately 4 cups provided by food and metabolism and the 10 cups lost, the average person needs to drink 6 to 8 cups of water every day just to stay healthy.

Here's How

Right now, reach for a glass of ice-cold water. Sip slowly.

Can you feel the energy reaction in your body and senses, a quick pick-me-up effect? Many people can. It happens that fast.

Make it a point to keep ice-cold fluids nearby. My wife, Leslie, and I use inexpensive insulated plastic water bottles. Our children carry water bottles with them to school and all outdoor activities.

When I travel, I carry an insulated liter-size water bottle. It keeps water ice cold for hours.

FEW WOULD DENY THAT THE CAPACITY FOR **HUMOR**, LIKE HOPE, **IS ONE OF THE MOST POTENT SOURCES OF ENERGY** AND RESILIENCE.

—George Vaillant, Ph.D., *Adaptation to Life*, 1995

heated or air-conditioned workplace, the air is often dry. Caffeine is also a factor since it's a diuretic, meaning that it causes you to lose fluids.

The benefits of sipping water may be even more pronounced when the water is ice cold. When ice-cold water reaches your stomach, it stimulates increased energy production throughout your body and increased alertness in your brain and senses. So as long as you're filling your glass, make it ice water whenever you can.

Get some bright light. Active energy can fade quite rapidly in the absence of light. But a quick burst of increased brightness can boost your energy, often dramatically.

More than half of your body's sense receptors are clustered in your eyes. Studies show that your eyes act as light harvesters, firing neurological impulses in a direct stream to the pineal gland and the higher centers of your brain. With more stimuli, those light harvesters act more rapidly, getting regular doses of novel images, beauty, and brightness. The impact of that steady flow of new images can produce invigorating, antidepressant effects, according to studies done by researchers at Harvard University.

Many people report that when they're exposed to bright sunlight, they experience a strong sense of calmness followed by a surge of energy. Even some extra indoor light, not much more than the intensity level of normal room lamps, can increase your energy level. During each strategic pause, take a few moments to expose yourself to more light. Either step to a brightly lit window or turn on some extra lights in your work area.

Reengage. Active energy is highest whenever you feel most involved with an activity or task, that is, whenever you're doing something that is meaningful and exciting to you. On the other hand, "whenever work is boring or monotonous, energy and alertness fade," according to Martin Moore-Ede, M.D., Ph.D., associate professor of physiology and director of the Institute for Circadian Physiology at Harvard Medical School.

At the end of each strategic pause, reengage with what's most meaningful and exciting to you. This kind of focus is an essential component of alertness. Ask yourself, "Why am I doing this? Exactly where is it leading me? Should I shift my focus? How can I make more of a difference?"

You may not have all of the answers to those questions. But as you return to the task at hand, those questions will automatically raise your active energy and keep you more aware of what you're doing—and why.

Reset Your Pace

The biological force that we call active energy is powerfully affected by time. In the intriguing field of scientific exploration known as chronobiology, scientists have been mapping and measuring the natural energy rises and falls that we each experience throughout the day. They've thoroughly studied circadian rhythms, the sleep-wake patterns that are repeated in 24-hour cycles. But there are also ultradian rhythms, rises and falls of energy that occur many times in each 24-hour cycle.

Ultradian rhythms occur in 90-minute to 180-minute cycles. The current understanding of ultradian rhythms is based on hundreds of biological and behavioral studies conducted in laboratories throughout the world.

These regular rhythms of activity and rest that occur every 1½ to 3 hours involve complex patterns of communication caused by messenger chemicals. The messenger chemicals connect all the activities of your senses and nervous system. Via these messenger chemicals, your brain activity is connected with your body and activates a wide range of functions that raise your alertness and sharpen your perspective and focus in life. Ultimately, these messenger chemicals help regulate your energy levels.

The repeated, detectable patterns of ultradian rhythms suggest that messenger chemicals ebb and flow in predictable sequences. No matter what else is going on, you'll have a sinking feeling when energy seems to be at low ebb. If you just take a few key minutes to manage the downswing, rather than fight it, you can essentially get in sync with your body's chemical signals. This resetting gives you a better chance of recovering smoothly amid the continually shifting challenges and pressures of life.

I call such a resetting an essential break because that's just what it is, a break that's crucial to reestablish the best biological rhythm in your body and to fully restore your sense of well-being.

Get with the Rhythm

If you're unaware of your ultradian rhythm and don't take essential breaks during the downturns, you may pay a steep price. Escalating tension levels and health stresses can turn, over time, into constant fatigue and illness.

Throughout the day, your energy surges, then declines, then surges again in a steady rhythm of chemically controlled messages that gives you the energy advantage at certain times but causes you to struggle at other times. If you've ever tried to swim against oncoming ocean waves, you know what it's like to fight your ultradian rhythm. Imagine that you could swim *with* the waves all the time, moving strongly when you're at the top of the wave, then taking a moment to gather your strength while the next surge builds underneath you.

When you reset your pace with essential breaks, you automatically make the mental and physical adjustments that get you in harmony with this rhythm. This has a powerful effect. With just a few moments of mental or physical adjustment, your mental and physical rhythms are more in sync with what's happening in your life and your environment. You stop wasting strokes and emerge from the moment feeling more in tune and more powerful than you did a few minutes before.

Taking an essential break to resynchronize your rhythm is quite different from taking a strategic pause. You can easily plan a strategic pause, and it doesn't take more than 30 seconds. But knowing when you need to take an essential break is more intuitive. You need to recognize the upswings and downswings that you experience during the day and, instead of fighting those waves by drinking coffee or using increased tension or time urgency to wake yourself up, figure out how often you need to take essential breaks—mid-morning, lunchtime, and mid-afternoon?—and how long they should be.

Should each essential break be 2 minutes, 5 minutes, or something in between? Should you get right back to what you were doing? When the break is over, do you return to peak alertness?

The timing and lengths of your essential breaks are highly individual. You may need to experiment with different lengths of breaks and different intervals between the breaks to find out what's right for you. While you may not be able to take your essential breaks exactly when you want to, it's helpful to know your ideal daily pattern and time your breaks accordingly.

When you do take an essential break, you may feel like a rebel. In nearly every workplace, there are norms for essential breaks, and the person who breaks out of those norms may end up feeling guilty.

But science is on your side. More and more people are realizing that pushing nonstop and skipping breaks creates a wide range of preventable problems.

In a number of workplaces, the prevailing theory seems to be that there's no need for breaks—they're just a waste of time.

Research tells us that the reverse is true. Short breaks actually speed up work and increase energy, according to Etienne Grandjean, M.D., Ph.D., an expert on productivity at the Swiss Federal Institute of Technology. When people take short breaks, he discovered, they have a greater number of total accomplishments per day. Not only that but they also exhibit less distress and fatigue.

Once you get used to taking essential breaks to reset your pace, you'll find that they actually save time rather than waste it. Dozens of scientific studies support this observation.

When you learn to take 2- to 5-minute essential breaks to reset your pace, you experience natural, powerful waves of biological energy that generate a continual stream of active energy for up to 3 hours. This can strongly influence your thoughts, feelings, and actions, biologically lifting you up. But if you skip a break, your active energy level will fall, unavoidably.

If you take all these breaks, will you ever catch up with all the chores you have to do or the assignments you have to complete?

It isn't fatalistic to accept the fact that the answer is no. You'll never complete everything. It's just good common sense to accept that condition. Instead of rushing and pushing harder to catch up, the better strategy is to take essential breaks that will allow you to respond to your natural energy waves. That way, you can work with them rather than constantly opposing them.

Perfect Timing

Reset your pace at mid-morning, at lunchtime, and again in the middle of the afternoon, when the dips occur in your ultradian rhythm. You should consider these the minimum requirements. Remember, the cycles can occur as frequently as every 90 minutes. So it makes sense to notice other signs or symptoms that tell you when to take a break. Here are some of those signals.

- Feeling a need to stretch or move
- Finding yourself yawning or sighing
- Becoming distracted or finding that you're unable to concentrate
- Feeling increased tension or fatigue
- Hunger pangs
- Feeling anxious about pressures or progress
- Becoming increasingly frustrated with a task or obligation
- Increased errors in judgment
- Having trouble with such basic skills as spelling, counting, or typing

In terms of time, the breaks don't need to last very long. As little as 2 to 3 minutes at each break may be enough to get you in sync with your ultradian rhythm, though some people take as much as a 20-minute break when they have the chance.

However long you take, breaks are vital activities needed to reset your basic level of active energy. Each break is really the key for getting the most out of the 90 to 180 minutes that follow it.

Where Breaks Are the Norm

The idea of taking a break to reset your rhythm can be found in many cultures. In fact, the instinctive need to pause, consider, and share with others is probably as old as mankind.

Everywhere I have traveled in the world, I have seen the essential break woven into social life with a variety of customs. In fact, I have made friends and gained insights in many cultures when I've shared these brief chances to slow down and rekindle vitality and humanity. No matter what the custom, each formal break is an opportunity to restore active energy.

In Tibet, for instance, the people instinctively and traditionally pause many times a day to make tea and unwrap a favored serving of food.

Each person, while enjoying each sip and every single bite, looks into the eyes of those nearby, then gazes off toward the horizon. Each shares a few minutes of warm conversation or reflection about the path just traveled.

Through these reminders as well as the discoveries of modern science, I have come to know that one of the simplest and healthiest of human pleasures is not forgotten. Indeed, many people like the Tibetans recognize it as a necessity and make breaks a part of their daily lives. Such breaks provide great immediate and lasting rewards, especially in a world that seems to be moving faster each day.

Find a Refuge

As soon as you change your mental pace, you immediately generate a measure of internal restoration and renewal. Research suggests that you have to disengage, that is, step away from the place where you're working or doing your chores.

"A brief period of time—even just a few minutes—away from the normal influx of work and mental information will allow your brain to do some of the filing necessary to sharpen your memory," says Michael D. Chafetz, Ph.D., neuropsychologist and author of *Smart for Life: How to Improve Your Brainpower at Any Age*. "Anything that stops the normal flow and lets your brain redirect . . . is worthwhile."

You can feel an on-the-spot surge of energy whenever you take the kind of break that Dr. Chafetz is talking about. In your workplace, that may mean leaving your office for a few minutes. If you're at home, maybe you need to step outside. If you have a nearby deck or garden, one of these may be a good place to take your break. Or a nearby park could become a favorite refuge.

Just Imagine

Can't get away physically? Surprisingly, you can still get some energizing benefits by simply imagining that you are elsewhere, according to Winnifred Gallagher, psychology editor of *American Health* magazine. "The basic principle is simple," Gallagher explains. " A good or bad environment promotes good or bad memories, which inspire a good or bad mood, which inclines us toward good or bad behavior."

That can happen whether or not you are consciously aware of it. "We needn't even be consciously aware of a pleasant or unpleasant environmental stimulus for it to influence us," says Gallagher.

"There is mounting evidence that even brief exposures to a natural scene can be an excellent antidote to mental fatigue," note physician David Sobel, M.D., and psychologist Robert Ornstein, Ph.D., in the journal *Mental Medicine Update*. Reviewing studies of people who hold desk jobs, these researchers found that satisfaction ratings doubled when workers had access to views of natural scenes. When people could enjoy these scenes, they felt less frustrated and more patient.

Dr. Sobel and Dr. Ornstein also found that people felt more involved in their work if they were surrounded by natural settings or reminders of outdoor scenery. In these environments, people were more likely to say that they found their jobs challenging and interesting. They also expressed greater enthusiasm for their work and reported greater overall life satisfaction and health.

Something as simple as a cool, fresh breeze or a splash of cold water on your face may be the ticket to this enhanced perspective on your work. That may not be a cold mountain stream, but it may well be close enough. On each break, make it a point to step closer to a window if possible, both for the view and for a dose of sunlight.

Jump on Exercise

Most of us still view exercise as an all-or-nothing issue. Right there, you have a reason for not doing it. Even if you enjoy various kinds of exercise, that doesn't necessarily mean that you want to devote yourself to it. It's even worse when you subscribe to Mark Twain's simple but discouraging point of view. "Exercise is loathsome," teased the author of *Tom Sawyer* and *The Adventures of Huckleberry Finn*.

But maybe it doesn't have to be that way. The truth is, you don't have to get out there and do a full-scale, formal workout every day. And that's a good thing. In a worst-case scenario, where people drive to and from a health club for their exercise, that little workout can easily tie up a couple of hours.

The truth is, you really don't need to commit that much time to physical exercise. Just add a few active minutes here and there. In fact, one study showed that a single brief set of muscle-toning exercises is nearly as beneficial as a workout session that lasts three times as long.

A review of 14 major studies indicated that exercise can be an effective treatment for mild to moderate depression and is up to five times more cost-effective than other treatments. Medical research at Harvard University Medical School's Institute for Circadian Physiology suggests that every time you get up and move, causing even brief muscular activity, you increase your energy and alertness. That means that even if you engage in just a few minutes of activity, you get a metabolic boost. And as a bonus, you feel more alert and clearheaded.

According to researchers, the foundation of all strength and much energy production in your body is your abdominal region. When strong and balanced, your abdominal muscles flatten your waist, help hold your internal organs in place, and stabilize your lower back at

IF EXERCISE COULD BE PACKAGED INTO A PILL,

IT WOULD BE THE SINGLE MOST PRESCRIBED
AND BENEFICIAL MEDICINE IN THE NATION.

—Robert Butler, M.D., Mount Sinai Medical Center, New York City

its most vulnerable point. Weak abdominals contribute to poor posture, shallow breathing, weakened resilience to stress, and low active energy.

I admit it: I actually like a few stomach-toning exercises. I've modified them so that I don't need a gym or workout room. I can do them anywhere, a few at a time, several times a day. And I feel the results right away.

In addition to increasing your active energy, these exercises are also very effective for weight loss.

When I started to develop these exercises, it was with the realization that the traditional, popular abdominal exercises, situps and leg lifts, often cause or aggravate lower-back pain by pulling on the front of the lower spine. When this happens, your back sways inward and your lower abdomen pushes out. Apart from the way that this can harm your back, such a pelvic tilt also contributes to a potbelly appearance.

As an alternative, I recommend a pair of stomach-flattening exercises called the trans-pyramid exercise and the abdominal curl. You don't need to do hundreds of fast repetitions for these exercises to have an effect. Abdominal muscles are small. Slow, controlled movements of at least 10 repetitions per exercise are all you need.

To do these right will require some mental concentration as well as physical effort. The more you focus your attention on exactly which muscle areas are working, the more your brain activates those muscles— and you get improved results.

TRY THIS NOW!

Even if you increase your physical activity for just a few minutes, you condition your body and brain to create more active energy.

When you exercise, you stimulate the production of a powerful messenger chemical called catecholamine. This is the same hormone that is released by your nervous system to increase energy and responsiveness. When you take an extra minute or two for increased physical activity, your body releases catecholamine. Essentially, you're training your body to make more energy available.

Here's How

Here's a simple breathing technique that has been used for years by fitness experts to firm and slenderize the midsection. It takes just a few minutes to try it out.

Breathe in, then out, taking normal breaths. Then repeat, but with the next breath, forcibly expel all of the air from your lungs. As you do this forced exhalation, put extra pressure on the two key muscles that allow your lower abdomen to come in and up as much as possible. This should take about 10 seconds.

Sometimes, it takes a few tries before those two lower-abdominal muscles wake up and start working again. But before long, you'll feel the response in your body and senses.

When you do this exercise, you're developing your active-energy-generating power. Practice this forced exhalation several times throughout the day. This simple exercise can literally change your body's capability to produce and sustain high levels of active energy.

A GREAT PIECE OF ADVICE FOR THE 30 TO 50 MILLION
MOSTLY SEDENTARY AND UNFIT AMERICANS IS
'TURN OFF THE TELEVISION, GET UP OFF YOUR FANNY,
AND **MOVE AROUND A BIT**.'

—Steven N. Blair, director of epidemiology,
Cooper Institute for Aerobics Research, Dallas

Trans-Pyramid Exercise

The trans-pyramid exercise is a simple breathing exercise that can be very effective in helping you build a toned, fit lower abdominal area. "These are the most important exercises you can do to flatten your abdomen," according to Lawrence E. Lamb, M.D., an exercise expert and national medical columnist. As the trans-pyramid works its magic, you'll automatically feel your active energy rise.

To learn this movement, you may find it helpful to begin by lying on the floor in a comfortable position. But once you've mastered the exercise motion, you can do the trans-pyramid either sitting or standing.

Place your hands on your hips with your thumbs pointing to your back. Spread your fingers across your abdomen. The index finger of each hand should point toward your belly button, without touching it. Keep your shoulders relaxed. If you're standing, your knees should be comfortably bent.

Take a deep breath, then exhale. As you breathe out, notice which way your lower abdomen moves. When the transveralis and pyramidalis muscles of your lower waist are involved as they should be, you'll feel your lower abdomen moving inward toward your spine at the end of each exhalation.

(continued on page 178)

Speeding on the Train to Weight Loss

If you've been nagged by overweight and would like to be trimmer, you've probably heard as much about exercise as you have about diets. The fact is that all of the strategies for active energy will also help you lose weight. These strategies include moderate kinds of exercise.

To understand why moderate exercises can aid weight loss, we have to take a close look at the tiny compounds that cause so many problems when it comes to weight gain. These compounds, called fatty acid molecules, are extremely small and very mobile. They pass easily through the membranes of cells. They can also pass through capillaries, the tiny blood vessels threaded throughout your body. Fatty acid molecules are in regular motion, sometimes being released from fat cells, sometimes being deposited into fat cells, sometimes passing into muscle cells to be burned as fuel. That's why they're sometimes called free fatty acids.

Free fatty acids can blithely move out of your bloodstream into muscle cells. But they're not always happy with muscle cells. If a muscle cell is underused or lacking in tone, the fatty acids don't really have a reason to be there. They just move back into the bloodstream and travel to fat cells for storage. In other words, those highly mobile free fatty acids, which are the basic fuel for energy, will just be stored as body fat if you don't burn them.

When you stay active and tone your muscles, you make it easier for your muscle cells to keep burning free fatty acids as fuel. That means that fewer fatty acids are sent to your fat cells for storage. With a variety of physical activities throughout each and every day, your body-fat stores will be reduced.

Similarly, scientists have learned that the fat-burning enzymes that help your muscle cells use the fuel that comes their way function well only if they're used regularly. This is another reason why long stretches of time without frequent, moderate periods of physical activity and muscle toning invite weight gain. During periods of inactivity, your body's biochemistry shifts toward fat forming and fat storing, and away from fat burning.

Research indicates that regular physical activity and exercise can produce body-fat losses even without caloric restriction and may be the single most important factor in maintaining weight-loss success. In one study at the University of California, 90 percent of the individuals who reached and maintained a goal weight reported exercising regularly, compared to only 34 percent of the relapsers.

Exercise may also help you reduce dietary-fat intake by offsetting your natural cravings for high-fat food.

Even if you don't want to be more active for your own sake, perhaps you'll want to do it for your children or grandchildren. According to research from the Framingham Children's Study that was presented at the 1992 National Institutes of Health Conference on Physical Activity and Obesity, when both parents are active, children are nearly 6 times more likely to be active and energetic than are children of two inactive parents.

You can lose a pound of fat a week just by ratcheting your activity level up a notch or two, according to Janet Walberg-Rankin, Ph.D., associate professor of exercise physiology at Virginia Polytechnic Institute and State University in Blacksburg. She suggests activities such as walking, mowing the lawn, chopping wood, cleaning the basement, or climbing stairs.

On the inhale, notice how your belly tends to pop outward against your fingers.

To make a very clear distinction between the inhalation and exhalation, exaggerate both movements. When you exhale and finish expelling your breath, use your lower abdominal muscles to press that area inward even more. Then, as you inhale, consciously release your abdomen so it presses out against your fingers. (For muscle-toning, the exhalation phase is the most important part of the exercise.)

You'll get even better results if you try the exercise in a sitting position. Slowly exhale and, as you reach the point where you normally finish breathing out, smoothly and forcefully breathe out even more. Make sure that you use the full power of your lower abdominal muscles. You can emphasize the upward movement of your lower abdomen by using your hands to help push upward as you finish the exhalation phase.

This exercise is ideal for a work break since you can practice it while you're sitting. (No one will even notice.) You'll increase energy and muscle tone if you can do a total of 5 to 10 repetitions each day. Once you've started to fit it in during the day, you can also make it part of your morning routine, doing one or two before you get out of bed in the morning. If you have a commute, you can do several repetitions when you're stopped at a red light. Or fit in a few repetitions before meals.

Abdominal Curl

For this type of abdominal exercise, you really have to be lying down. But otherwise, it's simple and convenient. The abdominal curl is an easy, effective exercise for toning your upper abdominal area.

As shown in the illustration, lie on your back with your lower legs placed on a chair seat or bench or your knees bent. Just make sure that your feet are free. (You shouldn't tuck them under a heavy object or hold them in place, as this lets your powerful hip-flexor muscles take over the movement and stresses your lower back.) Cross your arms on your chest, or clasp your hands with your fingers loosely intertwined behind your head.

Don't let your arms whip upward, since this may cause injury to your neck.

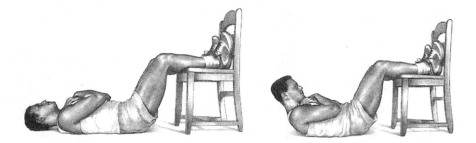

Keeping your middle and lower back flat on the floor, slowly raise your head and shoulders off the floor about 30 to 45 degrees. Keep your lower abdomen flat. (Do not let it "pouch out" during the upward movement.) If your hands are interlocked behind your head, don't try to yank your head up when you start the lift, as that could injure your neck.

Pause for a second at the top of the motion. Then, using your abdominals for support, slowly lower yourself to the original position.

If you haven't been doing abdominal exercises regularly, it's best to begin gradually when you start practicing abdominal curls. But if you don't feel any serious discomfort or pain, you can steadily increase the frequency of repetitions. After a few weeks, you may find that you can do up to 100 total repetitions each day.

The exercise is even more effective if you introduce a slight torso twist at the top of each curl. Instead of keeping your hands on your chest or behind your neck, reach both hands toward one knee and slowly twist your shoulders in that direction. Alternate on each repetition so you reach and gently twist toward the left knee, then the right, at the top of each curl. But be sure to go back to straight curls if you feel any pain when you twist one way or the other.

Take Everything in Stride

When you take an essential break, it's an ideal time to release any accrued muscle tension.

Exercise physiologists used to subscribe to the belief that people had to do intense physical exercise to get measurable health benefits. With further study, that assumption has faded.

"It's not the intensity of physical activity that leads to better health," says John Duncan, Ph.D., exercise physiologist at the Cooper Institute for Aerobics Research in Dallas. "It's the total number of minutes that you spend each week exercising."

In the past, doctors believed that you had to improve a factor called aerobic capacity before you would gain any health benefits. They thought that this capacity, labeled max VO_2, would increase only if you walked very briskly or did some other kind of hard-driving exercise.

That thinking has changed, Dr. Duncan observes. "We now know that metabolic changes occur very quickly at very moderate exercise intensities and that those metabolic changes confer health benefits."

You even get some benefits by moving around in your chair when you're at work, stuck in a meeting, or sitting and reading. "No matter how good the chair," says David Thompson, Ph.D., ergonomist at

Stanford University, "human beings weren't designed to sit in one position for extended periods." Nutrients inside your spinal column are moved around by a muscular, pumplike mechanism that exchanges fluids in the spinal disks. When you shift your posture, that "pump" goes into action, helping to move the nutrients to the nerves that need them.

Take a physical break at least once every hour, advises Dr. Thompson, and if you're reading at a desk or computer, "make it a habit to stop and stretch your arms and do a couple of shoulder or head rolls every couple of pages."

"Even the most ideal posture can lead to musculoskeletal 'loading' if it is maintained too long," warn occupational-health experts Jeanne Stellman and Mary Sue Henifin, "because the human body is designed to move. Static positions are contrary to biology."

Have a Cool Drink

It's common to mistakenly perceive thirst as hunger. If you make that mistake, you're likely to eat high-fat snacks such as cookies, potato chips, candy bars, or pastries when you're really just thirsty, not hungry. These high-fat foods create an energy blockade, draining vigor and causing tiredness.

"Drinking generous amounts of water is overwhelmingly the number one way to head off food cravings, boost energy, and reduce appetite," according to George L. Blackburn, M.D., Ph.D., director of the Center for the Study of Nutrition Medicine at Beth Israel Deaconess Medical Center West of Harvard Medical School. A good rule of thumb is to sip a glass of ice-cold water when you feel hungry and then wait for 5 to 10 minutes. If you're still hungry, go ahead and eat an appropriate light snack.

During every essential break, head off the symptoms of mild dehy-

Energy-Boosting Activities for Busy People

Nearly any type of muscular activity can immediately increase your level of active energy and alertness. If you stand up, move your arms and shoulders, or walk up a flight of stairs or down a nearby hallway, you're actually creating active energy, according to Martin Moore-Ede, M.D., Ph.D., associate professor of physiology and director of the Institute for Circadian Physiology at Harvard Medical School. "You do not have to be running a mile or lifting weights. Taking a walk, stretching, or even chewing gum can stimulate your level of alertness," he observes.

Here are some other ideas for low-level activities that can increase your active energy.

- Take a 2-minute walk before breakfast, right after lunch, and right after your evening meal.
- Park your car a row farther away from the office or grocery store.
- Have the bus or cab drop you off an extra block from your destination.
- Move your wastebasket off to the side of your work space so you have to walk to it to discard trash. (The key here is to walk there instead of shooting baskets, which my wife and children love to do.)
- Stand up and stretch, or do a few pushups.

dration by making a point of sipping a tall 16-ounce beverage. Drink more or more frequently whenever the air is noticeably hot or dry, or when you're engaged in active physical work.

By keeping the liquid ice cold, you help boost your active energy, and you'll probably burn more calories since your metabolism will increase to warm the water to body temperature.

Want something besides plain water during your break? A lot of cold beverages can spark your vitality, fend off fatigue, and provide benefits in

- Make active dates with friends and family that include enjoyable physical activity.
- Plan some errands that require walking a bit farther on your lunch hour.
- Sweep your sidewalk and patio, balcony, or deck.
- Plan a short evening stroll to take in the sunset or gaze at the stars.
- Walk in place or jump rope for a minute or two.
- Put on some of your favorite music and move your feet (even just tapping your toes can boost active energy).
- Walk and talk with your love partner, your children, or a friend.
- Walk your dog instead of just turning him loose in the backyard.
- Take your neighbor's dog—or your neighbor—for a quick walk.
- Walk somewhere that's at least 2 minutes from your workplace to eat your lunch so that, afterward, you can enjoy a 2-minute return walk to work.
- Three or four times a day, climb a flight or more of stairs instead of taking the elevator. (You rev your energy level up to 10 times higher by climbing stairs than you do by sitting motionless.)
- Stand up and move around while reading mail or talking on the telephone.

terms of long-term health improvement and body-fat control. On each essential break, plan to drink a full glass of fluid. By evening, your total fluid consumption should reach 6 to 8 glasses. Fluid options include:

- Water with natural lemon, lime, orange, berry, or peppermint flavoring
- Carbonated mineral water, with natural lemon, lime, orange, or berry flavoring, if you like
- 100 percent fruit juice

- Vegetable juice
- Iced green tea, sweetened with a maximum of 1 teaspoon of sugar or honey, if you like
- Iced green or black tea with a dash of milk or soy milk
- Iced black tea, sweetened with a maximum of 1 teaspoon of sugar or honey, if you like
- Iced decaffeinated coffee, with fat-free milk or soy milk, and a maximum of 1 teaspoon of sugar or honey, if you like
- Iced decaffeinated cappuccino with fat-free milk or soy milk, and a maximum of 1 teaspoon of sugar or honey, if you like

The Question of Caffeine

What about caffeinated beverages? First of all, remember that downing stiff doses of caffeine in any form may stimulate stress hormones. That stimulation may create an illusion of energy, but messenger chemicals are depleted and your health and performance suffer.

On the other hand, it's probably fine to have an occasional cup of coffee, tea, or caffeinated soft drink. As long as you don't overdepend on caffeinated beverages, they can sometimes be refreshing. Yet they have a side effect that most of us don't take into account. All caffeine-containing beverages—and also alcoholic drinks—act as diuretics. That means that they cause increased urine production and loss of fluids. To some degree, they counteract the beneficial effects of the fluids that you take in.

In addition, caffeine has mood effects that you might not like so well. According to a study published in the *New England Journal of Medicine*, when people consume even moderate amounts of caffeine on the job, they can end up feeling out of sorts. On weekends, when caffeine consumers are likely to cut back, they may find themselves doing fewer invigorating or rejuvenating activities.

The Negative Stimulus

As for the long-term health effects of caffeine, findings are still unclear. Data from a study at the University of Geneva in Switzerland suggest that, for some adults, a moderate intake of caffeine may increase energy production and metabolism. However, in other individuals, caffeine may increase symptoms of stress or either increase or decrease appetite.

But what about the claims that caffeine revs up your energy or metabolism? "Caffeine stimulates in a negative way," says Judith Rodin, Ph.D., former professor of psychology and psychiatry at Yale University and current president of the University of Pennsylvania in Philadelphia. When you drink caffeinated beverages, you increase the release of insulin, which promotes the rapid movement of fat into your cells. So caffeine consumption may also promote fat storage, she observes.

Many women drink caffeinated diet sodas to help them through days when they're fasting or eating very little because of diets, Dr. Rodin notes. But this practice is probably counterproductive. Caffeinated diet drinks actually make people feel more hungry.

Get Some Energy Bites

Each and every essential break requires food.

I know, I know. Millions of Americans have learned to starve themselves between meals, assuming that it is a weight-control habit. It's not. Eating low-fat between-meal snacks can actually increase your active energy and metabolism. With what I call Energy Bites, you trigger a process that scientists call the thermic effect of food. This is a heat-producing, energy-revving, and calorie-burning process.

Here's why. During the day, when you go for 4 to 5 hours at a stretch without eating, your blood sugar levels drop and your energy wanes. It may take a dose of willpower just to get out of your chair, let alone to do some daily exercise.

Research published in the *New England Journal of Medicine* and the *American Journal of Clinical Nutrition* suggests that you'll reap all kinds of health benefits if you spread out your food intake. That is, you're really better off if you don't sit down to two or three meals a day where you quite possibly overeat and overstuff yourself. It makes far more sense to eat less at each meal and also to eat more often.

If you have moderate-size meals plus small between-meal snacks, you increase your levels of energy and alertness, lower your blood-cholesterol levels, and reduce your body fat. With smaller and more moderate meals, you also enhance food digestion, lessen your risk of heart disease, and increase your overall metabolism. One study showed that people who ate more frequently had lower cholesterol levels despite eating more food.

Snacking on low-fat, high-fiber foods throughout the day has considerable energy-producing advantages, observes Dean Ornish, M.D., founder and president of the Preventive Medicine Research Institute in Sausalito, California, and assistant clinical professor of medicine at the University of California, San Francisco, School of Medicine. In part, this is because eating low-fat, high-fiber snacks in mid-morning and mid-afternoon makes you less likely to be fatigued when you sit down to main meals or get a snack in the evening.

If you skip Energy Bites, your blood sugar falls and you experience increased fatigue and tension. When you're tired, you tend to overeat, which means that fatigue can cause you to eat too much at main meals or to lapse into stress-related food binges in the evening. Energy Bites can help keep your metabolism going strong and can minimize the blood sugar drops that can trigger overeating.

When you eat late in the day, it's essential to choose the right kinds of food. That's because your energy gradually starts to decline in mid- to late afternoon. Your brain, along with the rest of your body, has a strong tendency to lose energy and begin to crave high-fat, high-sugar foods.

With a combination of moderate meals—and I emphasize *moderate*—and the right kinds of Energy Bites, you find that you're better able to sustain steady energy production and fat burning. Smaller, nutritious meals and snacks, while helping to stabilize blood sugar levels, also help optimize memory, learning, and performance.

Snacks to Live By

I suspect that many of us skip snacks and then overeat simply because it's hard and often inconvenient to find great-tasting, energy-boosting snacks. But if that's the case, it just means that you have to take steps to make those snacks convenient. Your active energy depends on it.

Research indicates that adults make an average of 20 to 30 food decisions a day, according to Dr. Blackburn. That being the case, it's critical to have Energy Bites readily available to make your between-meal food choices as easy as possible. Otherwise, if you are unprepared, you may grab what's convenient but not at all energy producing or healthful. That's how you end up munching potato chips, sipping sodas, picking up a candy bar, or stopping by the coffee shop for a creamy cappuccino.

Grab the wrong kinds of snacks, and you may end up consuming 50 to 60 grams of fat—that's more than 1,000 calories—all at once. Your energy will take a sudden plunge soon afterward. Planning makes the difference. What you choose to eat can influence the production of brain-messenger chemicals called neurotransmitters, which affect your mental alertness, concentration, attitude, mood, and performance.

Whether you find your stomach growling at 10:30 A.M. or 2:30

P.M., you need to have Energy Bites available. Whenever you take an essential break and enjoy a few bites of this kind of great food, you are more likely to find ingenious ways to have other great-tasting foods available for your next break. For ideas and some recipes, see Energy Bites: Foods That Stoke Your Energy Furnace.

The Lift of Protein and the Calming of Carbs

According to some leading nutritional scientists, there's compelling evidence to support the power of food over mind and mood. Just a few bites of healthy, high-protein food can contribute to increased energy. After eating high-protein food, you may notice that you can pay greater attention to detail and also that you're more alert. These effects can last for up to 3 hours.

Your options among high-protein foods? You might have a sandwich with chicken breast, turkey breast, or fish; a cup of bean or lentil soup; or a small serving of nonfat yogurt or cottage cheese. Nonfat cream cheese and fat-free milk are other options, along with some fruit.

When you're on the run, try a small handful of almonds, raisins, or figs, You might have a whole-grain cracker with a very small portion of lox. Or cut a thin slice of low-fat, low-salt cheese and put that on the cracker.

In recent years, one of the surprise findings in nutritional research has been that, in many cases, eating carbohydrate-rich snacks can actually help alleviate feelings of impatience or distress. So, one of the simplest ways to reduce mental distress and tension is to eat something that is low in fat, low in protein, and high in carbohydrates. This kind of snack influences the production of neurotransmitters and may help produce a calm, focused state of mind and relaxed emotions—a state that can last for up to 3 hours.

All in Good Taste

The best between-meal snacks are, to put it plainly, those that taste great to you. For most of us, these snacks must also be high in complex carbohydrates and fiber and low in fat.

Options include low-fat cookies or a low-fat muffin, bagel, or English muffin. Other good high-carbohydrate foods are cooked whole grains. Rice, wheat, oatmeal, corn, buckwheat, and barley can be delicious with fruit or a sweetener rather than with milk. Also good (and good for you) are low-fat pasta salad with fruits or vegetables, bean salad, whole-grain bread, or low-fat baked potato chips. If you like rye crackers, have some topped with your favorite all-fruit preserve.

Your success in choosing the right foods and combinations of foods to help you manage your emotions and mind depends on careful observation of your body's responses and habits. Over the next few weeks, take notes on your state of mind and mood 10 to 15 minutes before meals and snacks. Do you feel alert and motivated? Calm and focused? Tense and irritable?

One hour after eating, reassess your state of mind and emotions and quickly and honestly write down your observations. Review your appraisals to create a list of the food choices that seem best for you. Then, you can use that list as a helpful tool in monitoring your day-to-day eating patterns.

Snatch a Bit of Inspiration

Late one night on a street corner in a small Irish town, I was accosted by a friendly old man who was eager to talk. Before many words had passed between us, he asked me if I'd found my "bit of inspiration" here and

(continued on page 192)

Favorite Energy-Boosting Snacks

Here are more than two-dozen healthy snack options that can be a convenient and valuable part of a high-energy lifestyle. These low-fat, high-fiber snacks generally have less than 6 grams of fat and fewer than 400 calories. I recommend one portion at one of your essential breaks in the mid-morning and another in the mid-afternoon.

• A blender smoothy made with ice-cold water or juice, ice cubes, and fresh fruit; add yogurt or soy milk or soy yogurt, blend, and enjoy
• A thick piece of 100 percent whole-grain bread with 100 percent all-fruit preserves and nonfat or low-fat cream cheese
• A whole-rye cracker or bagel with nonfat or low-fat cream cheese, served with or without fruit
• A whole-wheat English muffin or bagel with all-fruit preserves and nonfat cream cheese
• A whole-wheat English muffin with nonfat or low-fat mayonnaise and a thin slice of low-fat cheese such as Jarlsberg Lite Swiss
• One slice of whole-rye or whole-grain bread with nonfat or low-fat cream cheese and all-fruit spread
• Two or three whole-grain cookies
• Fat-free bean dip served on whole-rye crackers or other 100 percent whole-grain crackers
• 1 cup of nonfat or low-fat yogurt with canned, frozen, or fresh unsweetened fruit
• ½ cup of nonfat old-fashioned whole-oat granola, served with fat-free milk or yogurt
• 1 cup of fruit-juice-sweetened nonfat or low-fat yogurt
• 1 cup tomato soup (made with fat-free milk) and two whole-rye crackers
• 1 cup of non-instant oatmeal with fat-free milk and 1 teaspoon of brown sugar
• A fat-free or low-fat whole-grain muffin

- A small container of whole-oat granola
- One to three pieces of Ry Crisp, Wasa Crispbread, Scandinavian-style bran crispbread, or other whole-rye cracker with all-fruit preserves or nonfat or low-fat cream cheese
- Whole-grain bagel with 1 teaspoon of dijon mustard, 1 teaspoon of nonfat or low-fat mayonnaise, and two slices of turkey breast or two thin slices of low-fat cheese such as Jarlsberg Lite Swiss
- ¼ cup of nonfat ricotta cheese topped with a handful of nonfat whole-oat granola
- 4 ounces of low-fat frozen yogurt
- ½ cup of nonfat cottage cheese with canned, frozen, or fresh unsweetened fruit
- Tapioca pudding made with fat-free milk: I've loved this my whole life
- 1 cup of nonfat or low-fat vegetable soup, bean soup, or lentil soup
- A variety of fresh-cut mixed raw vegetables and fruit with several whole-grain crackers and a nonfat or low-fat dressing or dip for dipping
- 1 piece of angel food cake with fresh unsweetened berries
- 1 piece of whole-rye or whole-grain bread with 1 teaspoon of nonfat mayonnaise and 2 ounces of water-packed albacore tuna
- 8 ounces of unsweetened orange juice with a small, whole-grain, very low fat muffin
- One celery stalk stuffed with 1 tablespoon of nonfat or low-fat cream cheese or cottage cheese
- One apple or other piece of fresh fruit with several whole-grain crackers
- Sliced fruit and berries in ½ cup of nonfat or low-fat plain yogurt or cottage cheese
- Air-popped, very low fat popcorn

there throughout the day. "You can't wait to have it all at once," he cautioned, with a glimmer of lifelong wisdom in his eyes.

He was right. I've pondered this often since then. On each and every break, we all need a dash of inspiration, a thought or feeling that lifts us and calls us to be our best. As you will discover throughout the rest of this book, neuroscientists are discovering that the mind and heart are great generators of human energy.

So end each essential break by taking a few final moments to savor one of your dreams. Steal a glimpse of where you're headed. Remember one of the mentors or teachers who had a great influence in shaping what you have become. Recall a genuinely supportive word or note that you have received lately. Or stop to gaze at a favorite photo of your loved ones, for whom your sustained active energy may count the most of all.

Have a Vigorous Lunch

Lunchtime should be a break, right? It should be a chance to grab a sandwich, sneak out the door, and find a shady spot in a green glade for a snack, a chat, or a snooze.

Sure, sure.

It's more likely that you've gotten into the habit of considering lunch a very inessential part of the day. There's no time. There's so much to do. And why bother, if you're not that hungry and you're feeling swamped?

Here's the crux of the problem: For nearly all of us, the lunch hour lands right in the middle of an active-energy downturn. If you ignore this chance to renew your vitality, researchers have shown that you lose out in some very significant ways. Not only do you experience that slump at midday but you also have measurably less attentiveness and productivity throughout the afternoon.

You can try to fight back with caffeine, increased tension, and more willpower, but these don't work well, if at all. Eventually, you'll run out of steam and good health. What's called for here is skillpower, not willpower.

Furthermore, when you skip lunch, you arrive at the evening meal more famished and with a greater tendency to overeat high-fat foods. Those are the kinds of foods that blunt your senses and bog down both your body and mind.

But the urge to overeat at the evening meal and the resulting feeling of grogginess don't just suddenly appear in the afternoon or evening. It's more likely that they started at noon, with skipping lunch. If you want better afternoons and evenings, look first to lunch.

Taking a Break

When I think about the ideal lunch break, I don't think first of food. I think of an expanded essential break.

During your lunch break, you have some extra time to reenergize. It's more than just a chance to grab a bite of food. I'd rather call it a vigorous lunch. It's the ticket to having more energy for the rest of your day.

Here's the four-part vigorous lunch that deepens and expands on the essential break and can take as little as 20 minutes.

1. Find more breathing space.
2. Eat a smart, easy meal that tastes great.
3. Do "1 + 1 = 10" aerobics for energy.
4. Seek a fresh vantage point.

1. Find More Breathing Space

Your transition into the lunch break can be brief, usually less than a minute or so, but make sure that it happens. With some practice, it's easy and enjoyable.

First, step away from whatever you have been doing, physically, mentally, and emotionally. Head to a window. Walk outside. Shift your thought stream. Begin to get excited about something totally different. From time to time during the day, the human brain needs you to deliberately unlock it from habitual focuses, says Ellen J. Langer, Ph.D., professor of psychology at Harvard University.

2. Eat a Smart, Easy Meal That Tastes Great

Only on the surface is skipping lunch palatable. Deep inside your cells, in the energy-production processes, the notion of abandoning the noon meal is something akin to a plane losing a jet engine in midair. It's even worse than losing just one engine, actually. You're also losing your cabin oxygen. Sure, you might still manage to fly. But it's unnerving and survival-driven.

Eating a good lunch is highly recommended "for both health and work efficiency," says Etienne Grandjean, M.D., Ph.D., an expert on productivity at the Swiss Federal Institute of Technology.

Researchers concur that skipping lunch is no solution for busy people who see it as a possible time saver. On an empty stomach, performance scores plunge. People who have skipped the midday meal soon feel more tense and anxious. Skip lunch, studies show, and you'll be less likely to exercise or take specific energy-boosting actions in the afternoon.

And skipping lunch can be one of your most costly metabolic mistakes, leading to a ravenous appetite late in the day and heightened cravings for high-fat foods, says C. Wayne Callaway, M.D., clinical professor at George Washington University School of Medicine and Health Sciences in Washington, D.C. "People who skip breakfast or lunch tend to get more tired and binge in the evening, instead of eating moderately and having more energy throughout the day."

When you overeat in the evening, often on high-fat foods, you're left feeling tired. You get pushed into a daze of further inactivity—the

TRY THIS NOW!

As neuropsychologists point out, when you keep pushing yourself through natural break times such as lunch, your brain's physiology changes. Brain cells constantly engage in concentrated, complex activities, exchanging ions and other messenger substances between their inner compartments and fluids. It takes vast amounts of energy for them to do this. If brain cells keep conducting too many messages or if too many of the same messages come traveling through over and over, the cells fail to recover. Nerves become fatigued, unable to replenish vital energy. The result is that numbness sets in, and then tension.

Can a grande coffee or monster cup of caffeinated soda prod your brain back into full function?

Not a chance. The rush from a tankard of caffeine can somewhat mask the deterioration and make you feel "energized" enough to skip lunch. But brain fatigue at midday and other times is not something you should overlook. That fatigue is a signal that your brain is shutting down. In a way, your brain cells are trying desperately to tell you how exhausted they feel.

evening slump—as your metabolism drops to its lowest zone of the day. No wonder so many people feel numb at night.

The right kind of lunch is actually quite easy to prepare, and it produces even more energy when the food tastes great to you. This is key: Foods that you love actually increase your metabolism. Conversely, foods that don't taste good to you, no matter how healthy they may be, don't provide the same energy-boosting power.

According to researchers, lunch is the largest and most important meal of the day for many of the world's healthiest peoples. But you've prob-

You have to attend to your brain's needs. Maybe all you need is a brief change of pace, a moment of rest, or a bite or food to restore active energy.

Here's How

When you move from one task to another, don't rush. Instead, *shift* what you're doing and how you feel.

If you stop one thing and instantly jump up to do something else, the quick, jumpy change can be tiring rather than energizing.

Right now, practice taking a break from reading. Stand up slowly and stretch for a moment. Blink your eyes and refocus them.

Now, before you turn your attention back to the words on this page, think about the next thing you plan to do today. Take a deep breath or two, enjoying the extra few moments of transition.

With practice, you'll be able to extend this simple exercise—and the feeling that goes with it—as you make any kind of shift in your task, attention, or routine.

Don't rush. Flow. It's a crucial and simple way to bring some extra energy into each midday renewal period.

ably discovered that you don't choose nutritious food just because it's good for your health. There have to be some real taste temptations. Therefore, the single most important factor in enjoying lower-fat lunches and all other meals and snacks is taste. To an astonishing extent, "the brain is more interested in what's happening on the tongue than in the body," says Harvey Weingarten, Ph.D., chairman of the psychology department at McMaster University in Hamilton, Ontario.

Take a few moments to reconnect your imagination with the great tastes ahead. What are you planning to eat? Here are some of the basics.

TRY THIS NOW!

Do hot, spicy foods have an energizing and fat-burning power? It appears that they do, at least for some people.

When it comes to food, what warms you up may help slim you down, according to some Canadian medical studies. In particular, hot spices may help increase your after-meal metabolic rate. They may also make you less likely to stuff yourself, because the flavor is so intense.

Here's How

Whether you're having soup, a sandwich, or a salad today, bring some spices into the picture. Hot mustard lends distinction and adds dimension to any meat or cheese sandwich. Chili powder or hot-pepper sauce adds zing to soups. You might also look for low-fat dishes that contain hot spices, such as Mexican, Thai, and Indian foods.

Go light on the fat. Many lunchtime problems arise from the fact that what you think is a good food choice could be loaded with hidden fat. Beyond the obvious weight-gain problems, one of the main reasons to avoid high–fat lunches is because they cause fatigue. "Fat seems to slow other processes, like thought or movement," says Judith J. Wurtman, Ph.D., a nutritional researcher in the brain and cognitive sciences department at the Massachusetts Institute of Technology in Cambridge. "It makes people very lethargic. During the long digestive process that follows a high–fat meal, more blood is diverted to the stomach and intestines and away from the brain."

Choose ice water or iced tea. The best noontime beverages are water, preferably ice water, and brewed tea, which you can enjoy iced. Research indicates that brewed black or green tea may provide valuable protection of some key brain fuctions, and this effect may last for up to an hour and a half.

Include some protein-rich food. At MIT, Harris Lieberman, Ph.D., and Bonnie Spring, Ph.D., did a study to determine whether people function better in the afternoon when they've had high-protein lunches. The test group consisted of 40 college students. Some were given high-protein turkey sandwiches for lunch; others got high-carbohydrate sandwiches that had the same number of calories as the turkey sandwiches. Those who ate turkey sandwiches performed faster and more accurately on tests of coordination and mental skills throughout the afternoon.

Go light on dips and be picky about the chips. Say no to mystery dips and traditional high-fat chips. Instead, substitute fat-free bean dip or nonfat sour cream dip. I also like ultra low fat cheddar cheese. This goes well on top of rye crisps or thin rye-crisp crackers, 100 percent whole-grain crackers, or, on occasion, fat-free tortilla chips.

Soup it up. Research suggests that soup increases your energy while also reducing fat cravings. According to scientists at Johns Hopkins University in Baltimore, soup is the most satisfying kind of appetizer you can have. Their research showed that people ate significantly less during their meals if they had soup beforehand, especially tomato soup. For variety, go for fresh gazpacho. Just be sure to avoid beef-base, pork-base, or cream-base soups.

If you're headed for the salad bar, think whole foods. There's increasing evidence indicating that you'll have more vibrant health and highly sustained energy if you sidestep large amounts of typical refined or fat-laden processed foods. Instead, select more whole grains, beans and legumes, low-fat or nonfat dairy products, and fresh fruits and vegetables.

If this represents a real diet change for you, make the change gradually rather than plunge in all at once. For starters, visit the salad bar more often, and really explore the produce section at the supermarket.

A vast array of interesting new foods is showing up in supermarkets these days. Look for such new stars as fresh arugula, Bibb lettuce, bok choy, Boston lettuce, red cabbage, chard, cilantro, cress, cucumber, dill, and Belgian or curly endive. Other great choices include escarole, fennel, garlic, scallions, hot peppers, kale, kohlrabi, mushrooms, mustard greens, red onions, Vidalia onions, parsley, bell peppers, pimientos, radicchio, radishes, red-leaf lettuce, romaine lettuce, shallots, spinach, tomatoes, and watercress.

Many supermarkets have premixed, prewashed bags of mesclun greens, a tasty variety of many fresh greens that makes an instant salad.

Pick high-taste salad dressing minus the fat. A garden salad can be part of a great lunch, but when you pour on regular salad dressing, you add a whopping 25 or more grams of fat. At once, your energy will plummet.

High-fat salad dressing is now the number one source of fat in the diets of American women ages 19 to 50, accounting for almost 10 percent of their fat intake, according to the National Cancer Institute and the USDA Human Nutrition Information Service.

Choose the nonfat, low-calorie dressings that you like, and make sure that you keep them on hand. Or make your own nonfat vinaigrette. So many flavored vinegars are available that this is easy to do.

Bypass full-fat dairy foods. Ask for alternatives to whole milk, cream cheese, cottage cheese, or traditional cheeses. Low-fat or nonfat cheeses, such as Jarlsberg Lite Swiss, are popular choices. Look for nonfat cream cheese or cottage cheese. And if you drink milk or pour it in your tea or coffee, make sure that it's fat-free.

On sandwiches, use all-zest, zero-fat sandwich spreads. Fat-free spreads include mustard, hot-pepper sauce, and fat-free salad dressing. Be sure to stay away from butter or margarine. If you love mayonnaise, buy

CLOGGED WITH YESTERDAY'S EXCESS,

THE BODY DRAGS THE MIND

DOWN WITH IT.

—Horace (65–8 B.C.), Roman poet

the low-fat or, better yet, fat-free varieties. Regular mayo is loaded with fat calories—a whopping 11 grams of fat per tablespoon.

Savor some fresh pasta with nonfat sauce. It's easy to avoid cream, oil, or cheese sauces on pasta. Just make sure that you choose tomato-base or wine-base pasta sauce. If you opt for pasta salad, get a fat-free dressing to go with it. Skip the olives or chunks of cheese.

Skip the croissant sandwich. If you love deli-made sandwiches, carefully avoid a croissant in favor of a whole-grain bun or slices of whole-grain bread. The croissant can torpedo your energy by delivering up to 50 grams of fat. By comparison, in two slices of 100 percent whole-grain bread, you get only 4 to 5 grams of fat, about one-tenth that of the croissant. Better yet, have old-world whole-grain thick rye or pumpernickel bread.

As for the fixin's, have the sliced turkey breast instead of high-fat ham, bologna, or sausage. Fresh vegetables are also good, though they don't have the protein of turkey. But whatever you do, be sure to hold the mayonnaise (unless it's fat-free), and decline the olives, cheese, or oil. Feel free to add fat-free extras such as lettuce, tomatoes, green bell peppers, jalapeño peppers, sprouts, pickles, onions, a dash of spicy mustard, and a splash of vinegar.

Be picky about pizza. Pizza is a great lunch choice if you get the order right. When possible, get a whole-grain crust. Go light on the cheese and hold the olives, which are almost pure fat. Also, stay away from high-fat meat toppings like sausage, pepperoni, ham, and ground beef. If you're going for extras, add vegetables and a dash of fresh pepper on top.

Be choosy about Mexican and Tex-Mex. South-of-the-border favorites can be fine if you choose nonfat bean burritos or nonfat bean soft-shell tacos. As with pizza, go light on the cheese and get extra vegetables. Add plenty of salsa. Watch out for fat-packed favorites that drain your energy. Nachos and taco salads are particularly fat loaded. A single taco salad can contain 55 grams of fat and 800 calories.

Bump the burger for something else. If you think it's a hamburger that you want, consider some better choices. You can keep your energy high and cut way back on your fat intake by choosing a grilled chicken breast or ground turkey-breast burger. (Try seasoning these with steak sauce.)

Better yet, have a garden burger. One popular version of this no-meat burger is now available at such popular chain restaurants as T.G.I. Friday's and Hard Rock Cafe. The garden burger is low in fat—but again, be sure to use mustard or nonfat mayo instead of regular mayonnaise.

If it's beef, keep it simple. If you must have a hamburger, get a plain one with mustard or ketchup and pile it high with fresh vegetables. Stay away from the version that includes such fat-dripping add-ons as bacon, mayonnaise, and cheese.

Ban the batter-fried foods. Any food that's cooked in batter or breading is a magnet for fat. Think of the breading or batter as a sponge that soaks up fat and grease and drains away your energy for hours to come.

Hold the fries. I know that this is hard. But from an energy perspective, it doesn't matter what kind of oil they're fried in—french fries still hit the snooze button in your brain. Instead, say yes to several whole-grain breadsticks. Or order a low-fat bean salad to have on the side.

Skip the "Best Deal"-size sodas. A single mega-cup can add up to 800 calories to your lunch. Far from giving you a lift, the big soda can make you tired. During the afternoon, your blood sugar rebounds from the sugar or sweetener in the soda, and your metabolism drops.

When your sweet tooth demands dessert, have two or three bites.
My wife, Leslie, teases me about this. How can I eat just a few bites of a delicious dessert and stop there? I wish I could say that I am genetically programmed to do that, but I'm afraid that's not the case. It's a practiced, healthy habit—and one that you can acquire. In fact, Leslie now does the same thing. We leave a lot of desserts behind; but on the other hand, we've been able to really savor some wonderful desserts without the downside of feeling bloated, overfed, and lethargic when we get up from the table.

Even if you aren't dining out but just want something sweet to end your meal, there are many good choices. Fresh fruit is ideal. Or have a whole-grain nonfat brownie or a small cup of frozen yogurt or nonfat regular yogurt. Another good dessert is a single chocolate mint. Or have some mint gum. I also like a nonfat whole-grain granola bar or nonfat pound cake, but take just a few bites when you choose these.

Whatever dessert you're having, chew each bite very slowly, savoring the taste. Then, immediately brush your teeth before you head into your afternoon. That final brushing helps end the meal and prevents further cravings for more sweets.

3. Do "1 + 1 = 10" Aerobics for Energy

Getting some key minutes of exercise after your midday meal can significantly increase your energy for the rest of the day. The 1 + 1 represents eating plus activity. But when you calculate the total, 1 (eating) + 1 (activity) = 10, not 2. This is because the energy-producing, heat-generating effect of physical activity adds a vast amount to the effect of food alone. And that increased effect, also called a thermic reaction, is the critical process in your body—it leads to more energy.

This exercise may turn out to be one of your key energy-revving actions of the entire day. In controlled scientific studies, Robert E. Thayer,

Ph.D., professor of biological psychology at California State University, Long Beach, found that as little as 10 minutes of brisk walking leads to very significant increases in energy. After 10-minute walks, some people in the studies reported that they felt like they had reached their peak energy levels for the entire day. And the effect was more than short term. The energy boost lasted for at least an hour and for as long as 3 hours.

Apart from the direct and immediate physiological boost, there are other good reasons to engage in $1 + 1 = 10$ exercise after lunch. There's a real brain-clearing factor. A brief walk is a good antidote for frustration or anger, both of which can wear you down and drain your energy as the day goes on.

As the result of research with more than 400 men and women, ages 16 to 75, Diane Tice, Ph.D., a psychologist at Case Western Reserve University in Cleveland, reports that going for walks helps people step back from irritations and detach themselves from feelings of anger or frustration. After walking, she found, people's empathy increased. That is, the active respite gave them the opportunity to begin seeing things from other people's viewpoints.

Even in light doses, exercise is one of the best protections against energy loss and memory loss and may even make you younger, according to René Cailliet, M.D., chairman of the department of physical medicine at the Santa Monica Hospital Center in California and former chairman of the department of physical medicine and rehabilitation at the University of Southern California School of Medicine in Los Angeles. "Researchers are finding that moderate exercise can not only retard the effects of aging but can actually reverse them," says Dr. Cailliet.

Now that you know the positive effects of $1 + 1 = 10$ exercise, you may still be wondering if exercising after lunch will just make you hungry again. Perhaps so. But it's the right kind of hunger. "Research is showing that exercise may enhance your preference for fruits and veg-

Does Your Doc Need to Know What You're up To?

It's always a good idea to check with your doctor before beginning an exercise program, particularly if you've had heart problems or if there's a history of heart-disease in your family. Your doctor may decide that you should take an exercise-tolerance test (ETT) or maximal graded exercise test (MaxGXT).

According to the American College of Sports Medicine, any healthy person under age 45 with no major coronary risk factors can usually begin an exercise program without undergoing an ETT or MaxGXT "as long as the exercise program begins and proceeds gradually and as long as the individual is alert to the development of unusual signs or symptoms."

But you should consult your physician if you have any medical symptoms, are undergoing treatment for any ailment, or have one or more major coronary risk factors. These risk factors include:

• A history of high blood pressure, heart attack, or cardiovascular disease in family members prior to age 50
• A history of high blood pressure above 145/95
• An elevated total cholesterol/high-density lipoprotein cholesterol ratio (above 5 for men or 4.5 for women is considered elevated)
• An abnormal electrocardiogram
• Symptoms suggesting metabolic, pulmonary, or coronary heart diseases

"People often ask, 'Should I have a medical checkup before I start training?'" says Per-Olof Åstrand, M.D., Ph.D., director of the Karolinska Institute in Stockholm, Sweden. "The answer must be that people who are in doubt about the condition of their health should consult their physician. But as a general rule, moderate activity is less harmful to the health than inactivity."

etables," says Diane Hanson, Ph.D., a lifestyle specialist at the Pritikin Longevity Center in Santa Monica, California. This decreases the chance that you'll instinctively reach for energy-blunting high-fat fare.

Exercise is a fairly simple matter—just put your body in motion, as we

TRY THIS NOW!

After-lunch exercise turns out not only to rev up active energy but also to be a real calorie-consuming, fat-fighting strategy that can give you a big boost in reaching weight-loss goals. According to research, you can get up to twice the usual calorie-burning benefits for each minute of activity if you exercise within 30 minutes after eating lunch.

In fact, if you don't exercise during that time frame, you may actually be encouraging your body to store fats. That's because, in the absence of muscular activity, messenger chemicals in your brain and body respond by conserving energy. If you don't use the carbohydrates or fats for ener-getic activities, the food is directly stored as body fat.

Research indicates that your body's metabolic rate goes up by about 10 percent after a meal or snack as a result of the chemical processes that are activated to digest food. Evidence shows that your metabolic rate can be further increased—sometimes even doubled—if you do 5 to 20 minutes of moderate physical activity such as walking while initial di-gestion is going on.

When you choose pleasurable ways to be physically active, "food can be made to burn hotter, in a sense, with fewer calories being available for fat storage," according to Bryant A. Stamford, Ph.D., exercise physiol-ogist and director of the health-promotion and wellness program at the University of Louisville. Essentially, you're "pulling oxygen into the body," he explains.

all do every day, and you're engaging in some form of exercise. But as scientists have been telling us, there's something special about aerobic exercise, the kind of exercise that you need to make the $1 + 1 = 10$ formula work for you.

Here's How

Within a half-hour of finishing lunch, get in 10 to 20 minutes of light aerobic activity. Going for a walk is only one way to do this. You can also climb stairs or pedal a stationary bicycle. At the very least, stand up and move around while talking on the phone or poring over your mail.

To make do-it-anywhere energizing activities too convenient to ignore, take a moment to figure out which equipment you may want in your home or office. It needs to be in a convenient location and readily accessible. If you have only a few extra minutes here and there, you don't want to waste them taking equipment out of the closet to set it up or trudging to a distant corner of the basement. Even if your fitness equipment doesn't match the decor in the "action area" of your home, keep in mind that this discrepancy may be well-worth accepting: Research indicates that the happiest people, at every age, tend to be those whose bodies stay healthy and fit.

Whenever you can, make this post-lunch exercise session last for 10 to 20 minutes, but if you can squeeze in only 5 minutes, then by all means do it. The point is to keep moving, not just after lunch but throughout the day. To a significant extent, "inactivity fatigue" and "creeping obesity"—two common complaints of many people over 40—are both the result of "creeping inactivity" that zaps energy and piles on excess weight. By making after-lunch activity extremely convenient, you prevent the "creeping inactivity" from ever getting started.

As scientists and exercise physiologists have been striving to understand the different kinds of exercise that we're capable of doing, they've taken steps to determine the impact of exercise on our muscle cells and nerve cells. As a result, we now understand a great deal about the ways in which our bodies create and use energy when we're exercising.

Two terms are especially important in understanding this science. The first term is *cardiovascular endurance*, which is a measure of the sustained ability of your heart, lungs, and blood to perform optimally. The second term is the one that you've probably heard bandied about quite frequently, *aerobic exercise*. In aerobic exercise, oxygen intake, transport, and utilization are improved with regular training. As a result, your cardiovascular fitness and endurance are likely to increase.

The fact that aerobic exercise is a flourishing pursuit can be largely credited to preventive-medicine specialist Kenneth H. Cooper, M.D., founder and president of Cooper Aerobics Center in Dallas. His research team has supervised nearly 52,000 program participants during a 20-year period, recording and assessing their performance during a total of 1.25 million exercise hours.

Here are some of the benefits you get from exercise.

- When you do aerobic exercise, you safely and comfortably increase your breathing and heart rate for an extended period of time, usually at least 20 minutes. Dr. Cooper has found that aerobic exercise increases the amount of blood in your system and the amount of oxygen-carrying hemoglobin in your blood. Your blood becomes, in a word, richer: It can bring in more oxygen to each cell while taking away more carbon dioxide and other waste products that are the outcome of your cells' energy burning.

- With more aerobic exercise, your muscle cells have greater ability to more efficiently process oxygen and eliminate wastes like carbon dioxide. At the same time, aerobic exercise makes your blood vessels more flexible, so they don't tend to accumulate deposits of artery-harming plaque as readily. The result is less resistance in your blood vessels and less work for your heart.

• Aerobic exercise also increases the number of tiny blood vessels, or capillaries, that form a network throughout your body. New vessels may appear from nowhere, their growth stimulated perhaps by increased circulation or chemical trigger. Lung capacity also increases. Some studies have linked this increase with greater longevity.

Other benefits are that your heart muscle grows stronger and is better supplied with blood. It also attains increased stroke volume, which simply means that it can pump more blood with each beat.

• With aerobic exercise, your quantity of high-density lipoprotein (HDL, the so-called good cholesterol) increases and your total cholesterol/HDL ratio decreases, which is a welcome sign of improved cholesterol level. Overall, there is a reduction in your risk of developing atherosclerosis, or hardening of the arteries.

• Your resting heart rate is lower when you do more aerobic exercise. Elite athletes in endurance sports can become so well-conditioned that they have resting heart rates between 30 and 45 beats per minute. People who have developed good cardiovascular fitness from regular aerobic exercise generally have hearts that beat 45 to 50 times a minute when at rest, pumping at least the same amount of blood as does an unconditioned person's heart beating 75 to 80 times a minute. Over the course of a day, the unconditioned person's heart must beat 50,000 more times than a conditioned person's heart. In a year, that's 17 million extra beats that an unfit person's heart must provide.

If you want to feel good about aerobic exercise and also avoid injury, it's important to warm up gradually, pace yourself sensibly, exercise for a reasonable amount of time, and, above all, enjoy yourself while you're doing it. Here are my guidelines for a great, energizing aerobic session.

Warm up. Precede each aerobic session with at least 5 minutes of gentle warmups. Mimic the activity or sport that you're about to do, but move around at an easy pace. It's fine to stretch, but do it gently, without bouncing movements, *after* your muscles are warmed up. That's important because if you go right into stretching without warming up first, you may injure your joints.

Use major muscles at a rhythmic pace. Exercise at a rhythmic, comfortable pace using major muscles such as your thighs. Begin gradually. Listen to your body. Stop if you feel any pain at all.

Choose safe, sensible low-intensity exercise. Choose an exercise intensity that's reasonable. There's an easy way to measure that: If you can exercise steadily and talk at the same time without gasping for breath, you're at a good pace. This is known as the talk test.

To be more exact, you can adjust your level of exercise so that your target-heart-rate zone is 60 to 75 percent of a number known as your predicted maximal heart rate (PMHR). Here's how to calculate your PMHR and then figure out what your target-heart-rate zone should be when you exercise.

1. Subtract your age from 220 to get your PMHR.
2. Multiply your PMHR by .60 to find the lower limit of your target-heart-rate zone, measured in beats per minute.
3. Multiply your PMHR by .75 to find the upper limit of your target-heart-rate zone in beats per minute.

Take your pulse at your wrist shortly after beginning to exercise, again at a midway point in your aerobic session, and once more when cooling down. Starting the count with zero on the first beat, continue to count each beat for 15 seconds. Then, multiply by four to get an estimate of your heart rate per minute.

You might also consider using an electronic heart rate monitor to accurately measure and guide your individual cardiovascular and physiological response to exercise. A heart rate monitor provides you with biofeedback, "feeding back" to your eyes and ears. You wear an elastic chest strap, with a monitor on your wrist that gives you audible and visual information about your number of heartbeats per minute. Using this monitor, you get a continuous reading of your heart's responsiveness to variables such as stress, intensity, thoughts, and tension levels. Taken together, these are keys to regulating the intensity and quality of aerobic fitness.

If you can precisely monitor and refine your exercise, you can then maximize each and every individual workout, getting the greatest benefits per minute. This measurement must be tailored to your unique needs and condition, which means that you'll need to consult with a trainer or exercise physiologist. (And if you have a history of heart problems, of course it's essential to consult with your doctor.) This is the key to the most effective conditioning to increase both your exercise performance and your overall health.

Go for 20 to 30 minutes. When it fits your schedule, plan to do 20 to 30 minutes of low-intensity aerobics three or four times a week. But remember, if you can't find the time some days, don't worry about it. Just go ahead with a few 5- to 10-minute mini-walks, or climb several flights of stairs once in the morning and again after lunch. Even with these lighter exercise periods, it helps to begin at a slow pace with a warmup and finish off with a cooldown.

Keep things fun and noncompetitive. Here's a finding that may come as a surprise: Competitive thoughts during exercise can increase harmful stress. According to a study at Shippensburg College in Pennsylvania, levels of stress hormones such as norepinephrine, which normally increase a moderate amount during strenuous activities, rise dramatically when you drive yourself with words like *harder* and *faster*.

Psychologist Kenneth France, Ph.D., who directed this study, examined the effects of thoughts on norepinephrine levels. He monitored athletes who participated in a wide range of sports and gave them sets of mental cues during identical workouts. France first used the words *calm, relaxed,* and *steady,* then shifted to more competitive words like *faster, harder, better.* Both types of mental signals produced equal pulse-rate changes, but the aggressive words caused norepinephrine levels in the athletes' urine to more than double. After completing the study, France recommended that people "abandon competitive thinking during workouts. Performance may even improve when you take pressure off yourself."

In short, keep things lighthearted and, yes, fun. While *fun* is not a word that's heard in rigorous exercise circles, it's the key to high levels of active energy. Besides, from a scientific perspective, it's essential. Begin thinking of exercise as time for something special for yourself, and include friends in your fitness sessions if that's enjoyable to you.

As your fitness improves, consider adding a few easy speedups. Can you fool your body into burning more body fat as a fuel when you exercise? There's one way to find out. Use your daily exercise as a test program.

If you want to increase your energy level and at the same time increase your fat-burning power, try elevating your activity level in short spurts. If you've been doing aerobic walking, for instance, speed up your pace for a few minutes during each walk. The pace shouldn't be too intense; make sure that you're still comfortable.

With just that little spurt, researchers say, your muscle cells get ready for more intense exercise and draw on more of your body's fat reserves. During that interval, you use up more fat-burning enzymes in your blood and burn off more fat molecules. As a result, you get the maximum out of that exercise and you end up feeling healthier and more energized.

It's important to note that, ideally, a brief, higher level of activity must

OF ALL THE **CALORIES** BURNED IN THE BODY,
50 TO 90 PERCENT **ARE BURNED BY YOUR MUSCLES—**
EVEN WHEN YOU SLEEP.

—Covert Bailey, *Smart Exercise*, 1996

be followed by prolonged aerobic exercise that will burn up the liberated fat. "Just step up the pace or even jog a bit now and then to boost adrenaline output," advises Dr. Stamford, then follow this with a period of slower, steady exercise.

The fat loss from aerobics may occur primarily in the abdomen. To test this theory, a 1991 study at the University of Washington in Seattle had 15 men—average age 68—follow an aerobics program that totalled 30 to 45 minutes a day, 5 days a week. After 6 months, the men had lost fat preferentially from their abdomens.

The cause of this preferential fat loss may be the release of adrenaline during exercise, according to Dr. Stamford. "One of the jobs of adrenaline is to increase the free fatty acids in the bloodstream so the body can use them as fuel for activity," he observes. "A prime location for that to occur is the stores of fat in the abdominal areas." Possibly, those abdominal fat cells are particularly sensitive to adrenaline.

Cool down. At the end of each aerobic activity, keep moving for enough extra time to allow your heart rate to slowly return to normal. The cooldown period, brief though it is, is critical from a health standpoint because it allows your body to return gradually to its pre-exercise state.

To avoid shocking your whole system—and possibly encouraging heart attack—the main rule is that you should never stop exercising suddenly. The drop in blood pressure that occurs during the cooldown period should take place gradually, so keep moving, swiftly at first and then at a slower pace. During your cooldown period, you can talk to a friend or review project notes or just take a break—but don't stand still. Keep moving.

4. Seek a Fresh Vantage Point

As you wrap up your lunch break and get ready to go back to work, take another quick breather. Before you return to your desk or chores, reconnect with the big picture. What's your reason for working in the first place? Why does it matter? How much more of your ingenuity and attentiveness can you bring to the projects, tasks, or challenges ahead? If your present efforts are more drudgery than excitement, how can you finish them earlier so you have more time and energy for whatever you love to do?

These final thoughts and feelings serve as a healthy transition that sustains and builds on the energy that you have gained from your lunch break. They also help rekindle your innermost drive to do whatever you can in the afternoon to make more of a difference, not just make a living.

Active-Energy Switch #4

Go Home Feeling Better

I n the late afternoon, as you look ahead to evening, there's a danger
zone in front of you.

This is one of the most crucial times of the day for active energy.
What you do or don't do has a tremendous influence over the quality
and energy of your evening hours.

It's common to rush from work to home and to end up feeling like
it's all work. When that happens, regrets build and dissatisfactions gnaw
away at you. You lose energy from the struggle and feel like you've lost
any chance to recover along the way.

Instead of feeling relief as they head home, many people report feeling
numb, like they're on autopilot. Chronobiologists, scientists who study
the influence of time cycles on human beings, refer to this late-afternoon
slump as the breaking point.

But it doesn't have to be. You can build your own lifeline of energy
to help carry you through this demanding period. You have the skills to
navigate the danger zone of late afternoon with more energy and atten-

tiveness than you may have had for many years. It's up to you to make new choices and build your own bridge away from the intensities and urgencies of the day's efforts. That way, when you finally arrive at home, you reap your fair share of the timeless benefits that have always awaited us there but that so few of us receive anymore.

A Plummet Position

For many of us, late afternoon is the time when energy plummets to the lowest point of the day. Don't be surprised if this is when you feel most vulnerable to tiredness and frustration.

In late afternoon, we're coming to the end of a workday and the beginning of . . . well, that's for you to determine. Some of us are anticipating a long ride home. For others, the afternoon ends with transporting children or waiting for other family members to arrive at home. But whatever lies ahead, these minutes are a vital time to unwind and shift gears, staying active while thinking ahead and giving your mind and heart a boost.

Studies show that late afternoon is when people make the most mistakes. Negative thoughts can predominate; molehills appear as mountains. Misunderstandings, arguments, and disputes frequently occur.

Even if you've been home all day, you're not free from the afternoon slump. Your body's inherent and ancient metabolic patterns are poised for a wavelike downturn from about 4:00 P.M. on. This common dropoff in active energy, alertness, and fat-burning power sets up a high-stress fatigue-and-fat-storing zone that can last all night.

A New Track

You can reverse this low-energy pattern, but it may take some thinking ahead to do so. If you're in a workplace environment and preparing to head home, you need to make some key choices. The rhythm of your work is considerably different and probably more intense than the pace of life at home. None of us wants to be fatigued and distracted when we get home. But often, that's what happens, and then we spend much of our evenings on autopilot.

Afternoon preparation for the evening is just as challenging for someone who has been at home caring for family members or doing errands all day. You still have some pivotal choices to make.

This is the time of day when your body and mind may be most in need of an energizing boost. At work, thoughts turn to the snack machine. At home, you may feel compelled to start snacking. Exhaustion is a factor to deal with.

In the midst of these pressures, however, there are some simple, practical ways you can create a late-day burst of active energy.

Dealing with the Real

Millions of us are sensing that grueling hours and ever-greater demands are not just a bad patch that we'll eventually get through. Economic recoveries or recessions have little to do with the degree of stress that many of us are feeling right now. That pressure is probably here to stay. And, according to a number of business analysts, it's going to keep stress levels at a record-breaking high.

The clash between job and home has never been more pronounced. Nationwide surveys report that 72 percent of men and 83 percent of women experience "significant conflict between work and family."

The stress cycle can be very hard to break. If you don't manage your on-the-job pressures with active energy, there's a good chance you'll create or magnify problems at home. Conversely, when there's no active energy at home, stress there may readily cross over into your work performance. There's reason to be concerned about interrelated stress

ALL YOU HAVE TO DO IS PAUSE....

IT'S OUR IMPATIENCE THAT SPOILS THINGS.

—Molière (1622–1673), French dramatist

and the way that it can mount up. Researchers have found that relationship problems can also lower your resistance to disease and even shorten your life.

Workaholism is just as damaging. People who value power over family and friendships appear to have a harder time fighting off disease and get sick more often. In addition, this high-tension pattern can leave a trail of personal bitterness. Many divorces seem to be the direct or indirect results of workaholic lifestyles. Children feel alienated from parents who seem consumed by work. Workaholism touches everyone. How you manage your active energy can make a big difference.

Can you clearly draw the line between work and home? If so, there is compelling evidence that you're less likely to suffer from energy loss and burnout. You're more likely to have physical exhaustion and stress-related health problems if you have trouble separating work from home.

Doing things at home to generate active energy can help you draw the line. It can also relieve some of the stress patterns that tire you out. Turning on active energy doesn't mean you have to turn your whole evening upside-down. But there are a few easy strategies you can use as you make the transition from work to home.

Changing Tempo

I've mentioned some of the common, tension-producing problems that confront many of us when we're unprepared for the shift from work to family. You can easily be knocked off-balance. As you're greeted by loved ones at the door, perhaps it seems like everyone is talking at once: "This happened; that broke; he got sick; her feelings got hurt; blankety-blank called; and you-know-who forgot to pick up you-know-what on the way home." It's easy to get rattled, especially if you've been looking forward to a peaceful homecoming and a quiet place to retreat from the day's stresses.

Appropriate questions to ask yourself are "Where do I begin to change things? How can I leave work problems at work? How do I stop the stress of home from infiltrating the office? How can I balance these two phases of my life so that each is positive and neither is in conflict with the other?"

For people who work at home all day, the end-of-the-workday challenges can be just as intense. But we can't wish away those challenges. Practical steps are needed. That's why researchers suggest that we begin with some minor adjustments in daily routine. Take some small, well-focused actions to alter several of the common counterproductive habits that influence work-family balance far more than most of us realize.

Turnaround Strategies

In the discussion of Calm-Energy Switch #5, I mentioned some calm-energy tactics that you can use to help decompress from the day. Here are several ways to tap into your active energy as well before you leave work.

Catch some extra afternoon light. Researchers at the Harvard Medical School have discovered that one of the quickest and simplest ways to give a quick boost to your brain's alertness and your overall vigor is to turn up the light.

Today, as you wrap things up at work, turn on some extra lights or open the blinds as wide as possible. If you get a moment to spare, step outside for a minute or two of late-day sunlight. It doesn't matter whether you rely on indoor lighting or get a good dose of sunlight; either way, light offers an ancient and powerful way to lift your late-day energy and mood.

For many of us, the workday restricts us to limited indoor space. Stepping outdoors at the end of the day is literally a step into the outside world. Relish that moment. It's like returning to your physical body after a day in which you were wrapped up in many of the typical office problems, such as schedules, deadlines, meetings, phone calls, and memos.

Free up your shoulders, free up your energy. Why do so many people finish the workday slumped over and then stay that way on into the evening? There's no reason for that to happen.

Take a few moments to do some stretching. Use gentle physical movements such as neck rotations, shoulder shrugs, torso turns, wrist circles, and knee bends. Any of these freeing motions will help increase bloodflow throughout your body. All of these motions make it easier to shake off the mind-set of work.

Pause to ask yourself, "Where am I feeling tightness or tiredness?" Then respond by loosening and activating those areas, smoothly, slowly, and in circular or front-to-back, left-to-right, and right-to-left motions. It's a fast and easy technique that works.

What's Your Rush?

Today, more and more of us rush home, hurry to prepare dinner, flip through the newspaper, eat quickly, and then either collapse in front of the TV or plunge into another round of scheduled activities. Do you have nightly errands? Parental duties? What about the paperwork that you need to catch up on? Do you need to prepare reports or pay bills?

What's missing is a brief time-out when you can shake off stress and tension and start the evening with a dose of extra energy and excitement.

TRY THIS NOW!

It makes sense to arrange for some kind of brief transition time or decompression period between your workday and your downtime. If you've been in an office all day, devote the last 5 to 15 minutes of your workday to your least pressured tasks.

Here's How

At the end of your next workday, try this simple way to begin the transition toward home. As you move for the door or step outside your work area, draw in a very deep, smooth breath and let it out slowly.

Imagine yourself being home. Begin to experience the sights and sounds of what waits for you. Will there be hugs and smiles? Go ahead and recall an ideal day, when you were immediately surrounded by the feelings of caring and comfort. Think about how you'll wind down and experience the love and laughter that you find at home. Maybe great food is waiting for you. Maybe great sex.

As you're focusing on this homecoming, leave your work worries behind. This mental release is powerful. In a matter of moments, you'll find that your mind and mood begin to settle into the slower rhythms of home. Those feelings will help make the journey feel less rushed and the arrival less hurried.

Here are some active ways to take an evening time-out.

Dress down. To help make the break between your workday and evening, change into comfortable clothes as soon as you get home. The ritual of putting away your suit or work clothes and putting on a comfortable flannel shirt and sweatpants is a way of "coming home" again. With comfortable clothes on, it's easier to be active, too.

Relish some indoor chores. It may be more tempting to you to pour a drink or switch on the TV than to take out the garbage or put the laundry in the dryer when you get home. That's certainly understandable if these are chores that you don't like to do. But tackle the small chores that you may enjoy for a few minutes, like spinning the lettuce for the dinner salad or setting the table.

Take care of outdoor matters too. We tend to think of outdoor jobs as big ones, like mowing the lawn, raking leaves, sweeping the walk, or weeding. But these chores are a lot less onerous if you spend just a few minutes doing them in the evening. Don't even think about finishing the job. This is just a quick opportunity to flex your muscles and get your blood moving.

Pamper the pets. Is there a household pet that would be glad to have some attention? If you have a cat that enjoys playing cat and mouse with a stuffed animal, go ahead and meet the challenge. This is a good time to take the dog for a walk or spend a few minutes throwing a ball for a game of fetch.

Play around. Part of the American landscape is a classic image of dad arriving home from work and playing a quick game of catch with his kids before the sunlight fades. Apart from the Little League hopes pinned to this activity, it's a great way to restore your active energy. For children and parents, there are hundreds of activities that can be great energizers. It all depends on the children's ages, of course, but a few of the things that you can do close to home include walking or running, jumping rope, or playing basketball, darts, Ping-Pong, croquet, or badminton. No matter how long you spend playing or how often you engage in these activities, you'll reap the benefits of active energy.

If you have tennis courts, a pool, or a fitness club nearby, there are dozens of activities that you can enjoy with your kids or spouse, especially in the evening. Naturally, these activities take more planning. But if you can do them once or twice a week, you'll find that any of these activities helps banish end-of-the-day fatigue and boost your energy.

See the sights. For some reason, porches and lawns seem to be vastly underutilized. If you walk around many suburban neighborhoods, you're unlikely to see much outdoor activity, even on a balmy summer's evening. Of course, there's a chance that you'd rather be indoors than out. But if you like your neighborhood, why not get out and enjoy it? Here are some easy ways to get a few minutes of activity.

- Walk once around the edge of your yard, noticing changes in trees and flowers.
- Stroll up to the end of the street and back again.
- Collect the mail.
- If you have a porch swing, outdoor rocking chair, or hammock, take a few minutes to swing or rock and just enjoy the view.

Trade some massage. Know how stiff and tense your neck and shoulders can feel at the end of a long, hard day? Well, you're probably not the only one in your household who feels that way. Take a few minutes to give a back rub or neck massage to your spouse. You can ask for the same in return, of course, but maybe you don't even have to. Some interesting studies have shown that a person who gives a massage gets just as many benefits in terms of stress relief and muscle relaxation as the person who gets the massage. Not only do you get to work your muscles and relax them, you also get the benefit of physical contact, which is calming and stress-relieving.

The Good of Humor

As you plan your evening, be sure to include some simple ways to increase your active energy from now until bedtime. One of the most important is humor. While you may not think of the physical, active-energy aspects of humor, they're there. Researchers have found that laughter can affect everything from your hormones to your body temperature. With a belly laugh or two, you can transform the whole chemistry of your evening—and of your family's too. That's the active-energy boost of humor.

If there are children in your household, they can probably teach you everything that you need to know about laughter. In my house, we love to laugh. Our children know that they can take the lead when the spirit moves them. Life at all ages is filled with funny antics and experiences. If you have friends, relatives, or kids who have ready wits and quick senses of humor, you've probably noticed how much you love to spend time with them.

I consider this one of the most rejuvenating and energy-revving aspects of together time. Humor is one of the simplest and most effective ways for the human brain to switch gears. If you really want to free up your attention for the evening ahead, have a good laugh.

Need some help in that department? (Most of us do.) One way to ensure laughs is to bring home a funny story or to keep your eyes open for

IF YOU WISH TO GLIMPSE INSIDE A HUMAN SOUL, JUST **WATCH A PERSON LAUGH AND PLAY**. THOSE WHO LAUGH AND PLAY WELL ARE THE MOST ALIVE.

—Fyodor Dostoyevsky (1821–1881), Russian novelist

the levity that so often arises naturally during commute time. Or just look around your household to see some of the antics.

Needless to say, we don't all have lighthearted temperaments. But we can acquire the skills to create a relationship that contains light-heartedness.

In part, this involves collecting memories of what's funny to you. Start doing that in the afternoon, and you'll brighten your whole evening.

Get Evening Relief

I'm a great believer in the importance of invigorating family rituals. Research indicates that rituals have a lot to do with shaping and deepening relationships. This can have a significant effect on our energy levels, health, and mental outlooks.

By rituals, I mean many simple things such as sharing meals together, saying hello and goodbye, exchanging a warm embrace, or bidding good night at bedtime. These reveal how we honor the wondrous possibilities of family life.

Such rituals are especially important in the evening. "Daily rituals give us a sense of the rhythm of our lives, help us in making the transition from one part of the day to another, and express who we are as a family," say family therapists Evan Imber-Black, Ph.D., and Janine Roberts, Ph.D. "They are not just routines. They are meaningful actions, often including symbols that can express far more than words. . . . Every time we participate in a ritual, we are expressing our beliefs, either verbally or more implicitly."

Purposeful Rituals

Research indicates that many common arguments between partners arise because they have unspoken differences about rituals. If you think of how you enter the home space at the end of the day and what that first encounter means to your spouse, it's apparent how misunderstandings can arise.

If you take some of the steps that I suggest to switch on active energy, you may change some of your evening rituals, and you and your family will need to discuss why and how those rituals may change. When I suggest walking the dog, taking a stroll around the yard, or swinging in a hammock for a few minutes, all for the sake of active energy, I'm not suggesting that everyone in your household will instantly understand what you're up to.

You can't assume that family members will automatically agree with the day-to-day rituals that give you active energy. But if you openly discuss why you're changing your daily rituals, maybe you can find better ways for each family member to connect with what you're doing. In fact, you may discover that the discussion revitalizes your whole family life.

Take a few minutes tonight to talk about your daily rituals and what you need to do to maintain active energy. If you want more active time in the evening, how can you get it? If television gets in the way, what about a night without it? What are some of the activities that your spouse or children would enjoy, and how can you do those things together? If you discuss your options and make it clear why you need more active energy, you'll probably find that your spouse is willing to respect that need and that many school-age children will accept that you want to change some of the family rituals from what they used to be to what they could be.

If everyone in a family sits down to dinner together, that's an expression of a belief, Dr. Imber-Black and Dr. Roberts point out. Without words, that family is saying that they value shared time together.

Nightly bedtime rituals, when parents sit by the bedsides of their children, provide necessary moments when parents and children tell each other what they believe about all kinds of matters. "The bedtime ritual expresses a certain kind of parent-child relationship where warmth and affection and safety are available," the therapists report.

Apart from dining together or talking at bedtime, there may be other ritual moments that you and your family share. Do you drive a child to school or take your spouse to the train station? Do you gather to watch a favorite weekly television show? What about special activities on weekends, such as going to ballgames or meeting with other families for picnics, games, or entertainment? These daily rituals confirm over and over again how we relate to each other and what we value.

And of course, it's not just families that have daily rituals. If you're a single adult, you need rituals too. With symbolic daily actions, you have the opportunity to create a comforting as well as comfortable environment and quiet space for yourself in your home.

Get Your Second Wind

With just a few changes in your evening routine, you may find yourself getting a second wind of energy. The benefits are tangible: more attentiveness to personal and family matters, a greater tendency to stay active and excited about your evening, a new surge of fat-burning metabolism, and increased likelihood of deeper sleep and rest.

How can you get these benefits? Six steps matter most.

1. Eat before you eat.

2. Enjoy an early, light dinner—and go for tastes that you love.

3. Get up and get going within 30 minutes after the meal.

4. Have a delayed dessert.

5. Put the day in perspective.

1. Eat Before You Eat

I know that it sounds unlikely, but to rev up your evening metabolism and vitality, it's often essential to have some munchies before dinner.

According to scientists, when you stay active in late afternoon and early evening and munch on a few bites of high-taste, low-fat food before your meal, chances are that your energy and mood will stay higher. There are long-term benefits too. You'll end up eating less for dinner and, consequently, storing less body fat.

By the way, there's another little-known payoff. When you take time out for a pre-dinner snack, you're likely to feel less argumentative at the end of the day. That's because eating helps stabilize your blood sugar levels, which influence your mood. Evidence indicates that simple hunger-related tensions contribute to fading energy, negative emotions, and late-day arguments, according to William Nagler, M.D., psychiatrist at the University of California, Los Angeles, School of Medicine, who specializes in effective relationship communication.

Reach for energy-boosting bites. But here's the twist: Those bites have to satisfy. A fat-packed pastry or monster cookie may numb your senses and drain your energy. And if it also contributes to weight gain, that's an additional, long-term energy drain.

The right pre-meal snack, on the other hand, is just what's needed. It's a good idea to choose a beverage such as hot tea, juice, or a healthy drink on ice. Then, help yourself to a small, low-fat, high-fiber appetizer. Have some fresh vegetable pieces with low-fat or nonfat cream cheese or bean dip and a whole-grain cracker or two.

Even a slice of healthy pizza or small serving of pasta can be a good choice. Or you might try several whole-grain, low-fat cookies with a half-glass of cold fat-free milk or ½ cup of low-fat or nonfat yogurt. (For more suggestions and recipes, see Energy Bites: Foods That Stoke Your Energy Furnace.)

Best of all may be a cup of tomato soup with several whole-grain crackers. Research suggests that soup can reduce fat cravings and total calorie intake. When scientists at Johns Hopkins University in Baltimore interviewed people who had eaten many different kinds of appetizers, they found that soup was the most satisfying and invigorating.

The least invigorating and least satisfying? Surprisingly, it was cheese and traditional snack crackers.

2. Enjoy an Early, Light Dinner—And Go for Tastes That You Love

For years, health researchers have puzzled over the finding that the French, compared to Americans, are considerably less likely to die of heart disease. Experts in population studies have looked at all of the distinctive differences in eating and exercise patterns that separate the two lifestyles. Many have remarked on the fact that the French drink more wine with their meals. Could organic substances in red wine account for the differences in heart attack statistics?

That has been identified as one factor. But another factor seems to be even more significant. According to researchers, the French are considerably more likely than Americans to consume fruits, vegetables, and fiber-rich whole grains. They also tend to eat less meat. They generally eat their main meal earlier in the day than Americans do. And the

AVOID LARGE INTAKES OF FOOD AT ONE TIME....
THIS REDUCES THE HORMONAL SIGNAL
THAT CAUSES FAT CELLS TO DIVIDE AND MULTIPLY.

—Peter D. Vash, endocrinologist,
University of California, Los Angeles, Medical Center

French are more likely to follow up their main meal with physical activity.

The French are accustomed to having their largest meal at midday. In one preliminary study, R. Curtis Ellison, M.D., a scientist at Boston University School of Medicine, showed that many French men and women consume 57 percent of their daily calories before 2:00 P.M. and then do a wide variety of physical work activities that last until evening.

In contrast, Americans take in a total of only 38 percent of their daily calories before 2:00 P.M. Most of us eat dinner, the largest, highest-fat meal, in the evening. And what do we do in the hours before bedtime? Usually, sedentary activities like watching television.

And here's a related problem: When we eat late in the evening, we're inclined to skip breakfast, say researchers.

In a study conducted at the University of Minnesota in Minneapolis, researchers compared groups of people on 2,000-calories-a-day diets to find out which groups had the most energy and lost the most weight. Specifically, they compared people who ate most of their calories early in the day with those who ate most of their calories late in the day. The study showed that people who ate earlier in the day had the most energy and lost weight. People on the same diet who consumed most of their calories later in the day gained weight and felt the most tired. The difference in weight loss was astounding—an average of 2.3 pounds per week.

Given this evidence, it just makes good sense to eat your evening meal as early as you can. Between 5:30 and 6:00 P.M. would be ideal, and 6:30 to 7:00 P.M. is probably fine, at least occasionally. But if you end up eating later than 7:00, make it a point to eat less, to eat more slowly, and to eat more vegetables and grains and less protein-rich or fat-rich foods. On weekends, try for 5:30 to 6:00 whenever that's reasonable; or, better yet, eat your main meal at midday.

What's the ideal evening meal? It may be a lighter meal than you're accustomed to, but that doesn't mean that you need to skimp on taste or flavor. Here are some guidelines.

Lose most of the dinner fat. One of the simplest ways to gain energy by reducing the fat in evening foods is to steadily shrink the portion sizes of the higher-fat foods that you eat and to simultaneously substitute lighter servings of lower-fat or nonfat alternatives. Be sure to emphasize those that are high in complex carbohydrates and fiber. Here are some options.

- Use plenty of nonfat, delicious salad fixings topped with fat-free dressings.
- Poach, bake, or steam vegetables, fish, and other foods instead of frying them.
- Increase your intake of fresh and steamed vegetables and whole grains as side dishes or in bread.
- Cook or lightly sauté with vegetable broths and a very small amount of oil.
- Help keep the fat content low by using cooking sprays and no-stick pans.
- Drink fat-free milk or 1% milk instead of whole milk; and choose

nonfat yogurt, cream cheese, cottage cheese, and sour cream, and nonfat or low-fat cheeses.

• Eat less red meat and pork. Substitutions include beans, peas, lentils, pasta, potatoes, vegetables, fruit, and low-fat cottage cheese.

• Instead of meat, go for small servings of fish (all finfish, canned salmon, water-packed tuna, and shellfish), turkey (skinless breast, drumstick, or thigh, or ground without the skin), or chicken breast without the skin.

• Enjoy tasty international recipes—Italian, Japanese, Mexican, Chinese, Greek, and Middle Eastern, for example—that combine vegetables or fruits with whole grains, beans, and little or no meat.

• Eat more 100 percent whole-grain foods such as breads, crackers, rolls, bagels, tortillas, or pastas. On occasion, eat whole-grain, low-fat muffins, waffles, or pancakes.

Emphasize taste. The mere sight, smell, and taste of low-fat food that you love may help increase your metabolism. You'll stimulate your body to burn more calories than you do when you eat bland, boring food.

Medical researchers in Quebec performed repeated studies, first on rats and then on people, to compare nutritionally identical meals, one tasty and one bland. They found that the smell and taste of flavorful food seemed to stimulate the thermic effect of food, which is the number of calories burned while digesting, absorbing, and utilizing food.

Accentuate recipe tastes and help reduce the need for fat as flavoring by seasoning foods with pepper, parsley, basil, oregano, jalapeño peppers, garlic, onions, shallots, curry, ginger, horseradish, tarragon, and other fresh spices and herbs.

Turn this taste challenge into a family affair. Get everyone involved. If the focus is first on savory flavors and second on lowering the fat, everyone should have more energy and fun along the way.

TRY THIS NOW!

Surveys show that most of us are amazingly unaware of what we consume from 5:00 P.M. on into the evening, according to research by Albert F. Smith, Ph.D., a cognitive psychologist who studies memory at the State University of New York at Binghamton. Ask anyone what they've been eating and how much, and you'll get some very incomplete information, according to Dr. Smith.

Despite that selective memory loss, however, it's essential to have a good idea about what and how much you eat during those all-important evening hours. To avoid weight gain, improve your energy, and reduce heart attack risk, research suggests that you need to limit your evening meal to 500 to 700 satisfying and energy-boosting calories. "The first, and perhaps most important, lifestyle behavior is to keep records," says Kelly D. Brownell, Ph.D., director of the eating and weight-disorders clinic at Yale University.

Here's How

Grab a pad of paper and a pen. Write "Evening Foods for Energy" across the top of the pad.

During the coming week, jot down everything that you eat from 5:00 P.M. until bedtime. It's essential to keep this list near the kitchen or dining room, where you can make notes right away. If you wait until the end of the evening and try to remember everything, you could be way off.

At the end of the week, keep this list as a basis of comparison as you begin changing your evening menu for best energy and sleep.

What are your favorite main courses, side dishes, fresh vegetables, fruits, soups, breads, and pastas? Pinpoint the tastes that you love and start searching out or creating recipes that accentuate those tastes while gradually reducing fat, refined sugar, and cholesterol.

Spread the heat. You can get an energy-boosting benefit from liberally sprinkling your food with spices like hot chili peppers and mustard. In a study published in the journal *Human Nutrition/Clinical Nutrition*, people ate meals that had identical numbers of calories, but some of the meals contained 3 grams of chili peppers and 3 grams of mustard sauce, while the others were spiceless. When researchers tracked the people's post-meal metabolic rates, they found that the spicy meals boosted metabolism by an average of 25 percent during the 3 hours after eating.

Start your meal with a few bites of protein-rich foods. One of the main reasons for eating supper is to give you the fullest surge of renewed energy to enjoy your evening. Yet typical high-fat fare does the opposite. Oil-drenched salad, cheese dips, or "killer" nachos give you a full dose of dietary fat that can plunge you into an extended period of mental and physical fatigue. To make matters worse, the fat calories can, at least indirectly, leave you feeling too tired for evening physical activity or even sex.

You can turn dinner into a more energizing experience by eating a few bites of low-fat, protein-rich food before you consume the rest of the meal. This is certainly worth a try. According to a number of neuropsychologists and nutritional researchers, protein has been shown to stimulate the natural production of neurotransmitters, or messenger chemicals, known as catecholamines. These chemicals activate your brain to provide feelings of alertness and energy for up to 3 hours.

AS LIFE'S PLEASURES GO,

FOOD IS SECOND ONLY TO SEX.

—Alan King, *The New York Times*, October 28, 1981

Your choices of low-fat, high-protein foods include favorites such as tomato soup, bean soup, and lentil soup. Bean or lentil salads or casseroles are also good. You can also opt for low-fat or nonfat yogurt or cottage cheese, a small glass of fat-free milk, or a few bites of a low-fat entrée that features beans, legumes, skinless chicken breast, turkey, or fish.

3. Get Up and Get Going within 30 Minutes after the Meal

What you do in the 15 to 30 minutes after eating your evening meal sends powerful signals to your metabolism. You'll set the stage for more vigor throughout the evening hours along with a night of deep sleep if you stay active after your meal. Make sure that you don't stay seated, particularly with the TV on, for long periods of time. That's the kind of "relaxation" that promotes fat forming, fatigue, and grumpiness rather than fat burning and a pleasant rush of positive evening energy. If you exercise at this time of day, you'll elevate your metabolic rate just as it's winding down.

There's also a weight-loss benefit to exercising shortly after you eat. "Exercise after eating seems to give a double boost of energy, so it burns more calories," says Bryant A. Stamford, Ph.D., exercise physiologist and director of the health-promotion and wellness program at the University of Louisville. The combined metabolic lift of both eating and exercising within a half-hour time frame can extend the energy renewal process for more than 10 hours.

Research indicates that a lifestyle filled with frequent physical activities also helps lessen your odds of becoming or staying depressed or overwhelmed by stress. Depression and stress deter many people from engaging in active evenings. Numerous surveys report that physically fit people who exercise regularly are more likely to be self-confident, self-disciplined, and psychologically resilient. Light evening exercise may also help ease late-night cravings for high-fat foods. If a craving does hit, you may be better able to choose a nonfat alternative and bypass the tendency to binge.

Make certain, however, that your postmeal activities are low intensity. Your digestive tract needs steady bloodflow after a meal, and if you exercise hard right away, your muscles will compete with your digestive tract for bloodflow. Digestion will be slowed as a result.

In my household, right after the evening meal is when we do some relaxed, low-intensity aerobic activity. Sometimes, we go for a brisk, short walk or bike ride. It's a time to shoot a few baskets, do some gardening, or head to the playground with the kids.

I guess we're lucky to have an old stationary cycle, Ping-Pong table, and stairclimber in the basement. That's where the family goes after dinner when it's too rainy or cold to do much outside. Sometimes, my wife and I do easy calisthenics while the girls practice their gymnastics or dance steps, which they love to do.

Our goal is always to make this time fun, not a chore. And if you have young children, you don't really need exercise equipment. With our girls, it's easy to spend 10 minutes playing chase, and we've created a few other get-up-and-go games that they enjoy. If there are household chores to be finished, we do those, too, during this active time,

The Love Dividend

My wife and I have noticed that an evening active time helps bring our family closer together. It also helps to improve our love life. Maybe that's because, when we're doing active things together, this helps align our wavelike ultradian rhythms, rises and falls of energy that occur in 90-minute or 180-minute cycles.

The bond is especially strong when we go walking together. If you share an after-dinner walk with your love partner, you'll have a chance to talk. Hold hands while you're walking. Get back in touch with each other. All of us have wavelike brain-body cycles that may be either in or out of sync. When you're walking and those cycles are in sync, you and your partner have a great opportunity to relax together and experience feelings of strong affection and sustained sexual attraction.

gathering and folding laundry, vacuuming the floor, and cleaning up the kitchen.

Among many possible activities, walking is one of easiest ways to get some extra minutes of exercise after a meal. In fact, research shows that if you walk after a meal, you may burn 15 percent more calories than if you walked the same time, distance, and intensity on an empty stomach.

A single 10-minute walk may trigger a 2-hour boost in your sense of well-being by raising your energy levels and lowering tension. In addition, a walk can make evening family time more enjoyable and invigorating and may also help prevent cravings for high-fat foods.

A Cool Sleep Benefit

There is some compelling evidence, though it's not yet conclusive, that you may burn more calories if you "sleep cool" at night. While you want to raise your body temperature before bedtime with exercise or a shower, by the time you climb between the sheets, your body should be cooled down.

"Your body will burn significantly more calories each night if you sleep cool," explains Ellington Darden, Ph.D., a strength expert and exercise scientist who has been director of research for Nautilus Sports/Medical Industries in Colorado Springs for the past 20 years. "I'm convinced that most people bury themselves under too many covers when they sleep. This prevents their normal thermostats from kicking in and supplying natural body heat (and burning off excess body fat to provide that heat). If you tend to sleep with too many covers, try to eliminate one or two. Try to wean yourself from cranking up the temperature on an electric blanket or using flannel sheets during the winter months; and during the summer, try only a single sheet on top of you. Soon, you'll be burning several hundred more calories each night."

If you opt for a postmeal stroll, you may wish to include other family members or friends as well. It gives all of you the chance for some good old-fashioned talk and lighthearted fun. These walks are the kinds that bring you closer together.

4. Have a Delayed Dessert

Want to hold on to your active energy as late as possible into the evening? Postpone dessert.

Make it a habit to get up from the table without dessert. Later on, you can savor a small portion. After a light and early dinner followed by some exercise, a tasty, low-fat dessert can be just the right accompaniment to some great conversation, music, games, reading, or television. Postpone the sweet conclusion to a satisfying meal, and you give your tastebuds something to look forward to later on, once you've picked up the pace of your evening. Then, you will also more effectively digest and metabolize your delayed dessert.

Whatever evening treat you choose to eat, plan a small serving that generally does not exceed 6 grams of fat and that has fewer than 300 calories. Select one of your taste favorites and chew each bite very slowly, savoring the taste.

Active Time for Mom and Dad

This shouldn't require a reminder, but the fact is that you may need to remind yourself that physical intimacy is an important component of active energy. Once you and your partner have agreed that you need time together, you must be clear about how you're going to get it.

If you and your partner decide that your time together comes at the end of the evening, your children need to be aware of that. Your time alone with your spouse should be a respected family ritual. If you're a parent, you might get in the habit of closing your door after 9:30 or 10:00 P.M. to allow for sweet time with your partner. Explain to the kids, "Mom and Dad need time to talk and to feel close to each other."

When you set aside specific interludes to be with your partner, you are doing some very positive modeling. By example, you confirm that it's vital for all of the members of your household to achieve their own relaxation and rejuvenation.

Sweets Delayed

Here are some small, tasty desserts that add just the right touch of sweetness. But instead of having them with dinner, wait 1½ to 2 hours, then savor a small serving.

Baked Goods

- Fat-free angel food cake or sponge cake
- Low-fat multigrain brownie
- Whole-grain, very low fat or fat-free cookies (Health Valley is one brand)
- Nonfat, very lightly sweetened granola (Walnut Acres is our favorite)

Yogurt and Ice Cream

- Low-fat or nonfat unsweetened yogurt (add your own fat-free granola or fruit)
- Nonfat frozen yogurt
- Low-fat ice cream

Fruit

- Apple (or natural, unsweetened applesauce)
- Apricot
- Blackberries

6. Put the Day in Perspective

The last part of an invigorating and meaningful evening takes only a minute or two. Use a bit of your evening energy to put the day—and life—in perspective before you fall asleep. To do this, you need to think creatively while you take some sort of action, even something as simple as stepping outdoors, which provides fresh air and a boost to circulation.

- Blueberries
- Boysenberries
- Cantaloupe
- Casaba melon
- Cherries
- Figs
- Grapes
- Grapefruit
- Honeydew melon
- Kiwifruit
- Lemon
- Lime
- Mango
- Nectarine
- Orange (or orange juice)
- Papaya
- Peach
- Pear
- Plum
- Raspberries
- Rhubarb
- Strawberries

Other Occasional Treats

- Air-popped or very low fat microwave popcorn
- Fruit pie with very low fat crust and very little sweetener
- Tapioca pudding made with fat-free milk

My mom liked to tell me a story about President Teddy Roosevelt. Whenever he had guests, the president would take them for an after-dinner walk on the White House lawn. Pointing up at the stars, naming constellations, and savoring the view of the night sky, the president would lead his shivering guests on a lengthy stroll.

At last, he would turn to them and say, "There, now I feel small enough. Let's go get some sleep!"

Part 4

Sensory Energy

Your senses are the central bridge to life's richness and wonder. Each and every experience reaches you through sensory engagement.

At one point in our lives, each of us used our senses with passionate intensity to make discoveries about the world. Through our senses, we discovered the warmth and illumination of sunlight, felt rain on our skin and the breeze in our hair, saw the stars in the night sky and the morning grass glistening with dew, sniffed flowers, heard music, and experienced laughter and amazement in every part of our bodies. From infancy through child-hood, our senses were such an important link to the world that we gloried in the messages that we discovered.

As we grew into adults, most of us inevitably lost this ability to live by our senses. And with that loss came a sacrifice of wonder and a waning of our innate curiosity to learn and grow. We pay a far greater price for that loss than most of us realize.

A Bridge to the Mysteries

The greatest advances in human history have come about when people have recovered what was lost and fully explored what was yet unknown. Both of these processes require and produce heightened levels of sensory energy.

Traditionally, we've been taught that there are 5 senses: sight, hearing, touch, taste, and smell. But scientists have now discovered many more than that—more than 70, in fact. Seventeen of those senses are considered absolutely vital.

There are clusters of senses within newly discovered sensory systems, which include:

- The vomeronasal system, capable of detecting chemical signals given off to indicate such specific messages as fear, identification, and sexual receptivity (these signals are called pheromones)
- Noiception, a sensory system for pain that is separate from touch and temperature sensing
- Parallel but distinctive sensory systems for experiencing heat, cold, and the other sensations associated with touch
- Parallel but distinctive sensory systems for detecting visual contours, contrast, and forms as well as colors
- The pineal gland sensory system, for detecting light and using it to synchronize internal body rhythms

Each of these senses, plus others that may be as-yet undiscovered, connect the world outside you to the life within. There is energy in those connections, energy that helps keep you fully and vibrantly alive.

That's why sensory energy is so important. It's the primary source of vitality that enables you to reach out with all of your senses and more fully participate in every moment of your life and work. Sensory energy lets you move past the going-through-the-motions zone where so many people get stuck. It enables you to savor every experience more fully.

The problem is that with the pace of life moving so fast, we can easily lose this connection to the world. When that happens, a common kind of impairment sets in. In fact, it has become so typical that many of us scarcely even notice it. As our adult lives settle into a set routine, we become markedly less alive than the 2-, 3-, or 4-year-old who is immersed in discovery. But what can we do about it? A lot, actually.

Alert to the Possible

The year 1901 saw the publication of a small book by Stanford University neurologist Reuben Halleck entitled *The Education of the Nervous System*. Its central message, as the title implies, is that education goes beyond book learning, scientific exploration, and mathematical calculations. You can literally educate your nervous system, and Halleck set out to show how that could be done by stimulating all the senses.

But Halleck's lessons began with a warning. The person who has properly trained only one or two senses is, in his words, "a pitiful fraction of a human being."

"When it comes to exercising the full range of your brainpower, the more variety, the better," says Danielle Lapp, Ph.D., a memory-training specialist at Stanford University School of Medicine. In other words, variety is not only the spice of life, as the old adage claims, but also the spice of the human senses.

Biologically, human beings respond to two basic conditions in the world. First, we depend on the availability of life-sustaining substances including oxygen, water, light, and essential nutrients such as proteins, carbohydrates, fats, vitamins, and minerals. Second, we rely on the input and feedback that we get from our surroundings. The way that we evolve certain responses to the people and world around us helps determine our presence in these relationships. Internally and externally, human beings must be fed by the nutrients in our environments and the points of feedback that help us know ourselves and our internal and external capabilities.

But there's also a very harsh biological message with which we have to contend. The moment that we stop growing, we begin dying. A living human cell is not something that's fixed; rather, it's always *becoming*. As goes the cell, so goes the human organism. The more we restrict our alternatives for stimuli and enrichment, the more our growth stalls or regresses. Therefore, one of the keys to our lifelong growth is our senses—how engaged they are, how often and well we use them. Our senses respond to the world with energy. And the more our senses respond, the more opportunities we have to make more energy. Our senses challenge us to live more fully every moment.

Grow Young

When Ashley Montagu, Ph.D., professor in the department of anthropology at Rutgers University in New Brunswick, New Jersey, said, "The goal in life is to die young—as late as possible," he identified the challenge that we all face. As we age, how can we preserve, protect, and promote the youthful outlook that helps us get the most enjoyment out of every day? To live the richest life requires childlike qual-

Reaping the Benefits

Sensory energy will give you:
- Greater brain fitness and mental clarity at every age
- Exceptional awareness of and sensitivity to the inherent merit in people and the value of varied life experiences, beneath and beyond the obvious surface of life that others notice
- Increased creativity and inventiveness, even when under pressure
- Enriched heredity, turning back the aging clock to live a longer, younger life
- Increased activation of your brain's neuroplasticity to grow and change
- Enhanced ability to keep your life's priorities in better focus
- More fun as you do more of the things that you most love to do
- Heightened learning with less stress and greater memory power

ities such as a sense of wonder, playfulness, humor, and curiosity. How sad, he laments, that we lose these qualities in growing older and must—to look, feel, and live young—regain them. Indeed, we can, he says, but why would we also not take care to have our children retain them?

Marian Cleeves Diamond, Ph.D., neuroanatomist at the University of California, Berkeley, and author of *Enriching Heredity: The Impact of the Environment on the Anatomy of the Brain*, observes that sensory energy is essential to longevity and to growing young, or what she calls enriching heredity. In essence, the more you produce sensory energy, the more you are naturally inclined to learn and to stretch your senses. As a result, your brain's unused or little-used pathways begin to light up, and, in some specific and documented ways, you can become younger as you get older.

In the course of a lifetime, scientists have found, the average person may use only $\frac{1}{10,000}$ of their brainpower. At every point in our lives, there is lots of room for new energy and continued brain growth. We don't have to succumb to fatigue, tension, tiredness, or the well-worn ruts of everyday living.

Sensory energy is turned on and increased by a set of sensory switches throughout your body and brain. It serves as another primary source of feeling 100 percent alive. According to researchers, the full development and continued, energetic use of your senses can help promote lifelong physical, emotional, and mental well-being. In response to heightened sensory activity, the nerve cells in your brain's cortex apparently grow larger and become more resistant to certain aging processes.

"If we learn to modulate our senses," says neurosurgeon Arthur Winter, M.D., "and develop them even in advanced years, we increase our pleasure in living and we maintain normal function in the cells that receive and respond to sensual input. A decrease in sensory input due to changes in the sense organs or to social isolation is reflected in reduced metabolism and bloodflow within the brain."

No Ruts

The opposite of sensory energy is routine energy, or being stuck in a fixed routine or pattern. Many people defend this state, even crave it. But routine energy contributes to premature, accelerated aging.

So many people function on routine energy that it's sometimes difficult to fully understand its cost. But the cost is there. People resist learning, avoid new experiences, and age much faster than necessary. Worse, when you're functioning on routine energy, you fail to engage with either life's simple pleasures or its grandest possibilities. A big piece of the fun goes out of living.

Too easily, the nonsensical world of passive entertainment becomes the source and focus of routine energy. How much you miss if that happens. You need to awaken your full sensory energy and reach out to embrace more of life—quickly, before it passes through your fingers.

The following chapters are designed to help you gain control over some of the most important aspects of the energy that brings you into fullest touch with the world around and within you. The sensory-energy switches are quite simple to turn on, anywhere and anytime, once you clearly notice when and how your sensory energy wanes.

Mix Up Your Habits

Most of us have an instinctive drive to find the routines that are most comfortable. Having found those routines, we cling to the familiar. It's one of the roles of the amygdala, a tiny but important area of the brain. The amygdala, scientists have found, keeps pressing you to stay just the way you have been. Essentially, this is the part of your brain that keeps insisting that there's no need to change, venture forth, or try new things.

This insistent need for stability and continuity can sometimes be wise, but only up to a point. It's pleasant to have certain times of the day and week when you can enjoy your favorite activities and comfortably unwind from pressures. In today's stressful world, these moments provide a sense of stabilization and welcome rejuvenation. Yet this same instinct can paralyze your senses, tire your mind, block you from the richness of new experiences, and accelerate premature aging.

Stop for a moment to think about your daily routines. What do you crave? It turns out that the faster life rushes forward, the more likely you

TRY THIS NOW

African-American baseball star Leroy "Satchel" Paige once asked, "How old would you be if you didn't know how old you were?"

It's a good question. If you didn't have a clue about how old you actually are, how old would you feel? The differences between your chronological age and the age that you feel can be enormous. I know many 60-year-olds who feel younger than they did when they were 30. And, on the other hand, there are some 30-year-olds who feel like they'd like to retire tomorrow.

Here's something you can do to instantly feel younger.

Here's How

In just a moment, put down this book and look across the room or out a nearby window. Your assignment is simple: Extend your senses. Feel something new in yourself or in your surroundings.

To accomplish this, you need to forget how old you are—that is, forget the number of birthdays that have passed. Instead, imagine that you can choose to feel however old you want to be. All that matters, for this moment, is the present. Feel the air against your skin. Feel the texture of your clothing. Blink your eyes, and when they're open, discover some new colors in the room. Look at the play of light and shadow against a wall. Hear sounds from as far away as your ears can detect. Feel your heart beating.

Before you pick up this book again, feel its weight and the texture of the cover, and see the pattern of print on the pages.

Your perspective and sensory engagement will change, even though the change may seem slight. You have just used a departure from your routine to boost your sensory energy.

are to covet comfort and the status quo. That is, you'll want things to settle down and get back to normal. All of us are drawn toward predictable, autopilot ways of thinking, feeling, and behaving.

In some limited ways, stability gives you a platform from which you can venture forth with resilience and curiosity into life's uncertainties and newness. But familiar routines create another, dampening effect. Those routines can actually drain your energy and blunt your senses.

Based on the research of a number of scientists, here's one of the common dilemmas: If you get up each day and do the same kind of work, interact with the same people, and eat the same kinds of food, it's all but assured that you're aging at a premature, accelerated rate. If, on the other hand, you continually and actively thread your life with a mosaic of new experiences, your sensory energy is fully turned on and your brain continually changes and develops. People who experience life in this way are naturally smarter, younger, more vigorous, and more curious. As you grow older chronologically, you have the opportunity to actually grow younger inside. It's a physiological change as well as a mental one. You'll look, feel, and behave like a younger person.

Coming Alive

We admire people who are young in spirit, those with a sparkle in their eyes and a ready wit. Even when people aren't great at new things, those who love to try them are especially appealing. We marvel at men and women in their eighties or nineties who whistle while working in the garden. All the better if they can smile with joy. Or if they are always eager to go to a dance—and are the last to leave the dance floor.

No one wants to look and feel old, at any age.

Pets: A Nice Touch

Pets get a great deal of our affection, and dedicated pet lovers certainly feel as if they're getting a lot of affection in return. But whether or not our dogs and cats love us as much as we think they do, they certainly provide us with very tangible energy.

Maybe it's because we pet them and groom them regularly. Perhaps we draw something from the expression in their eyes, from their sometimes extraordinary and very nonhuman habits, or even from their barks and mews and purring. Whatever the reason, many studies have shown that people who live with pets are generally healthier than those who don't. Among one group of people who had suffered heart attacks, for instance, researchers found that those living without pets were much more likely to have subsequent fatal heart attacks than those who lived with pets. In fact, the pet owners had one-fifth the death rate of those without pets.

Pets provide moments of pleasure and solace during difficult times. They forgive us when we're angry. They also help us connect to nature and the larger world outside ourselves. All of these are rich sources of sensory energy.

So how does it happen that old age sneaks up on some people and not others? After all, it's not something that happens overnight, like a sudden change in the weather. Old age doesn't take hold like an early frost. It takes hold in stages. You can break its grip whenever you choose—and, of course, the sooner you slow down the aging process, the better.

Sensory energy is the kind of energy that helps you break out of your routines. You come at life's experiences and opportunities in new ways. When you stimulate sensory energy, you develop new brain pathways. It's a process that actually makes you smarter and more alive.

Growing Younger

The findings of a field of research known as neotony, or growing young, are helping scientists understand the biological processes that can extend our youthful years. National surveys by the Alliance for Aging Research in Washington, D.C., indicate that two out of every three Americans want to live for 100 years. The surveys indicate that most of us say that we're willing to "do whatever it takes to stay healthy and increase our chances of living longer."

How much longer? "We are designed to last a remarkable 120 years," says Walter M. Bortz II, M.D., former president of the American Geriatrics Society, cochairman of the American Medical Association Task Force on Aging, and a clinical professor at Stanford University Medical School.

But whether or not you want to look that far ahead, research shows that you can certainly extend your youth far beyond what was once thought possible. In fact, Dr. Bortz regards age 75 as nothing older than late middle age. That's because, to a surprising extent, how rapidly you age is up to you.

"Changes associated with growing older may be much more reversible and preventable than we recently thought," says John Rowe, M.D., president of Mount Sinai Medical Center in New York City.

But if our potential may be a 100- to 120-year life span, why do most people die when they're much younger? "Only one thing is certain: We are not dying of old age," says Dr. Bortz.

As You Age, Remember This

"The regular and 'irreversible' cycles of aging that we witness in the later stages of human life may be a product of certain assumptions about how one is supposed to grow old," observes Ellen J. Langer, Ph.D., professor of psychology at Harvard University. "If we didn't feel compelled to carry out these limiting mind-sets, we might have a greater chance of replacing years of decline with years of growth and purpose."

In a research project, Dr. Langer found that our fears of senility may be vastly overstated. Many young, middle-age, and elderly people held stereotypical views of what it means to be old, according to Dr. Langer. Among their assumptions were that physical deterioration causes memory loss, mental incompetence, loss of contact with reality, and helplessness. "A full 90 percent of elderly subjects felt that there was a good chance that they would become senile," Dr. Langer reports.

According to medical accounts, only 4 percent of people over 64 suffer from a severe form of senility. Only another 10 percent suffer from a milder version. In other words, most people dread a symptom of aging that is unlikely to be a problem for them. You may as well assume that you won't get senile, and there's a very good chance that you'll be right.

To a great extent, what lies ahead of you—at every age—will be the result of the choices that you make today.

Welcome the Little Moments

"Years steal fire from the mind," wrote the English poet Lord Byron, "as well as vigor from the limbs."

He was wrong. It's not years that sap our energy.

Regardless of our age, when we feel young at heart it's because all our senses are alive. We are in a continual process of waking up to the world around us, using all our senses to see, hear, and feel what's going on. While scientists are now discussing neotony and trying to understand how we can live long, young lives as we get older in years, I think that there are others who can teach us more about the subject. The real authorities are children.

Youngsters can be our greatest teachers. They can certainly teach us lessons about energy. Learning from them, there's a good chance that we can awaken and use our sensory energy more fully in everyday life.

Children have a sense of wonder that leads to curiosity, genuine imagination, and, above all, playfulness. By playfulness, I mean that they enthusiastically pursue interests that are not restricted to the attainment of a particular goal. Play is just for the fun of it. And if we can play more, we can dramatically broaden our perceptual horizons, prompt fresh insights and discoveries, and keep our priorities straighter.

Threaded within a sense of play is a sense of exuberance and humor. We have to hold on to the ability to laugh at ourselves and take ourselves lightly. Humor expands our perspectives of the world and gives us better inner perspectives about ourselves.

One of the simplest ways to put this to the test is by learning a lesson a day from children. This has been shown to contribute to turning back the aging clock. Every single day, make it a point to seek out a growing-younger insight from children. When you open yourself to these insights, you'll find that the learning is easy. All you have to do is let children share some of their experiences with you.

Watch for moments of exuberance or humor. Listen for exclamations of wonder and squeals of laughter. Then, pay close attention. Your senses cannot help but experience things in a new way. Children everywhere and anywhere give this gift.

TRY THIS NOW!

You can actually change your awareness of your brain and your senses and your body. Your central nervous system is capable of using sensory energy differently than it does now. There is evidence from psychologist Robert Masters, director of research at the Foundation for Mind Research in Pomona, New York, that a simple form of exercise can encourage your body's nerves to improve their sensory connections. You can try it right now as a demonstration of increasing the sensory connection between your brain and any part of your body.

Here's How

Stand barefoot with your feet flat on the floor, positioned about 12 inches apart. Notice how your feet contact the floor and how your toes are positioned. Pay attention to the parts of your feet where you feel most of your weight being placed. Do not move your feet during the rest of this exercise.

Focus on your right foot. Notice your big toe. Then, one by one, pay attention to each of your other four toes.

Can you detect a difference in size, position, and feeling among your toes? What does your right heel feel like? And the ankle above? Imagine raising all of your toes together, much as you would move your fingers.

Exercise your visual imagination. You've had your right foot all of your life, yes? Well, do you know exactly what it looks like? Can you visualize, without looking, the exact spaces between your toes, the shape of each toe, and the curves of your ankle?

Think about the simple act of walking. When you walk, how does your right foot move? Do you step down on your heel first or on the ball of your foot? Lightly or heavily? Can you think of the exact moment when your toes help with the stride?

Finally, compare the action of your right foot to that of your left during walking. Do they behave the same way?

You can also exercise your sensory imagery as you recall where your feet have been and what they have done. What does it feel like to bury your right foot in warm sand and wiggle your toes? What does it feel like to use your right foot during swimming? Or when gliding on ice skates or roller skates?

In your imagination, without actually doing it right now, can you feel what it's like to swivel your right foot from side to side? Can you envision making small and then larger circles with it on the floor or in sand?

Direct your attention to both of your feet. Do they still feel the same? Is there an increased sensation in your right foot? Can you sense it more clearly than before?

What happens during this simple exercise is that your senses and nervous system are connecting more attentively with your right foot, tuning in to it more closely. By comparison, this may make your left foot feel "worse," perhaps stiffer and less alive.

This sensory-engagement experience can be applied to your left foot, your hands, your legs, your arms, your back, your neck, and virtually any other area of your body.

How Kids Get Wrapped Up in Things

Children get absorbed in their surroundings more easily than adults seem to do. My son, Chris, is now 20. But as I'm writing this, I'm taken back to his youth and his periods of remarkable absorption in the natural world around him. At the ages of 5 and 6, he could get completely involved in sniffing flowers, moving from one to the next through an entire field of wildflowers, taking care to smell each one. When he saw birds, he mimicked their wing movements. When he worked in the garden, he had to take bites of the fresh fruits and vegetables, as if to assure himself that they really could be eaten.

He grinned, then laughed with glee, when he held a bouncy newborn lamb in his arms. I remember him buried under a pile of autumn leaves with just his feet sticking out. He needed two hands to hold an ice cream cone, and as he kept licking, it looked as though his face would end up covered with the sweetness.

I remember playing ball with him in our steeply sloping backyard and watching him dive to make one-handed catches. In the winter, we went sledding down the slopes, and we ice skated on the nearby lake. We took long canoe rides and hikes.

We studied the stars and gathered wood for winter fires. When spring came, we went swimming in the ice-cold water and watched the first wildflowers bloom.

Why am I remembering all this? Every moment that I shared with him and every moment that I remember is a sensory experience. I can't re-experience it, of course. And I can't expect Chris to remain an eternal youngster. (He certainly hasn't.) But I can remind myself that the opportunities for this sensory energy still surround me everywhere. There is something quite literal in the adage "Stop and smell the flowers." Every scent is a new one. Each one is a first-time experience because every scent and sight and situation is different.

THE GREAT PERSON
NEVER LOSES **A CHILDLIKE SPIRIT**.

—Mencius (ca. 380–289 B.C.), Chinese philosopher

I can't think of anything that could make us more youthful than taking each day as a fresh experience. This is the true source of sensory energy.

Stop the Car

Sometimes, it takes patience to experience things.

I know that this may sound like a contradiction because it's easy to feel like we're in motion much of the time. Here's what I mean.

One Saturday, my younger daughter, Shanna, came into the kitchen wiggling her loose lower front tooth. "It's killing me!" she said of the pain.

Trying to be helpful, her big sister, Chelsea, turned to her and said, "If you think that's bad, Shanna, all of your teeth have to come out." What a reaction on Shanna's face, to imagine that she was destined for something akin to dental prison . . . and no one had told her! Chelsea looked at me and said, "Dad, I don't think that what I said really helped her."

Later that day, we were driving in the car. Leslie, my wife, was in the front with me, and Chelsea and Shanna were in the backseat. All of a sudden, Shanna's tooth came out.

We were in a hurry to get somewhere. But I thought, "Time-out." A child loses her first tooth only one time.

I stopped the car, and we turned around to see her face. Her expression was awash with wonder as she sat gazing at the little white speck of a tooth that she held in her palm. She touched her gum in amazement, realizing that her mouth hurt a bit less than it had moments before. Would another tooth emerge where its predecessor had been? And now she knew, because her sister had just told her, that the tooth fairy would leave her money for this tooth!

A miracle was going on—at least, it was a miracle to her. What a delight it was to observe her for a few minutes, relishing the expressions of pure wonder. Shanna's smile was unforgettable. And Chelsea was smiling, too, nodding her head as if to convey what a wealth of knowledge and experience she had shared with her younger sister.

Can you find these kinds of moments? In the rush of this tense, technologically driven world, it's easy to miss them. Here's my advice: Don't drive on unless you have to. Stop the car.

Children provide us with the essence of sensory energy. They offer needed chances for us to play, to act without a goal, and to appreciate the simpler things in life. They invite us to look outside and inside ourselves. They link us to a seamless human progression through history.

Watch the Ruts

One late-autumn day near the headwaters of the Mississippi River in Northern Minnesota, an old man was pounding a stake into the ground at a sharp bend in a muddy road that served as a county highway. On the stake was a small but brightly painted sign that read, "Be careful of ruts. Once you get in one, you may be in it for a long time."

"By Thanksgiving, the muddy roads begin to freeze hard for winter," the elder said, gripping the stake tightly with his lumber mitts. "Then,

Sweat Equity Builds Sensory Energy

In recent years, a number of scientists have reported that regular exercise may help keep your brain sharp as you age, enhancing your memory, sensory acuity, learning abilities, and emotional control.

In a study of 55- to 70-year-olds conducted by Robert Dustman, Ph.D., and his colleagues at the Veterans Affairs Medical Center in Salt Lake City, 3 hours of exercise per week for 4 months led to clear improvement in intelligence-test scores. These studies were extended, with similar results, by Theodore Bashore, Ph.D., associate professor of psychiatry at MCP Hahnemann School of Medicine in Philadelphia.

Research at Scripps College in Claremont, California, showed that very active men and women from ages 55 to 91 did substantially better on cognitive and reaction tests than did a similar group of nonexercisers. The researchers suggested that "cardiovascular benefits from exercise may help forestall degenerative changes in the brain associated with normal aging."

When medical researchers in Texas studied 90 healthy subjects who had reached retirement age, they found that regular physical activity helps to sustain cerebral bloodflow, which reduces the risk of stroke. Over the 4-year study, the researchers noticed that people who were generally inactive exhibited a steady decline in cerebral bloodflow, so they had increased vulnerability to stroke and other cerebrovascular disorders.

This study also supported the findings of other research showing that people who remain physically active are more mentally agile compared to those who avoid physical activity. It seems that insufficient oxygen supply to cerebral nerve cells leads to a decline of certain neurotransmitters and diminished brain function.

as the logging trucks roll over the roads, the ruts get real deep and freeze solid until spring. Once a car or truck heads into one of these deep ruts, there's no getting out. The rut determines where you go and whether you can get out. You can accelerate all you want. It's no use. You may even be stuck until the thaw." And then he laughed. "The answer isn't to do what lots of people do these days—buy some big four-wheel-drive vehicle," he added. "They just let you get stuck farther from home and get in deeper."

"Many of us think we are thinking when we are only rearranging our prejudices," wrote William James, M.D., Ph.D., Harvard University's noted philosopher and psychologist. And it was Albert Einstein who said, "Insanity is doing the same things over and over again, but expecting different results." From both, the warning is clear: Watch out for ruts.

A good step in building sensory energy is to pay increased attention to your daily habits and to challenge them. Are you really trying new things, thinking new things, and experimenting with difficult approaches and possibilities every day? Or are you just "rearranging your prejudices"?

Instead of opening ourselves up to new ways, we often shuffle and re-configure our preset viewpoints and habits. We search for reasons to not truly change, rather than permit new ideas and experiences to arise.

And when we're just reshuffling, rather than experiencing the new, we're likely to get into pretty deep ruts.

Getting Unstuck

The essence of life and brain function is movement. This is also true of your senses—they are energized only when you keep moving through life in new ways, shifting perspectives and seeking fresh possibilities.

The philosopher George Ivanovitch Gurdjieff spoke of self-imprison-ment, describing how a person draws a circle around himself in the sand. Days pass. He adjusts. Soon, he believes that he is captive, barred from crossing over the line. "Take a step," Gurdjieff urges us. "It's simple. Go past the line."

Do you know what your "line" is? Sometimes, it's very difficult to see. Here's a quick quiz that may help. The questions are simple yet chal-lenging. Quickly respond either yes or no—the first answer that springs to mind.

	Yes	No
1. Are you doing the kind of work that you most love to do?	❑	❑
2. Is your work this week different in some specific ways from the work that you were doing last week?	❑	❑
3. Are you making new friends?	❑	❑
4. Are you tasting new foods?	❑	❑
5. Are you reading new kinds of books and going to new kinds of movies?	❑	❑
6. Are you taking once-in-a-lifetime vacations?	❑	❑
7. Do you change what frustrates you?	❑	❑
8. Are you genuinely curious about others' opinions and views, rather than being quick to make assumptions or judgments about them?	❑	❑

For this quiz, you don't need to count up your answers. Just reflect on them. For some people, even one "no" may be a sign that they are in a rut and want to change their choices and shift their habits. For others, many "yes's" and just a few "no's" may be enough variety to keep them challenged and keep their sensory energy at a high pitch.

But be honest in your evaluation. If some of your answers suggest to you that you're in a rut, think of a way that you can change. It may be a change of attitude, such as letting go of the frustrations that you've had

THE TRUE OBJECTIVE OF **ALL HUMAN LIFE IS PLAY**.

IN OUR FUN WE REVEAL

WHAT KIND OF PEOPLE WE ARE.

—G. K. Chesterton, *All Things Considered*, 1908

over past events. Or perhaps you need to be more lenient in your judgments of people, trying harder to understand their points of view without leaping to the conclusion that they're right or wrong. It could be a change of setting, a decision to take that once-in-a-lifetime vacation. Or it could be a new choice about your work, such as choosing to pursue an avocation or even modifying your career path. Whatever you decide, the course of action that gets you out of the rut can boost sensory energy.

Invigorate Yourself with Sensory Cross-Training

Sensory energy deepens and expands whenever you approach life or work differently. If you can increase your self-observation, you'll begin to notice your most familiar mind-sets or routines. Then it's easier to choose alternative ways of thinking, viewing, interacting with, and experiencing your life and work.

One way to do this is to create variations on one of your favorite activities. Change your daily schedule, play tennis with your left hand if you're right-handed, read fiction if you tend to stay hooked on nonfiction.

Are you quick to judge others? Develop increased empathy. Pause for a few moments to imagine, "What if I were you? What if I had your background, experiences, views, challenges, responsibilities, hopes, and dreams? What would it be like?"

Are you quick to defend yourself or make excuses? Listen intently and seek threads of truth in criticisms.

Mixing It Up

Brain experts report that mental calisthenics can make your mind more alert and agile and help keep it that way. Learning actually changes the qualities of your nerve-cell endings and increases the strength of nerve-impulse transmission and your sense of vigor.

The following activities highlight some of the quick, varied ways to increase your sensory energy for the rest of your lifetime. Do them only at those times when you're feeling rested and ready. To be effective, these brief exercises must grab your attention and keep you focused in the moment, with a sense of enjoyment. Otherwise, say researchers, you probably won't give your brain the extra surge of oxygen and nutrients that help make the experience rewarding.

Here are some ways that you can increase your sensory energy.

• Build perceptual flexibility. Be more observant of the people, places, and objects that enter and leave your awareness during the day. Notice shapes, textures, colors, shadowing, movement, and the other distinguishing features of each image. To exercise your short-term memory, try sketching an image shortly after you see it. Or work on your long-term memory: At the end of the week, draw some of the images that you have seen.

• On the telephone, practice recognizing voices the moment that you hear them.

• Make quick and accurate estimates of areas, distances, volumes, and other proportions of things that you encounter. This is what I call visu-

TRY THIS NOW!

"The more words you know and recognize in English and other languages and the more words you can use intelligently, the greater will be your brain capacity," says Vernon H. Mark, M.D., a neurosurgeon at Massachusetts General Hospital in Boston, in his book *Brain Power: A Neurosurgeon's Complete Program to Maintain and Enhance Brain Fitness throughout Your Life*. "And all other things being equal, the more resistant your brain will be to injury and disease."

Whether or not you learn a second or third language, you sharpen your memory and brainpower as you broaden your vocabulary. The more precisely you can use your mother tongue in referring to concrete and abstract concepts, the more you strengthen your short-term and long-term memory.

Here's How

Exposing yourself to new words and new sentence constructions is the equivalent of having brand new experiences. Here are some ways to broaden those experiences as much as possible.

• Each time you meet someone new, practice coming up with an anagram of his or her name.

• Listen to audiobooks while you drive.

• Strive to be more accurate and descriptive whenever you write and speak.

• Play word games such as Scrabble.

• Fill out crossword puzzles—and try creating one.

• Practice distilling the key points of radio or television programs as briefly and clearly as you can.

• Whenever you come to the end of a chapter in a book, imagine that you must summarize it, aloud or in writing, for someone who has not read it.

ospatial activity. When you walk into a room, immediately notice the number and placement of people, furniture, and other objects. Later on, see if you can draw of map of what you've seen. Have fun mentally re-arranging the furniture.

• If a meeting or travel delay allows you some extra time, try doodling. What should you draw? Whatever grabs your interest. Sketch some geometric shapes. Draw irregular line contours, like the lines on a geological-survey map. For an added challenge, use your nondominant hand.

• If you have access to a personal computer, video games are another good way to heighten your visuospatial abilities.

• Be swift at integrating. You can sharpen your ability to create coherent wholes from divergent pieces. For example, select a sentence at random from a newspaper, book, or magazine. Using the same words in that sentence, try to construct a new one. Or practice fitting together jigsaw puzzles as quickly as you can. Or cut a page of a newspaper into various shapes, scatter them, and reassemble the page in as little time as possible, guided by the shapes and meanings of the words.

• Sing or play music—even poorly. Yes, something as simple as singing in the shower is fine; lots of people are passionate about that. Humming along in the car is good too. Music is one of the universal languages of humanity. It supercharges your senses and is both gratifying and soothing.

• Jump-start your creativity. Want to be more inventive or ingenious? Spice up your experiences by asking "What if . . . ?" questions.

• Write your own mysteries, either on paper or in your mind.

• Create limericks.

• Work on puns. At their best, they can help you escape from one pattern of thought into another, spurring you to think of words or word patterns that sound alike but have a humorous twist.

• Strengthen your body. You may wonder what strengthening your body has to do with strengthening sensory energy. But there is definitely

Could Sleep Help Your Senses?

Among the many other benefits of sleep, it helps protect your brain. According to some researchers, as you grow older, the blood-brain barrier, which helps protect your brain against toxic susbstances that may harm it, becomes more permeable. Irritants and poisons may pass through that barrier with little resistance. To promote peak brain function, you need deep, rejuvenating sleep that can help the blood-brain barrier remain intact.

There's another way that sleeping can help improve your brain and provide more sensory energy. While you're sleeping, your brain reinforces memories and makes sense of your daily experiences. This is a process that taps into "cellular memory," because it involves changes within the brain cells that hold messages and transmit signals.

"During this extra neuronal activity during sleep, proteins are manufactured by nerve cells. These proteins, like those produced by the stimulation from directed brain exercise, help restore cellular memories," explains Michael D. Chafetz, Ph.D., neuropsychologist and author of *Smart for Life: How to Improve Your Brainpower at Any Age*.

Sufficient sleep time is essential, Dr. Chafetz points out. When you get enough sleep, you allow more time for production of proteins. That's essential because the wear and tear of daily life leads to a continual breakdown of the cellular proteins. If the proteins in the brain were to decay without being replaced, all of your memory would gradually be lost.

a connection. The more fit you are, the more sensitive and active the surface of your body. The more fit your muscles, the larger the active involvement of the related areas of your brain and the greater your level of sensory energy. For example, you can augment the area of your brain that is assigned to your fingers simply by increasing and varying the use of your fingers.

• Give special attention to those physical activities that challenge your balance and coordination. Playing the piano, stacking coins, using tweezers to pick up small objects, and playing jacks increase your sensory energy.

• Complete puzzles. A number of puzzle exercises are recommended by some neuroscientists for improving hand dexterity and hand-eye coordination. Among the puzzles that do this are connect-the-dots and mazes.

Lighten Up

"Overwork is a prime cause of mental impairment," according to Monique Le Poncin, director of France's National Institute for Research on the Prevention of Cerebral Aging. "The brain, like the whole cerebral mechanism and the body in general, works better when it respects a certain biological rhythm. If we force it to work at an excessive rate for too long, it causes mental strain."

Beyond the mind-numbing problem of overwork is the daily onslaught of useless information. In essence, everything that you see, hear, smell, taste, and touch throughout the day bombards you with stimulation. We all need techniques that periodically free us from this assault that jams up our creative circuits, warns Richard Restak, M.D., neurologist in Washington, D.C. "Too much nonessential news . . . may be hazardous to your health," he says. "Much of the information bombarding us from our televisions and radios lacks redeeming nutritional value [for the mind], dulls our sensibilities, and leaves us, idea-wise, bloated with trivia yet at the same time intellectually deprived."

How can you help your senses recover? Dr. Restak suggests a kind of healthy, "enlighted illiteracy." He recommends periods of rest and re-covery each day.

What happens when you are exposed to mind-numbing subjects that you really don't need to know anything about? Neurobiologist Richard F. Thompson of the University of Southern California in Los Angeles demonstrated that these high levels of uncontrolled stress may create memory disruptions and learning deficits.

Jerome Yesavage, M.D., a psychiatrist at Stanford, and his colleagues have discovered that many people can restore their memories simply by learning relaxation techniques. "Anxiety clutters the channels of memory," says Dr. Yesavage. "Relaxation opens these channels."

Clearly, there's a link between calm energy and sensory energy. As in-dicated by the research of Dr. Yesavage and others, if you can switch on calm energy, you become more open to sensory input. It's like clearing the playing field so you can begin a new game.

Sensory-Energy Switch #2

Stretch Your Senses

L ook around you. Listen to the sounds. Touch the arm of your chair. Sniff the air. Notice that taste in your mouth.

Your senses are your doors and windows on the world. They give your life richness and coherence. The expression *to sense* means to draw upon all of your senses to create perception, to inform your mind about everything that you experience.

Scores of studies have proven the importance of our senses to our vitality. It is highly desirable and very practical for each of us to conscientiously train our senses throughout our lives, according to Marian Cleeves Diamond, Ph.D., neuroanatomist at the University of California, Berkeley, and author of *Enriching Heredity: The Impact of the Environment on the Anatomy of the Brain*. Her research suggests that the richer your sensory experience, the slower you will age.

Through varied sense-stimulating activities, the nerve cells in your brain can be expanded or enriched at every age. Studies "caution us against entering into inactive lifestyles that reduce the sensory stimuli reaching our brains, and they provide hope, if we continue to stimulate our brains, for healthy mental activity throughout a lifetime," Dr. Diamond explains.

The Sensory Experience

I recall a visit to my grandparents that occurred when I was 14 years old. I had just finished eighth grade. A summer storm was brewing. When I arrived at their door, the first rumblings of thunder were right behind me.

My grandfather came outside, and we stood on the front lawn watching the gathering storm. The air, sticky with humidity minutes before, became threaded with cool, tumbling breezes. All around the yard, the normally chattering birds in the old oak trees fell silent. The trees themselves began to creak and sway in the wind, leaves whistling and hissing.

We watched the last of the blue get blotted from the southwest sky as it crackled with lightning that streaked across roiling columns of black clouds. Thunder sounded, gathering into a near constant roar. Several times, lightning lit up the front lawn like sunlight, and here and there blasts of thunder seemed to suck the air out of the sky.

I felt an icy shiver. A few raindrops fell, then more, stinging full-force as they hurtled down from the heights of the sky. All of my senses were fully roused by the storm. I felt incredibly alive.

This vivid sensory memory has not left me. Nor has the memory of what my grandfather said that day.

My grandmother was in the front window, motioning anxiously for us to come inside. I knew that she was worried about tornadoes, and I wasn't immune to her concern.

"Shouldn't we go in and get down to the basement?" I yelled to my grandfather over the growing noise and bluster. My legs were trembling. I could feel prickles on the back of my neck.

My grandfather peered down into my eyes. His grip tightened on the two canes that helped him walk.

"Go on in if you want," he shouted against the wind. "I want to stay here . . . and see what comes."

I looked into his steel-blue eyes and saw calmness mixed with intense curiosity. My grandfather loved nature and being outdoors. I shared his awe. Deep down, I, too, wanted to see what came.

I stayed there beside him. It was almost as if we could ride the wind and touch the electrical pulses in the air.

It wasn't long before the thunderclouds began to break up and the roar in my ears subsided. My cheeks were flushed. I had goosebumps.

I do not recommend what we did; I am merely remembering it. Thinking back, it was one of the times when I learned to stretch my senses, as my grandfather called it. He knew, as I know, that this is a vital part of being 100 percent alive.

In Touch with Our Senses

As a boy, I used to wonder—as I sometimes still do now—what it would be like to be deprived of some of my senses.

I recall my grandmother's description of meeting Helen Keller. She said that Helen Keller touched people's lips to read their words. By my grandmother's account, Helen Keller seemed so exceptionally attuned that she was more vibrantly alive than most people of her generation. Blind and deaf, she was filled with a love of life that was far greater than many of those whose God-given biological faculties were intact.

WE DO NOT RECEIVE WISDOM,

WE HAVE TO DISCOVER IT FOR OURSELVES ...

A VOYAGE THAT NO ONE CAN SPARE US.

—Marcel Proust, *Remembrance of Things Past*, 1918

I was awed by the stories of this woman who could neither see nor hear. My grandmother described how, despite her losses, Keller became a sensory genius and an inspiration to millions of people.

She registered colors in terms of touch and texture. Grey, to her, was "like a soft shawl around the shoulders." Yellow was "like the sun. It means life and its richness of promise." From smelling and touching people, she could tell a great deal about them—their energy levels, their degree of vibrancy in living. Entering a house, she sensed it as layers of life, each carrying its own scent of history.

Asked what she knew about city life, Helen Keller described a brilliant sensory canvas: "Long streets. Tramping feet; smells from windows, tobacco, pipes, gas, fruits, aromas, tiers upon tiers of odor. Automobiles. A whir that makes me shiver, a rumble."

She could sense music through her fingers. When she put her hands on a radio, she could tell the difference between the strings and the cornets.

She "listened" to colorful stories of life along the Mississippi River by touching the lips of her friend Mark Twain.

Helen Keller told the rest of the world about the richness that she experienced through touch, taste, and aromas. This was the way that she influenced the world: with her senses. She learned to muster her vast sensory capacities in ways that left others humbled and amazed.

Using What We Have

Listening to my grandmother's recollection of Helen Keller, I tried to imagine the sensory experiences of the extraordinary woman who could neither see nor hear. What would it have been like to listen to my grandmother's stories without hearing her, to watch her without seeing her? The loss seemed incomprehensible.

It still does. And yet, from a different perspective, I have come to wonder whether most of us have actually lost touch with many of our senses. In some startling ways, we are blind and deaf to the people and world around us. We have learned to value technical rationality over the heart of experience. We retreat into our heads and away from life. That's what everyone else is doing too. So we assume that what is common is actually just life.

When I extol the senses, I am not pretending that we can live in a state of constantly heightened awareness. But I do believe that, as research shows, by using our senses to the fullest, we can be more energetic, more alive, and more fulfilled than we can possibly be if we let our senses become dulled or atrophied.

Of course, we do not all have equal sensory powers. Some of us enjoy keener sight or hearing. I have read about people who have extraordinary abilities of smell or taste. And there are unfathomable and immeasurable distinctions between our powers of touch. Yet if Helen Keller has taught us one thing, it is this: Whatever senses we have, we can use to the fullest. If we are shortchanged in some areas, we can still use all of our other senses to achieve the greatest possible awareness and contact with the world and the people around us.

Our senses are gateways to the richness of life. Sensory energy pours in endlessly through those gateways. The challenge is to keep them as fully open as we can.

Enrich Your Life, One Sense at a Time

Every time you fully engage your senses, you change. In some small yet very specific ways, you become a new person. I know for certain that the sensory experience of the thunderstorm with my grandfather worked some invisible but lasting change in me.

Consider how you can be changed by sensory experiences. Each one of the following occurrences evokes an emotion that would be impossible to imagine without the very particular, explicit experience.

- Feeling warm sand on your bare toes
- Seeing the smile of a young child just before she wraps her arms around your neck to give you a thank-you hug
- Breathing fresh, pure air and smelling wildflowers
- Cuddling your favorite pet
- Smelling freshly baked cookies
- Admiring a dew-sparkling flower garden by the sun's first light
- Hearing your favorite music as you relax in a lounge chair at the day's end

If some of the experiences that I have just listed are familiar to you, then you also know how these evocative, powerful sensations can become humdrum or almost unnoticeable when they're encountered routinely. If you had to trudge along a sandy beach to work every day, you might completely lose your appreciation for warm sand underfoot. A baker who has to produce the same kind of cookies every day can easily become less than enamored with the smell of them. Even listening to music can be dulled by repetition if you play the same tunes while sitting in the same chair every day.

But there's an instantaneous way to break repetitive, sense-dulling patterns, to engage your senses and increase sensory energy. I'm reminded of the biographies of the greatest physicists of our times, men such as Albert Einstein, Aage Niels Bohr, Werner Karl Heisenberg, Subrahmanyan Chandrasekhar, and Hans Albrecht Bethe, who completely reconfigured our understanding of natural laws, of the physical laws of matter, and, indeed, of the universe itself. When such great minds got together, what did they do? There may have been meeting-hall discussions and late-night chitchat over after-dinner drinks. But their most vivid moments of perception seem to have occurred during their long, invigorating hikes in the mountains or along lakeshores.

They spent nights under the stars. They had frequent chances to notice the uniqueness in the world. And without these excursions into new places, their enjoyment of new vistas, would their science have amounted to much?

"In our research," writes Jean Houston, a psychologist and the director of the Foundation for Mind Research in Pomona, New York, "we have found that there is a real equation between the ability to sustain complex thinking processes and the richness of sensory . . . awareness." It is probably no mere coincidence that these men of vast vision and extraordinary intuitive power were able to free their minds from the library, writing table, and calculator long enough to experience other views of the world, outside the realm of academics.

New Vistas

You probably know from experience that changes of scenery are one way to have new experiences and to see the world differently then ever before. A vacation is nothing more nor less than a chosen release from routine. If all goes well, you come back from it feeling refreshed and renewed. But what about the vacations that you need every day, week, or month, in the form of a change of landscape or perspective that provides you with rejuvenation in body and mind?

Whenever you notice novel features in a person or situation, your sensory energy increases. Almost inevitably, you can see distinctions more clearly. The ability to perceive more sides of an idea or issue further increases your involvement and sensory energy.

How often has a beautiful sunset filled you with awe or a starry night sky lifted your spirits? Are any two of these the same? When have you felt deeply moved by a piece of music, a meal, a compassionate or passionate embrace, or a fresh bouquet of flowers?

What soothes and sparks your senses sends distinct signals to your body and mind. As the perimeters of consciousness, your senses are the most ancient gateways to your nervous system and brain.

Overuse of Secondhand Senses

You might argue that we're living in the midst of a sensory extravaganza. In our information-packed existence, we have the benefit of cameras, compact discs, computers, and a multitude of other communication devices that allow us to gather secondhand sights and sounds. At first blush, this seems like a supreme extension of our immediate human scope, allowing us to see and hear the remotest fall of a raindrop or rush of a tidal wave. Why, then, do we often feel like we're wrapped in a blanket of numbness?

Day in and day out, we're exposed to the sights, sounds, smells, tastes, and textures of an information-packed existence. But in our scramble to keep up, I suspect that we're actually falling out of touch with our senses.

The sensory data that come to us courtesy of the electronic media are what I call secondhand experiences. Contrary to conventional thinking, we cannot fully engage our senses when we're having experiences that are conveyed by a camera, microphone, or computer. Not only is it nearly impossible to have real perceptions through these filters but their use can soon become extremely fatiguing.

If you've ever spent much time in front of a TV (and who hasn't?), you know what this fatigue factor is like. Even if you're looking at the most technologically advanced TV, your eyes are working overtime to interpret and process the barrage of tiny dots that make up the image on the screen. And the same kind of mental processing is required to interpret the letters and graphics that comprise the images on the computer screens that so many of us contemplate every day in our work. All this processing adds up to a kind of mental fatigue that you don't experience if you're contemplating a real-life object, person, picture, or landscape.

Research indicates that without regular, varied sensory stimulation, the brain slows and even stalls. Secondhand sensory experiences are not enough to sustain the mind's powers. On the contrary, when we live in an environment where so many secondhand images come to us in a flat, framed, two-dimensional, electronic format, our minds and bodies show symptoms of premature aging. Even our susceptibility to disease is increased by a sense of numbness or of remoteness from real, immediate, firsthand sensory experiences.

Thus far, few of us have the benefit of full sensory enrichment. But we've all had glimpses of what might be possible—through people like Helen Keller, the woman who so profoundly impressed my grandmother during a single meeting.

Get a Daily Dose of Healthy Pleasures

"All you have to do is pause," advised Molière, the 17th-century French comic playwright. "Nature herself, when we let her, will take care of everything else. It's our impatience that spoils things."

With his understanding of the vagaries of human nature, Molière points out that we're all likely to undercut the rewards that are at our fingertips by trying too hard to attain rewards that are somewhere far-off in the distance. To me, this is what Molière is saying when he warns, "It's our impatience that spoils things."

Of course, we all search for happiness. And when we do, we may go to extremes to get more money, improve our status, or gain more experience. But there's a real danger that in so doing, we miss what is most immediate and near at hand.

"Simple pleasures," Oscar Wilde pointed out, "are the last refuge of the complex." What Wilde called simple pleasures are a wellspring of sensory energy, which creates, and is created by, moments of genuine enjoyment and fun.

Whenever you have brief experiences that engage your interest, stretch your perspective, and produce feelings of wonder or delight, you're automatically increasing your sensory energy. In other words, those good feelings can actually generate significant amounts of energy.

Energizing the Pleasure Principle

Take a few minutes to think about the healthiest, most vigorous and vibrant people you know. And I don't mean the celebrities profiled in *Time* and *People* magazines. I mean some people whom you really know. What sets those unique individuals apart from the crowd?

While they may not be rich or famous and they may not adhere to the "correct" health advice, I suspect that those individuals share a generous viewpoint toward the world. While confronting the same pressures and hardships as the rest of us, they generally expect good things of themselves and the world. And they expect to discover or experience amazement or fun in much of what they do.

The healthiest people seem to be "pleasure-loving, pleasure-seeking, pleasure-creating individuals," according to extensive studies by physician David Sobel, M.D., and psychologist Robert Ornstein, Ph.D. The people interviewed by Dr. Ornstein and Dr. Sobel didn't say that success or wealth determined their joie de vivre. Instead, they talked about enjoying small, healthy pleasures, which they often described as stolen moments.

Their greatest memories were associated with experiences related to sensory energy. They took joy in witnessing sunrises and sunsets. Some studied the constellations. Others beaded jewelry, built model cars, or collected stamps. They indulged their musical passions just because they enjoyed it, even though some of them sang or played terribly. There were those who savored cooking their favorite meals or trying new ones, and others who were caught up in boating or hiking. Their special pleasures meant indulging in all-out games or sharing silly talk with their family members or friends.

Enjoy Your Awareness

Look up, and you have the mysteries of changing cloud formations in the sky. Catch the gaze of those around you, and you may find yourself rewarded with the beaming smile of a loved one. Breathe in the aromas, the smell of fresh-baked bread or the scent of blooming flowers.

When you down an icy drink on a sweltering August day, make sure that you enjoy the coldness of the glass in your hand as well as the taste of the drink itself. Or press the glass against the side of your cheek, and leave it there while you soak up the relief.

Every day offers the opportunity to enjoy such moments. They are easily within your reach.

The key here is to begin to sharpen your senses and turn up your self-awareness. To stimulate a greater involvement of all your senses, ask yourself questions: What, precisely, does this feel like on my fingertips, on the skin of my arm? How, exactly, is this sound different than it was before? How has the lighting changed the image that I see before me? In short, begin to "sense" more of what you experience each day, both the unusual and the mundane.

Get Closer to Nature

In the discussion of Active-Energy Switch #2, I mentioned the work of Dr. Sobel and Dr. Ornstein, who found that office workers tend to be much more contented with desk jobs if they have some views of natural settings. Writing in the journal *Mental Medicine Update*, the researchers concluded that "workers with a view of nature felt less frustrated and more patient, found their jobs more challenging and interesting, expressed greater enthusiasm for their work, and reported greater overall life satisfaction and health."

If you have an affinity for beautiful natural scenes—water, sky, trees, flowers, or green plants—you probably have an intuitive awareness of the power of nature. As Dr. Sobel and Dr. Ornstein found in the work environment, when people are surrounded by reminders of natural settings, they feel less anxious and more relaxed. They're also less likely to have negative thoughts or experience stressful physical symptoms. In addition to the emotional lift that you may get from these settings, you may work more effectively, the researchers found.

Do your work breaks offer opportunities to change the scene and get more in touch with natural settings? You might gaze at fish swimming back and forth in an aquarium. Or look out your window. Enjoy nearby trees or flowers if there are any within sight, and keep an eye out for birds and squirrels. Or just look up at the sky and let your imagination run away with the cloud formations for a little while. It also makes sense to take a daily or at least weekly mini-walk in your favorite nearby park. You may want to cultivate a window-box garden. At the very least, how about bringing some flowering plants into your work area?

Even photographs spark the senses. While a picture is only two-dimensional, contemplating it doesn't entail the processing that's required when you look at a video screen. And any picture of your favorite vacation or natural scenery can be rejuvenating. Hang some pictures of waterfalls, canyons, forests, mountains, or meadows brimming with flowers. More than half of your body's sense receptors are clustered in your eyes. When people view slides or pictures of bright, beautiful scenes of nature, they report much higher levels of positive energy and friendliness and reductions in anxiety and fear. Compared to pictures of treeless urban streets and modern architecture, pictures of lakes, streams, trees, and flowers produce lower levels of stress arousal and higher alpha brain waves, a state associated with calm alertness and wakeful relaxation.

Let There Be Light—Sometimes

For a mental and emotional lift, experiment with turning on some added lights. Or, if possible, move your work closer to a window. As discussed in Calm-Energy Switch #1, research indicates that many people report increased calmness or alertness when exposed to bright sunlight or some extra indoor light.

But bright light isn't always what you want. When your eyes are tired, respect what your senses are telling you. Why not draw the shades or turn down the lights so you can enjoy a restful pause during your break time?

Seek Out Pleasant Scents

The human nose, with training, may be able to discern more than 7,500 different fragrances. And the sense of smell is so powerfully connected to the brain that some scents elicit pronounced changes in energy, emotions, and memory.

Scientists have long known that pleasing fragrances prompt us to take slower, deeper breaths and become more relaxed and refreshed. Your sense of smell contains "all the great mysteries," says physician and essayist Lewis Thomas, M.D.

Researchers at Harvard Medical School's Institute for Circadian Physiology report growing evidence that the power of smell can, at least in some cases, strongly influence mental alertness. Every breath that you take passes currents of air molecules over the olfactory sites in your nose. Odors flood the nerve receptors in your nasal cavities where five million cells fire impulses directly to your brain's cerebral cortex and limbic system. These parts of the brain are the mysterious, ancient, intensely emotional areas where you experience feelings, desires, and wellsprings of creative energy. Certain scents seem to activate specific chemical messengers, or neurotransmitters, in the brain.

Controlled brain-wave studies by professors at Toho University in Japan have produced surprising indications about which scents tend to

TRY THIS NOW!

At Rensselaer Polytechnic Institute in Troy, New York, researchers showed that people who work in pleasantly scented areas performed 25 percent better than those who were in unscented areas. The people in pleasantly scented rooms carried out their tasks more confidently and more efficiently. They also showed greater willingness to resolve conflicts.

In discovering that certain scents seem to activate specific neurotransmitters, or chemical messengers, researchers have sought to discover which odors are the most stimulating. To date, the top scent for raising energy and attention seems to be peppermint, but lemon is also effective.

Here's How

Which scent is most likely to give you the best charge of sensory energy? To find out, just try both and test the results. Start with tea. Both peppermint tea and lemon tea emit strong, heady fragrances. At different times, try a cup of each, sweetened with honey if you like. See which one has the stronger effect. Be sure to enjoy the lingering, fragrant vapors as well as the taste.

Get a small bottle of peppermint extract and one of lemon extract. Leave one or the other open to test your enjoyment of the scent. Some people strongly prefer one to the other. Whichever gives you the most sensory enjoyment as well as the most energy is the right one for you.

stimulate, which relax, and which promote significantly fewer errors on the job.

Which natural scents do you enjoy the most? Which invigorate you? Which are calming? Research indicates the potential value of bringing fresh flowers, a potted evergreen, or some piquant herbs or potpourri into your home and work areas. Scent dispensers are a good way to subtly use essential oils for fragrance. Tests at the University of Cincinnati indicate that fragrances added to the atmosphere of a room can help keep people more alert and improve performance of routine tasks.

To raise your sensory energy with aromas, you can use all-natural essential oils, which you strategically place in your environment. Among the relaxing oils are chamomile, lavender, rose, geranium, sandalwood, jasmine, frankincense, and vanilla almond and apple spice, which have been shown in a number of cases to promote more restful sleep. If you want something more energizing, choose from peppermint, citrus (such as lemon, lemongrass, and mandarin orange), pine, and orange blossom.

Eucalyptus is particularly good for combating sensory fatigue, according to NBC medical correspondent Bob Arnot, M.D., author of *The Biology of Success*. And rosemary is reportedly effective for uplifting energy and enhancing memory. Rosemary shouldn't be used by women who are pregnant or anyone with high blood pressure.

Add Spice to Your Life

Which specific, lively scents and tastes do you love the most? Which ones are most likely to perk you up in the morning? Are there certain spices that help you feel refreshed or relaxed?

Taste augments smell, and together they form a vast sensory territory. Perhaps you've never thought of the ways in which different spices can affect your mood, your energy, and your alertness.

There are many health benefits to be derived from exploring a range of scents and tastes. Scents and tastes also make your sensory energy rise.

As noted in the discussion of Active-Energy Switch #3, Canadian medical studies suggest that when added to foods, certain seasonings may boost energy and at the same time help defuse the urge to stuff yourself. Besides a dash of hot-pepper sauce, potentially energizing add-ons include hot mustard, chili powder, ginger, and curry.

Another way to add energy to your food and drinks is through juicing and tea-making, according to Judith Benn Hurley, author of *Healing Secrets of the Seasons*. Orange juice, lemon tea, and peppermint tea are effective energizers, while chamomile tea can help you relax. (Remember to test whether you feel more energized after drinking ice-cold beverages.)

Stay in Closer Touch

Touch is the most urgent sense, and the significance of touch has made its way into our language. When we speak of something being "touching," it suggests a close relationship between touch and the emotional reactions of the heart.

To enrich your sense of touch, be sure to enjoy simple, healthful habits such as hugging loved ones or literally giving a friend a pat on the back. You can also get great rewards from patting or scratching the family dog or cat. It's one of the great enjoyments of owning a pet.

Have you ever exchanged back rubs or gentle massages with a

partner, family member, or friend? This kind of letting go is a powerful way to increase sensory energy. The soothing pressure of hands has a relaxing effect, of course. The human touch stimulates your circulatory system and awaken your senses. And the sensory rewards go to the person who is giving the massage as well as to the person receiving it.

Take Pleasure in Energy Music

Without question, music generates sensory energy. One survey indicates that many people find music more thrilling than anything else, including sex.

Anyone who has ever danced to the beat of a rock-and-roll song or been lulled by the strains of a sonata has experienced firsthand the physical, emotional, and spiritual overtones of music. Apart from its nostalgia-producing or romance-inducing powers, it has immediate, measurable physical effects. Music influences heart rate, blood pressure, respiratory rate, stomach contractions, and levels of stress hormones in your bloodstream. Research suggests that it may also help strengthen your immune response.

You don't have to be musically talented to enjoy good rhythm and vibrations. Listening to music that you love is like receiving a terrific massage from the inside. The right melody at the right time can bring you feelings of exuberance or joy. It can also soothe frayed nerves.

"The primary importance of your hearing is to charge your nervous system," says Alfred A. Tomatis, M.D., a French physician, otolaryngologist, psychologist, and educator who for more than 50 years researched the influence of music. A number of experts on the auditory system now agree that listening and hearing are powerful sensory pathways "for problems related to energy level (tension or fatigue), loss of enthusiasm, and depressive tendencies."

Your mind processes music in ways that are intertwined with perception, memory, and language. Music speaks to us so powerfully that some psychologists have theorized that it's actually a language that we're born understanding. "Music is a secondary 'language' system whose logic is closely related to the primary alpha logic of the central nervous system," suggests composer George Rochberg in the journal *New Literary History*. Unlike verbal or written speech that must be mentally interpreted to be understood, the "language" of music can produce an immediate physical response. "We listen with our [whole] bodies," Rochberg says.

While finding your musical favorites is important, it's not the whole story. As often as possible, you need to vary the music that you listen to. Some scientists believe that after 20 minutes or so of listening to a single tune, your nervous system may become oversensitized to it and react with symptoms of distress.

Among my personal favorites for energizing music are the compositions of Michael Hoppé. Both a composer and a performer, Hoppé has produced such albums as *The Yearning*—a 1994 CD of the Year—and *The Dreamer*. When I listen to Hoppé's music, I find that it energizes my senses, eases tension, uplifts my spirit, and opens my heart. It provides an experience that, to me, epitomizes the impact of sensory energy.

Undiminished Drive

Many people see sex as a source of shared joy. But others have come to view sex as an added source of stress, just one more area of life where they have to perform. Already tense and tired because of the many professional and domestic demands in their lives, people find that their ability to enjoy the sensual, pleasant, and joyful aspects of sex takes a sharp nosedive.

Perhaps the most insidious obstacle to sexual fulfillment is the image of the aging sex life. Some people believe that sex can no longer be particularly frequent, pleasant, or rewarding at the age of 45 or 50, and that sexual interest plummets from about the age of 60. These myths persist despite studies showing that many couples are able to enjoy sex two or three times a week even when they're in their nineties.

I suspect that many of us, trapped by misconceptions, never come close to realizing our lifelong potential for the sensory energy that we receive or express through sex. Nor do we comprehend our capacity for extraordinary sexual pleasures and deeply satisfying intimacy.

The good news is that research confirms that by making even small changes, you can effect big, positive changes in your love relationship. There's a growing awareness that great sex is not something that just happens. But it can certainly be learned, as long as the learning is shared in a sensitive, open manner.

Researchers have enough findings to begin developing a model of human sexuality that emphasizes pleasure, closeness, and self- and partner-enhancement, rather than performance. Few of life's experiences are more energy rich. As our intimate relationships become more vibrant and aware, so, in turn, do we.

Touchstones of Great Sex

Here are some of the approaches now recommended by researchers to help give and receive the greatest amount of sensory energy in your sex life.

Put your senses first, sex second. When most foreplay and stimulation occur on a few square inches of the body's surface or are limited to the genital organs only, they hardly suggest the natural ecstasy that's possible. "Touch may be the most powerful sociobiological signal of all," says psychologist and chronobiology researcher Ernest Lawrence Rossi, Ph.D. "When we are touched gently and rhythmically, our brains release the feel-good messenger chemicals called beta-endorphins, and we slip into the psychologically receptive state [where we're] open to increased intimacy."

Often, more mature partners are best equipped to achieve this kind of intimacy. From their late thirties on, women tend to develop their richest sensuality, reports biologist Winnifred D. Cutler, Ph.D. "It is then that the capacity for sensual expertise most often expresses itself," she says. For men, this age is often a time of life when youthful eagerness diminishes, but it is replaced by experience and control that offer richer rewards. "Men have become more patient, more capable of learning to control the timing of their own pleasure to enhance that of their partners," observes Dr. Cutler.

Use all of your senses. The most satisfying lovemaking combines all forms of sensual stimulation. The association of sights, sounds, smells, and tastes as well as touch can build to create the kind of overwhelming experience that's characterized by the total involvement of your senses. The choice, of course, is yours. But here are some of the sensations and images that can be part of that experience.

- Images. For some, this is intimate eye contact. For others, seeing their partners in erotic positions are the most arousing images possible.
- Erotic sounds. These include whispers, music, ocean waves, or the sound of rain.
- Tantalizing smells. Do certain scents or aromas evoke sensual images for you?
- Special tastes. Do you pay attention to taste of your partner during sex?

- Movement and touch. Are you aroused by the rhythm of massage? By having your neck rubbed or hair stroked? By the feel of the sheets on your skin? By the special sensation of your partner's touch in erotic places?

Learn preferences. If you can tell your partner what gives you the most pleasure and learn what most pleases your partner as well, you'll be able to focus on those areas of sensual discovery.

Find new ways. To enjoy super sex, it's essential to suspend judgment long enough to approach lovemaking in fresh, original, highly sensitive ways. Sex can become too much of a routine. You know that you're in a rut when sex is so comfortable that your own or your partner's sense of passion has vanished.

Researchers have found, for example, that "super sexual" women have "learned to approach each moment with an openness to experience" that is referred to as a beginner's mind. In other words, they view each sexual interlude as if it were the first.

All that this requires is a bit of practice. Don't jump ahead with your thoughts. Instead, just keep pace with the wonderful information that you receive through your senses. Let your senses and heightened sensory energy lead the way.

Teach by touch. "Touch can be difficult to discuss with words," says Linda Perlin Alperstein, Ph.D., assistant clinical professor in the department of psychiatry at the University of California, San Francisco, Medical Center. "What does it mean if I tell you I like 'light' or 'medium' touch? That can mean different things to different people. It's much easier to demonstrate. You let your fingers do the talking."

Dr. Alperstein favors what she calls a body tour, which is guiding your partner to all of the sensitive and responsive areas of your body. "Of course, you can talk while conducting a body tour," she notes. "But simple 'oohs' and 'ahhs' can be just as communicative as words. . . . If you feel ill at ease naming certain parts of the body, the body tour allows you to show your partner how you like to be touched there, without saying anything."

Some ancient Asian philosophers and physicians believed that exquisitely sensual, masterfully controlled sex replenished and strengthened the life forces, or energy, of both men and women. The prevailing idea was that sexual vitality and potency depended, first and foremost, on sensory awareness and sensual expertise. The body tour is a way to increase your awareness of your body's sensitivity as well as your partner's.

Do some macho housework. Pitching in with household chores increases intimacy. Studies show that men who help out with housework have better sex lives, better health, and happier marriages than those who don't. Doing the dishes, taking out the trash, and cleaning the bathroom may seem like trivial concerns when compared to sexuality, yet women need to feel physical and emotional support, closeness, and tenderness before wanting to have sex. Even though many men think that they do their share of the housework, research indicates that almost every man overestimates the time that he puts in at home.

Create an island of peace when you get home. A brief transition period when you get home from work may also be an essential prerequisite for great sex life. It allows time to release work tensions and be together to chat, stroll, hug, hold hands, and perhaps sip a glass of wine. "A few minutes of peace and quiet can be worth 4 hours of foreplay," says psychologist Bernie Zilbergeld, Ph.D.

Make time. When you find your life especially busy, you might resist sexual overtures from your partner, feeling that those advances are intrusions that waste precious time. The true waste of time, more likely,

What Some Guys Don't Get

Day-to-day involvement with your spouse, even in the most mundane chores, may have a lot of influence on your sex life. Studies show that many people require sensory and emotional closeness as prerequisites for sexual arousal and passion. Women often experience a strong need to establish and sustain this emotional closeness, and when this need isn't met, their sensory energy wanes and their thoughts and feelings can subdue or block sexual desire.

The sensory-emotional bond is generally formed at three levels, says Patricia Schreiner-Engel, Ph.D., director of the women's sexual-health program at Mount Sinai School of Medicine of New York University in New York City. The most basic is organizing—interacting with a partner to schedule and handle joint chores and responsibilities, such as dealing with finances, planning meals, taking care of children, cleaning, and other tasks. When these obligations are responsibly and consistently handled, the woman's emotional bond with her partner ascends to the next level.

Level two is sharing, that is, communicating feelings about your individual lives.

When this stage is satisfactorily explored—and only then—the third level is within reach. This is the level of intimacy, which means holding, kissing, and mutually passionate lovemaking.

When men fail to pay attention to these needs, women are offended by sexual advances, says Dr. Schreiner-Engel. Ironically, the more insistent the man's demand for sex, the less desire a woman feels, because her sexual needs, based on emotional closeness, are not being met at the first two levels, organizing and sharing.

is losing those warm, intimate, shared moments. Studies have shown that intimacy actually boosts vitality and feelings of well-being that, in turn, contribute to more effective work habits and a more steady, productive environment at home. The biggest wastes of time, most couples realize, are the arguments that so often arise from the injuries and disillusionment that can occur when one partner complains, "You never have time for me."

Breathe together, be together. There is evidence that matching or approximating the respiration cycle of your lover can be a strong factor in creating heightened sexual rapport and erotic chemistry. Experiment with the effect of gently becoming in sync with your partner's breathing rhythm.

Sensory-Energy Switch #3

Imagine or Invent

When he was beginning first grade, my son, Chris, would snuggle with my wife and me on the sofa at night and we would read children's books. One of his favorite stories was *I, Monty* by Marcus Bach. The opening line is "Do you suppose a caterpillar knows its future lies in butterflies?" There was always a light in his young eyes, even as bedtime came, whenever he tried to envision that. Imagine the future life of a caterpillar!

For a young boy, that simple act of imagining was enough to change his view of nature forever. After that, whenever he saw beautiful butterflies riding the wind, he also envisioned the crawling, furry caterpillars that preceded their metamorphoses.

To imagine or invent is to use your senses to envision the depths of life, instead of settling for what exists in the present. It was U.S. Supreme Court Justice Oliver Wendell Holmes who said, "Man's mind, once stretched by a new idea, never goes back to its former dimension."

Change is the fabric of life itself. Within moments of reading a passage in a book or having a meaningful conversation, you are changed. And the experience of that transformation is conveyed to you through your senses. In split seconds, new nerve circuits are formed and new perspectives are shaped. These are the structures of consciousness that serve as our guides to the world.

Just Imagine

When Pablo Picasso was a schoolboy, he was terrible at math. Part of the problem was that the number *4* had a nose. At least, it looked like a nose to him. And that, in itself, became a terrible obstacle. Whenever his teacher had him write the number *4* on the blackboard, Picasso would look at that unmistakable, protuberant nose hanging like a cliff off its face. And he couldn't stop his restless chalk from filling in the rest of the face.

If Picasso's imagination could have been reined in, his math grades would certainly have been better. But Picasso without his imagination would have been like a tree without leaves. Everyone else who looked at the number *4* saw a 4. Picasso perceived the start of a face.

Pablo Picasso, of course, ended up making a major contribution to art, and no one (with the exception of his math teacher) ever begrudged him his difficulties with the number *4*. But the evidence of his runaway imagination can be found in all of his works.

I especially love his so-called one-liners. Picasso's rule about these little drawings was that he could not lift his pen or pencil from the paper until he was completely done. These drawings, funny, inspiring, intriguing, make me smile whenever I see them. Who could dream up such a rule? And, having made that rule for himself, what was the imagination that could dart this way and that, with swirls and squiggles, never leaving the paper until a recognizable semblance of a scene or face appeared? I encourage you to try it just for fun.

Creativity requires this kind of sensory energy. A composer or musician links sounds together in expressive ways, putting energy into the notes and harmonies. Musical compositions are waiting to be written or played all the time, but it's sensory energy that brings these compositions to our ears. Music doesn't come alive by itself. Sensory energy is the added element that goes into the act of creation.

Similarly, a sculptor uses sensory energy to shape clay or chisel stone with his or her hands. Sensory energy goes into writing books or speeches, painting pictures, designing buildings, or any other creative act that brings a concept or idea into existence.

Fortunately, all of us can develop more of the sensory energy that we need for creativity. This might mean making up an idea, however absurd or odd it may be, and then following that idea to its logical or illogical conclusion. What emerges might be a one-of-a-kind drawing, a novel crossword puzzle, an extraordinary magic trick, or a bar of music that can be shaped into a wonderful composition.

Whatever the outcome, each act of creativity produces a fresh perspective or interpretation. It's a clean break from the gridlock of habit and cliché.

Be an Expeditionary

Throughout history, a number of individuals have accessed and demonstrated rare capacities. They have perceived possibilities that other people never saw, have invented the unexpected, and have ventured into the unknown. They have performed or witnessed acts of profound courage and selfless love, have seen or created things of unimaginable value or extraordinary beauty, and have glimpsed the heights of possibility in human experience. These are the men and women whom I call expeditionaries.

Expeditionaries have always captured the public's imagination. Inside every human heart is a yearning to light out for new territory and to savor distant vistas. Expeditionaries are the ones who fulfill that yearning. They are the quintessential travelers of the globe, the universe, and your own neighborhood. Above all, they have rich curiosity and a sense of wonder.

Though we may often feel removed from the expeditionaries whom I have described, it takes little effort to become a greater expeditionary in your own life or work. In our work rooms and living rooms, we could be more adventurous and alive.

We can call forth more courage and curiosity; we can light up our imaginations. One of the axioms of living is that you must be willing to give up a part of what you have been in order to reach for what you can yet become. The expeditionary takes that to heart.

However secure your desk or living room or kitchen table, you can move beyond, either in your imagination or in reality. Think of those physical spaces as launching platforms for your imagination. Whether you begin to plan a trip to Tibet or doodle a face on the number *4* or create an entrée that has never been eaten before, you're the master of your creative powers. Enjoy them more than ever.

Build a Memory Mansion

Show-and-tell was my favorite part of kindergarten. In fact, it may have saved me.

My mother reminds me that on my first day of school, I made a break for it and ran the whole way home. In fact, I outran the school safety patrol, which had been marshaled to stop me, and made it home with

TRY THIS NOW!

Studies indicate that the memory powers of people over 60 may be just as accurate as those of younger people. In one study of nearly 1,500 people in three age groups—under 60, 60 to 69, and 70 and older—researchers discovered that there was a high degree of memory accuracy in those over 60.

But there's more. In many circumstances, researchers found, people over 70 could remember things just as well as those under 60. Memory loss, often considered an unavoidable part of growing older, may actually be due to such relatively simple factors as lack of genuine relaxation or intellectual stimulation.

Here's How

A memory exercise is, literally, an exercise. It can boost your sensory energy and brainpower just as physical exercise boosts your muscle power. Here's one to try.

Think back to your youngest days. What funny incident can you remember? Recall every detail of being there. What did it feel like? Let each of your senses play a role in the remembering. Are you relaxed and smiling?

Next, try this. Who was your favorite teacher? Why?

If you let your mind relax and wander, you'll probably find that these memories come back to you more easily. When experiences have meaning and are shaped as stories, recall is powerful, rich, and easy. You probably can't remember the precise facts, such as the dates of these memories. But the more you can recall about the sights, sounds, and feelings associated with these memories, the more vivid they'll be.

These are the kinds of memories that can stay with you forever, if you just let them.

nearly a half-block lead. My flight, unfortunately, was to no avail. My mother promptly returned me to class.

The problem that led me to such dastardly flight was a set of rules that seemed intolerable. The teacher made it crystal clear that there was to be no playing in school. We were not to have fun. If we talked, it was to be only when asked.

Fortunately, after my ignominious flight and my return to class, my teacher managed to hook my interest. Her method was a kind of class-room amateur hour. During this time, my teacher said, we could share anything with our classmates. They, in turn, would show whatever it was they wanted to. Of course, everyone knows that venerable teaching tool as show-and-tell, but to me, then, it was all new. And it was terrific—better, even, than recess and lunch, both of which I loved. Show-and-tell was just what education should be, at least to my young mind. It connected to my life experience.

Rooms for More Memory

What hooked me on show-and-tell, it turns out, is a common lure of effective education. We need sensory experiences to place memories in our minds. Real experiences are what ultimately enable us to imagine and invent. As educator Mark Albert Van Doren once said, "Teaching is the art of assisting discovery."

Memory is a kind of palace with many rooms. You can explore those rooms in the vividness of your imagination much as you would explore the hidden and secret chambers of a long-lost edifice.

Just such a palace was envisioned by Matteo Ricci, a 16th-century Jesuit who revived a memory system that had been used in the West since the time of the ancient Greeks. The system, which he introduced to the Chinese, was elegant in its simplicity. To develop exceptional

MAN'S MAIN TASK IN LIFE IS TO

GIVE BIRTH TO HIMSELF,

TO BECOME WHAT HE POTENTIALLY IS.

—Erich Fromm, Ph.D. (1900–1980), U.S. psychologist

powers of memory retention, Ricci said, you can create a "memory palace" in which each room holds some hidden or almost-forgotten recollection. With practice, you could arrange the memories in these rooms so that the images would become vividly real. Then, all you have to do is close your eyes and enter the rooms. The front door of the palace becomes an entryway to all of the hallways and rooms of memory. The palace is a structure for arranging wisdom throughout a lifetime.

Every one of us is subconsciously building such a structure. As each of your experiences is transformed into memory, the memory takes up a room in the palace. With a bit of practice, the imprint of each new experience, transformed into a memory with its own room, keeps re-shaping the very structure of your being.

Make More Vivid Imprints

The blueprint of the palace of memory is sure to change, depending on how well you use your senses. As I've noted, it's less likely that your mind will deteriorate as you get older. But as I've also emphasized, exercising your mind is a fundamental way to boost sensory energy, preserve mental alertness, and expand your mental agility.

Research published in the *Journal of the American Medical Association* suggests that regularly exercising your brain is one of the best ways to help prevent loss of mental sharpness. Scientists have discovered that with a broad range of active intellectual interests and a vigorous lifestyle, your mind can keep developing while you're aging. Nearly all of us can be as sharp—or sharper—at ages 70, 80, and even 90 as at age 20.

How is this possible? Whenever your brain cells are activated, they take in more electrochemical energy, form new connections, remodel nerve endings, improve receptor networks, and revitalize brain function. Those cells can be stimulated by new sights, sounds, conversations, creative pursuits, or problem solving. The change is instantaneous. With varied neural stimulation, you become more capable, smarter, and more vibrantly involved with life.

"It doesn't matter what age you are when you start—improvement is always possible," says Michael D. Chafetz, Ph.D., neuropsychologist and author of *Smart for Life: How to Improve Your Brainpower at Any Age*. The key to age-proof living is brain fitness; you must regularly challenge all aspects of your brain to expand its performance and slow or prevent its aging.

And what about your memory power? It is now quite widely accepted that memory is not stored in a single cell but is spread throughout an extensive nerve-cell network. "Even the simplest memory is spread over millions of neurons," says neurobiologist Charles Stevens, Ph.D., of the Salk Institute in La Jolla, California.

Memory recall also seems to involve multiple parts of the brain. "Memory is like a piece of music," says Marcus Raichle, M.D., professor of neurology at Washington University in St. Louis. "It has lots of different parts that come together to create the whole."

Keys to Vital Memory

Your most important memory power is known as vital memory. Vital memory, sometimes called long-term memory, "is one one of the most

TRY THIS NOW!

Most of the stories that we experience today are told by novelists or screenwriters, acted out by actors and actresses. They are not real.

Want a real story? Look at your calendar. Imagine that you have to tell a child the funniest or most memorable thing that happened today. What would that story be?

Here's How

One of the most meaningful and revitalizing ways to greet family members is with a funny story of something that has happened to you. Do you get together with family or friends for a brief while, just to talk, laugh, and share stories?

If you don't have some time like that coming up, plan it now. When will you see your friends again and find out what happened to them during the week? What will they have to tell you, and you, them?

Plan to spend time with children. Devote at least part of a day to sharing great stories with them. Once the television and radio have been turned off, you may be surprised how much they want to hear from you.

basic and necessary functions of our brains," says Vernon H. Mark, M.D., a neurosurgeon at Massachusetts General Hospital in Boston and coauthor of *Brain Power: A Neurosurgeon's Complete Program to Maintain and Enhance Brain Fitness throughout Your Life*. "It is at the core of your being, representing the essential you, your personality, your feelings."

Here's a glimpse how vital memory works: Each experience produces a memory trace that is registered in your brain, and each trace comes in a certain sequence. The memory trace is transferred from your senses into your vital memory, like a reference note that's placed in a file. It may be stored there for quite a while or maybe even forever without being noticed again. But some of these traces resurface in your vital memory, where they essentially come alive again.

Whether a memory trace will be transferred into your vital memory depends on how intently you paid attention during the particular experience that produced the trace in the first place. If you have an apple for breakfast every morning, obviously you don't pay much attention after the one-hundredth or one-thousandth time. But if one apple out of many is purple in color or has an exquisite taste, that's the one you're likely to remember. And it's simply because your senses paid the most attention to it.

Share Life's Stories

When I was a child, people in my family and neighborhood used to sit around kitchen tables and tell their stories. I don't suppose that I'm surprising anyone when I say that there's a lot less of that going on these days.

But when we don't sit together and share stories, something gets lost. Those stories are more than a source of energy and entertainment. They convey wisdom, curiosity, and caring. Stories get our senses fired up, activating our imaginations. All that stimulation of our brains helps keep them younger as the years go by.

What happens when a story is told across a kitchen table? First of all, there's what scientists call eye-to-eye validation. The story is not being sent through e-mail, appearing as letters on a screen. When we tell the story, we're visible and we're heard.

Also, the story that's told by one living person to another produces a host of memory traces that are related to all our senses. One good example is a ghost story that's told beside a blazing campfire. When we think back to that ghost story, we remember not only the speaker's face and voice but also the taste of roasted marshmallows, the smell of the campfire, the sensation of the cool night air along our backbones.

When we hear a story from a live speaker in a memorable environment, we have eye-to-eye validation that tells us how much and how intensely the speaker is trying to communicate. It is through sharing such stories, told at close range, that we come to find our voices and to know who we truly are.

My grandfather Wendell Downing was a surgeon who once described to me what he thought made each of his patients memorable. "Every person who comes to me brings a view of the world," he said. He vividly recalled what it meant to hear stories from those who earnestly and eagerly wanted to communicate. "Even if they are worried or in pain," he said, "they want me to listen carefully. They want to tell me their stories well enough that I understand who they really are and, because of this, can treat them in the best way."

I felt that my grandfather was right. And I'm even more convinced by what I've seen and heard in the years since.

Research shows that we learn most and learn best through stories. Our understanding is rarely shaped by strings of facts. What we want is the fabric of experience, the stories that help remind us of who we are and where we come from as well as the amazement of what we can imagine. We couldn't survive with lists of details or bundles of facts. Give us the stories that leave us hanging and the ones that extend the boundaries of our inner knowledge.

Real Chat Rooms

As human beings, we are touched by stories, and they travel in our senses and imaginations, beyond the limits of our individual experiences.

The poet and physician William Carlos Williams once said, "Each

IF OUR FRIENDS ARE WORTH HAVING,

THEN **THE BEST THING WE CAN GIVE**, EITHER IN LIFE

OR IN OUR TALK, **IS OUR GENUINE SELVES**.

—Ernest de Selincourt, "The Art of Conversation"

person's stories—theirs, yours, and mine—are all we carry with us on this trip of life we take, and we owe it to each other to respect our stories and learn from them."

But there's a growing problem. We don't talk to each other as much as we used to.

Yes, on occasion we certainly share conversation. But we have to contend with a technologically driven, highly litigious world. Steadily, we are losing our voices and becoming invisible. In some cases, we know certain people only by their e-mail addresses and not by their names, hearts, or experiences.

Finding the story behind the person and the person behind the story takes sensory energy. It involves eye contact, listening to a voice, responding to inflection. It takes sensory energy to fight the trend toward technological communication, and the fighting back, in return, produces sensory energy.

Telling Is Touching

With the stories that we tell, we offer front-row seats on life itself. No matter how different the experience of another person or how far off the events that occurred, the stories that touch us have a familiar feel. They are about us, too. Stories allow us to see something familiar through new eyes.

Are you at a loss to say what your stories are or why they would appeal to another person? Here are some ideas about what you have in your repertoire.

- What is your funniest story of growing up? What is the childhood tale that reveals the foibles of your family members and closest friends?
- Have you met someone who has lost a great deal and yet has lived a meaningful life? Who is that person? Can you describe what he or she has been through?
- What is one of the greatest challenges that you have faced and overcome?
- What are the best stories that you've heard from family members and friends?

Whether you tell the funniest stories or the ones that have touched you the most, you are likely to have more listeners than you ever expected. The most powerful stories are those about who we are, what we stand for, and what we may yet become. Once told and heard, they resonate within us. We hear and perceive at a deeper level. They touch us in our hearts in ways that no rational arguments ever can. They change us. In fact, through the emotion of such stories, we shape the people that we are becoming.

Love It or Set It Aside

As humans, we're dreamers. We imagine the improbable: winning the lottery, orbiting Earth, retiring to the Riviera. Or we dream of the impossible: the car that never gets stuck in traffic, the child who always gets perfect grades, the stock that goes up but not down.

These imaginative flights may seem to be little more than flights of fancy. But actually, brief times of wishing and dreaming can help you realize the things you really want to do.

Research proves that people are most creative and effective when they love what they do. By "love," I mean something more than being distracted or amused by, or mildly satisfied with what you do.

Far too often, we follow a path that has been blazed by what other people want or expect. We may do efficient or good work on such a path, but we feel that something is missing if we're not passionate about what we pursue. Doing what other people want, we may get the job done. But it's rarely our best or most creative work.

What about the person who truly believes that they can do everything well? Their idea is probably based on the notion that anyone can accomplish anything that they set out to do.

But those kinds of directives can be overwhelming or exhausting or just plain wrong. Research on more than 250,000 men and women over the past 40 years indicates that none of us can do everything well. Instead, we can do three or four or five things better than any other 100,000 people.

You may be relieved to hear that. After all, it means it's probably futile to keep trying to pursue everything with full energy on all fronts. Instead, one key to a vigorous and productive life filled with enthusiasm and happiness is to focus on the greatest strengths and talents you have. That doesn't mean that you can ignore your weaknesses. But it does mean that you can acknowledge them and learn to manage them out of your way. When you do that, you have more energy left over for the pursuits that stimulate your imagination, make you more inventive, and touch your deepest reserves of creative power.

According to researchers, it takes an enormous amount of time and effort to raise an area of poor performance to mediocre performance. In contrast, it takes very little time or effort to raise an area of good performance to great performance as long as you're doing something that you enjoy. This is not to say that you must never do things that you don't enjoy. Of course, you must. But when you emphasize things that you must do and sacrifice things that you love to do, you deaden a part of your passion and drive.

Invent Your Own Way

President John F. Kennedy loved to tell the tale of small boys in Ireland who had footraces across the lush hills. When they came to a fence that seemed too high to climb, they threw their hats over first. After that, they had no choice. They had to climb over the fence to get their hats back.

Think about throwing your hat over a fence. Which fence? Which direction are you going? Those are good questions to answer. Because as soon as you start climbing that fence, your energy is going to soar.

Selection Research International in Lincoln, Nebraska, has followed more than a quarter of a million people for 40 years. The researchers have traced the thoughts, feelings, and behaviors of those who are successful, those who are happiest and advance the farthest or highest in their work. The study suggests that the essence of success can be measured by people's abilities to define their strengths.

From your strengths, the things that you do better than the next 10,000 people, you discover unique potential and purpose. In their study of very successful people, Donald O. Clifton, Ph.D., and Paula Nelson, authors of *Soar with Your Strengths*, came up with a number of recommendations.

- Be aware of a yearning. There's almost an inner magnet that can pull you toward one activity rather than another. What attracts you may not be glamorous, attention getting, or financially rewarding. But the attraction is strong and steady.
- Look for something that deeply satisfies you. If you get a kick out of doing it, you probably have strengths and talents in that area.

TRY THIS NOW!

New experiences can fill you with a rush of sensory energy. Maybe you're traveling or trying out a new sport or reading a kind of book that you've never read before or pursuing a brand-new activity that you find challenging. At the same time, you can make discoveries about yourself and the intensity of your interests, passions, or fascinations.

Here's How

There's actually a way to measure your new or renewed interest. Here are eight key factors that are worth considering each time you reflect on a new kind of effort or activity.

1. Does it fit my values?
2. How natural or easy was it to learn or do, on a scale of zero to 10?
3. How proficient was I in doing it, on a scale of zero to 10?
4. Did I get a kick out of it? How satisfying was it, on a scale of zero to 10?
5. How valued or valuable did I feel in doing it, on a scale of zero to 10?
6. How much recognition or intrinsic reward may I receive for doing it, on a scale of zero to 10?
7. How great could the results be?
8. Do I want to give this more of my energy and attention?

Based on this quick analysis, you can begin exploring more of the experiences and pursuits that pique your senses. In the weeks ahead, it's worthwhile to think about how you rated your experiences. Which ones brought you the greatest personal satisfaction? How can you reorient your efforts in ways that are more satisfying?

- Notice when learning is easy. You catch on quickly and it feels exciting.
- Recognize when something comes naturally for you. You may catch glimpses of yourself performing well in this talent area.

Accept the Fear and Awe

Psychology pioneer Abraham Maslow noted that we "tend to evade personal growth because this . . . can bring a kind of fear, of awe." Maslow called this a "denying of our best side, of our talents, of our finest impulses, of our highest potentialities, of our creativeness."

To pursue your strengths and talents, first be an observer of yourself and appreciate your own reactions. One of the simplest and most effective ways is by keeping a small notebook. Enter your observations about new activities or kinds of work. Begin to answer these questions.

- Is there one kind of work about which you feel most passionate?
- When you daydream, where do your thoughts lead you?
- If your wishes could come true, where would you channel more energy?
- When you reflect on your work or life, what activities do you consider of greatest worth or value?

Keep Some Big Ideas in the Air

Fixed mind-sets don't have to control our lives. Whenever we put big ideas into play, we open ourselves to creativity. This is called the Zeigarnick Effect, and it is based on research in Germany showing that sensory energy and success rise whenever we keep exploring big ideas—keeping them within view—rather than doing things the usual way just to cross them off our lists. The moment that we reach closure, there's a good chance that we dispel every bit of creativity that we've put into a project or devoted to an issue. It ceases to generate the kind of energy that is evoked when something is up in the air.

Yes, it's important to finish things. But what keeps us eagerly, vibrantly, and energetically alive are the big unfinished dreams. Keep a few of them in front of you each and every day.

Develop a LifeMap

What I call a LifeMap is one of the best visual aids that I know for building sensory energy. A LifeMap is essentially a 21st-century bulletin board. It's constantly evolving as you change its size, borders, and dimensions with your own hands. Every time you walk by this evolving LifeMap, your senses are sparked to creativity. This happens both consciously and subconsciously.

Here's how to build your LifeMap. Choose a 3- by 3-foot space on a wall in your office or kitchen. Make sure that whatever space you choose is highly visible, a spot that you often pass. The LifeMap could even be posted on the side or front of your refrigerator. Using large self-stick notes, display your ideas in three categories: big dreams, big ideas, and small changes. Here's how the three differ.

Big dreams are things like starting your own business, traveling the world, or writing a book. Or you might say that you'd like to plant a great garden, compose poetry or music, create a work of art, or pursue a hobby that you love. Other big dreams could include spending more special time with your loved ones, being a friend or mentor to those in need, or providing your own unique contribution to your community.

Big ideas could be inventing a new product or developing a new way of producing something. Other big ideas include specific ways to make life simpler or more meaningful, to regain your sense of humor or develop it further, to bring smiles to people, to redesign your mornings to provide time to exercise or reflect, or to restructure your evenings so you have time to enjoy the sunset and gaze at the stars.

Small changes are the clear, doable actions that help turn big dreams and big ideas into results by making more of the right things happen.

Under each of the notes labeled big dreams and big ideas, begin adding the small-changes notes that describe what, when, and how you are adjusting the way that you spend your time and energy. Small changes are like ongoing reports about what you're focusing on or how you're developing your strengths and talents while managing your weaknesses. You can also change the ways in which you listen to your own feelings, empathize with others, and take care of yourself along the way.

As you come up with questions and insights, jot them on the edges of the notes that you already have. Or post new notes under the different categories.

Almost immediately, you'll begin to notice unexpected connective relationships, including missing links or hidden opportunities. The reason for using self-stick notes is that they're movable. They help you get past thinking in lines and boxes. Any time you want to, you can change the positions of the notes. If you have questions, jot them down and stick them somewhere on your LifeMap. If you have ideas for improvement or a breakthrough, go ahead and insert them.

As the flow chart expands, you begin to visually and emotionally sense more of the hidden linkages and possibilities in your life or work. You can make intuitive connections. Any time, you can move or replace any note. You may use different colors for different purposes.

With this LifeMap, you can boost sensory energy by imagining the future and considering various outcomes. Then you can return to present circumstances and concerns. You can shift the positions of notes, realigning them to lead to a better future outcome. The LifeMap can end up taking any shape, eventually involving not only your own life or enterprise but also your friends' and family's lives. It reflects today, but it can also lead you far into the future.

Keep asking yourself how you feel about this picture, about the connections. What's missing or possible? The chart encourages being flexible not only in process but in time, and it sparks your senses to make unexpected links from idea to idea, from current problems to the realms of possibility.

Strengthen Your Sight Skills

True learning requires deepened perception, which is ignited by and ignites sensory energy. Your senses open you up to the richness of life as it is and to the wonder of what life may yet be, whereas your rational, thinking mind constrains you to habit and the mind-sets of convention.

For your senses to stay involved with learning, the process has to be fun and invigorating, not drudgery. When your mind engages in rapid, full-sense learning, creativity expands and both comprehension and recall are enhanced. You link new ideas to both context and perspective. You become more curious and inventive. Your memory sharpens and improves.

In contrast, most traditional learning comes in what can be called closed packages of information, which we take to be facts. You memorize these facts and are left with little reason to think about them. Such memorization practices cannot be considered true learning.

It turns out that virtually all of us can learn more quickly and remember very well without exhausting memorization work.

More Learning Takes More Sensing

The goal of being 100 percent alive has much to do with the energy that we continually receive from learning and how this learning power energizes the rest of our lives. Unfortunately, few of us have accessed more than a fraction of our full learning capacity.

When we approach rote learning the way that we are taught to in school, it virtually ensures that we are deprived of much of our learning potential. From kindergarten onward, we are told to pay attention. We never actually learn how to do this, yet we come to understand that it means to sit very still and focus only on the subject at hand.

If our minds begin to wander, a teacher calls that being distracted.

But being distracted is hardly a bad thing. In fact, research now shows that we learn fastest and best by being distracted. When we learn, it's the distractions that cull most of our attention. To learn with all of our senses, we cannot stare at one thing for long.

Our minds need to move. Images must change.

Try It the Einstein Way

"To learn, to raise new questions, to explore new possibilities, to regard old problems from new angles, requires creative imagination with all of the senses," Albert Einstein once said.

It's an understatement to assume that the man who developed the theory of relativity had to imagine, visualize, and formulate quite a few things at once. Somewhere in his imagination, he had to conceptualize mass, energy, and light, all intertwined in some astounding ways. He had to consider what would happen in a theoretical situation where objects

Trusting Your Brain

"The less we ask of our brain," says Monique Le Poncin, Ph.D., director of France's National Institute for Research on the Prevention of Cerebral Aging, "the less it gives us, and eventually there are signs of what I call cerebral hypoefficiency: memory difficulties, absentmindedness, little quirks, inability to handle certain details of everyday life."

I suppose that this is exactly what we fear will happen when we age. But when we use all our sensory powers to feed our brains, we combat the effects of aging. In fact, by using sensory energy as much as possible, you can help age-proof your memory and increase the size, number, and function of many types of brain cells.

"Contrary to widespread opinion, people are capable of good cerebral efficiency regardless of their ages," says Dr. Le Poncin. "As the myths of mental aging have been cast aside, we have learned that brain function is remarkably changeable and that we possess nearly unfathomable capacities for learning, achieving, and remembering. This quality is called neuroplasiticity."

"Throughout our lives, we use only a fraction of our thinking ability," wrote the prominent Russian scholar Ivan Yefremov. "We could, without any difficulty whatever, learn 40 languages, memorize a set of encyclopedias from A to Z, and complete the required courses of dozens of colleges."

actually moved at the speed of light. And, among other things, he had to decide how energy figured into the equation.

What senses did it take to do that? Part of the answer can be found in his remarkable education. As a young boy, Einstein was a poor student who seemed to resist conventional rote learning. When he applied for admission to the academically demanding Polytechnic Institute in Zurich, he was denied admission. As it turned out, that was probably the best thing that could have happened to him. Forced to apply to a lesser institution, Einstein spent a year in the provincial Pestalozzi Institute, founded in 1770 and named after the educator Johann Heinrich Pestalozzi.

The Education of an Observer

Pestalozzi had been a passionate advocate of learning with the senses. He believed that it was necessary to enlist all of the senses in each and every experience. Founded upon his teachings, the Pestalozzi Institute continued to pursue his philosophy even in Einstein's day. Einstein found himself in an environment where the teachers adhered to Pestalozzi's original assumption: that the absolute foundation of knowledge is the ability to observe.

The word *observe, anschauen* in German, encompasses far more than merely looking. As taught and practiced at the Pestalozzi Institute, observation meant intense concentration of all of the senses. Students were expected to do far more than read and write. They were asked to observe completely and intently by handling, smelling, touching, listening to, and looking at everything they encountered in their day-to-day or classroom experiences.

The impact of this kind of education is exceptional. Students didn't begin with the name of something and then learn its characteristics. Instead, they first absorbed all of its properties, using their ever-improving powers of observation, and then, finally, named and labeled what they were observing. This mode of learning was perfectly in line with Pestalozzi's philosophy that before we can understand something, we need to draw together all of the sensory information we can gather and form it into a coherent whole.

Einstein's approach to learning emerged out of this early educational experience. "The intellect has little to do on the road to discovery," he

THROUGH THE WINDOWS OF THE SENSES,

THE SOUL REGARDS THE WORLD'S BEAUTY. . . .

—Leonardo da Vinci (1452–1519), Italian painter,
sculptor, architect, and engineer

once observed. But if we're not using intellect, what are our resources? All of our senses. The fact that Einstein could integrate and use every part of his mind, the parts that could sense and feel as well as the parts that could conceptualize, indeed provided a rare richness and comprehensibility to his work.

Although Einstein did eventually go on to attend the Polytechnic Institute in Zurich, his "resistance against enforced instruction, far from ever being 'broken,' became a deep and basic character trait that permitted [Einstein] to remain free in learning," according to psychoanalyst Erik H. Erikson. Erikson notes that Einstein, in his later years, emphasized a concept called *begreiflichkeit*, which translates, roughly, as comprehensibility. Einstein held the view that an active and intuitive beholding is a necessary step in thinking. "One of his later most childlike and yet wisest sayings is that the most incomprehensible aspect of the world is its comprehensibility," Erikson says.

Absorb It All, Every Which Way

According to researchers, it is highly desirable for each of us to conscientiously train our senses throughout our lives.

The best learning comes when the subject is exciting or the experience is new. Leonardo da Vinci called this creative seeing, using the Latin phrase *saper vedere*, which means knowing how to see. When it comes to how we learn, most of us don't realize that we often fail to see.

One way to encourage and enhance your own *saper vedere* is with a very simple but effective process. Make notes.

In the 1920s, researcher Catherine Cox of Stanford University conducted a study of 300 historic geniuses, including Sir Isaac Newton, Thomas Jefferson, and Johann Sebastian Bach. Her exhaustive work revealed a pattern: One key sign of genius is making compelling and clear notes. All of the people whom she studied customarily recorded their thoughts and feelings in journals. Or they wrote diaries, poems, or letters to friends and family.

Many of today's business leaders—including Fred Smith, chief executive officer of Federal Express, and Richard Branson, chief executive officer of the Virgin Group—also credit note making with contributing to their success. Throughout history, such leaders as Thomas Edison, Albert Einstein, Benjamin Franklin, Marie Curie, and many other geniuses who have had a lasting influence on the world all kept notebooks or journals. Whenever they interacted with others, conducted experiments, or read something new, they recorded their thoughts, impressions, and feelings. These notes sparked additional ideas and gave them a record of the high points of each experience.

Take Note

The notebooks of Leonardo da Vinci are legendary. For reasons that we don't understand, his notes are all written from right to left, in longhand, in a tidy, page-cramming script that is interspersed with sketches of his extraordinary, futuristic inventions as well as of studies of nature and the human body. Browse through this amazing testimonial of a man's observing, doodling, questioning, and creating, and you will come across pictures of rearing horses, flying machines, elaborate instruments of war, and thousands of other inventive sketches. And surrounding it all, flowing in and out of the visual representations of a man's ongoing daydreaming, is the steady flow of words leading up to, around, and through the stream-of-consciousness feats of art and engineering.

For a more modern-day version of this obsession, we'd have look at the notes of Thomas Edison, inventor of the lightbulb and 6,000 other patented items that are less publicized but just as inventive. In the process of inventing things that changed the way we work, play, and live, Edison logged in three million pages of notes and diagrams.

There's an important distinction, however, between note taking and note making. Note taking is what you were asked to do in class. Record the facts. Recall what the teacher said. Copy the outline. Remember your assignments.

Note making is something quite different. When you're jotting down things in your own notebook or journal, let your own ideas and perspectives take over. You don't have to outline things. You certainly don't need to write whole sentences or spell correctly. Just pick up on some of what you're observing every day, and let that flow into your personal impressions, images, and imaginings.

In fact, this process is so different from conventional note taking that I use a different name for the notebooks. I call them NoteStreams. NoteStreams, unlike notebooks, are meant to be impressionistic, jumbled, and disorganized—unless, of course, you want them to be neat, precise, and highly organized.

Is that a contradiction? That's precisely the point. NoteStreams are all yours, and they should reflect the way that you see the world and the way that you organize things in your own mind.

Most of us, however, were probably taught how to take notes sometime in our educational or professional training. And since note taking is different from NoteStreaming, you may have to unlearn some of those habits before you can begin to unleash and enjoy some of the pleasures of NoteStreaming.

Get a small notebook, lined or unlined, that's easy to write in, something that's slim and light enough to tuck into your purse, briefcase, or pocket. The next time you have a wait or a few free minutes, take out your book and begin writing or doodling.

Don't think. Well, of course you'll think about something. But if you've never tried this kind of writing or doodling before, it's important to let your pen or pencil do the walking for you. Glance to your left and write down the first color that you see. Glance to your right and sketch the first shape that you see. Recall what you had for breakfast and describe what it tasted like.

Does this seem nuts? It is, at first. The human brain has vast organizational capacities, but most of the time it's helping you to take the next step without toppling over while it picks up the sounds of oncoming traffic, copes with that argument that you had yesterday with the ticket taker, cooks up vacation plans, lists the phone calls that you have to make, flashes images from your childhood, registers the ache in your right elbow where you bumped it last week, and tries to figure out how to get to the dry cleaners before it closes. And that's only about one-billionth of what's actually going on in that brain of yours.

So just catch some of it, a few fleeting moments. Scribble away, make notes, make sketches, and most important, don't reflect on what you've just written down or go back and conscientiously review yesterday's notes. Just keep going till your hand stops. Then, close the NoteStreams and put the book away.

But keep that notebook with you, and return to it here and there throughout the day.

Reading: The Riot Act

Woody Allen joked, "I took a speed-reading course. We read *War and Peace*. It's about Russia."

This is an apt summary of what many people fear about so-called speed-reading. They figure that they won't comprehend the material if they don't stick to the cumbersome word-by-word approach that they're used to.

Skimming is what some people imagine speed-reading to be. And if you're just going to skim a book, well, why bother?

I think it's important to take a few minutes to pay attention to how you read. Reading is one of the most powerful interpretive devices that you have at your command. After all, it's a skill that can actually change and heighten all of your senses, alter your views of the world, and open up your imagination and intellect to vast new experiences. And it's all done with little squiggles of black type on a series of pages.

Reading, like the other uses of your senses, is also a great energizer. Time and again, you will hear about adventurers who trekked to the farthest corners of Earth because they had read some tantalizing account of some far-off place. Men and women of action, from the studious Marie Curie and Thomas Jefferson to the enterprising Steven Spielberg and Oprah Winfrey, are vastly stimulated by what they read.

Why not soak up more if you can? After all, you constantly learn from reading, and why not get as much as you can from the quadrillions of squiggles that can stimulate your mind and imagination?

Word Absorption

Here's an interesting thought: If you feel that you recall very little of what you read, could it be that you're going too slow instead of too fast?

Your brain, linked to your senses, has the proven capacity to read up to 50,000 words a minute with more than 90 percent comprehension. However, the average person reads about 250 words a minute with less than 50 percent comprehension.

What's getting in the way? Here are some likely suspects.

Habit. Most of us learned just one way to read when we were children, and that way happened to be relatively slow. After we got the hang of it, we stopped learning new ways to read.

Word-after-word pacing. Chances are that when you open a book and glance at a page, your eyes focus on a word or two right away. Just for the fun of it, turn the book so the page is upside down. Look again. What is your focus now? It's likely that you see large blocks of print. But if you turn the book right side up again, your focus will again zoom in on a few words.

Why? From a very young age, you were taught to narrow your senses to read one word at a time. Yet you are capable of absorbing much more: those larger blocks of type that you saw when you upended the book.

Linear subvocalization. This is the way that we learned to read, by saying each word silently to ourselves as we see it with our eyes. The problem with this is that we can only read as fast as we can talk. Hence, the 250-words-per-minute limit that many people experience. But your brain has the ability to grasp huge chunks of visual input, and you can substantially increase your reading speed and comprehension by picking up whole phrases or sentences every split second. This also frees your mind to grasp ideas, images, and concepts, rather than burying itself in the word-after-word progression that paralyzes creative thinking.

Regression. This is the common process of backtracking to re-read words, sentences, and entire pages. Most regression is unconscious; you instinctively guess that your learning will improve when you keep stopping and going back over sentences. However, instead of increasing com-

Catching the Read Eye

Obviously, you read with your eyes, so to understand the process of reading it's helpful to know a little bit about these information-gathering extensions of intelligence. When light enters your eye, it is focused by the lens onto the retina, the light-sensitive inner surface at the back of your eye. In the retina, a mosaic of nerve cells gathers information and transfers it to the optic nerve. From there, impulses rocket to the brain, which picks up the signals and interprets them.

At the very center of the retina is a small spot called the fovea. A dense area of light-receptor neurons, the fovea provides an area of perfect focus. But the amount of perfectly focused information that you can gather at any one time is minute, only about $1/40,000$ of the visual field. That means that when you look at a page crowded with words, only two or three letters in a single word are in perfect focus.

Needless to say, if your sight had to crawl down the page three letters at time, *War and Peace* would be a lifetime's worth of very slow entertainment. But of course, that's not what happens. Your peripheral vision, the area outside the tiny range of the fovea, picks up huge chunks and gobs of impressions. True, they're not quite as clear as the images viewed through your foveal vision. But they're clear enough to reach your brain for quick and easy translation into words, impressions, and meanings.

When you read faster, you just make more efficient use of your peripheral vision. That's why concentrating harder or becoming more focused is not the objective when reading. Instead, you want to let your peripheral vision engage in the kind of image collecting and word connecting that it likes to do. It's the difference between using the whole playground and using just a single swing.

prehension, regression actually undermines and reduces it. Your brain's learning is repeatedly disrupted, and your brain becomes fatigued and distracted. This further slows down reading speed.

There is evidence that the more you stimulate your senses, the more information your eyes can deliver to your brain. This enables larger chunks of words and images to be conveyed faster. Numerous studies have shown that the "better" readers, those who read far faster and with greater understanding of what they read, do not read word by word, but instead take in groups of words or sentences with each visual fixation.

Take a Visual Pause

You'll have more energy for reading, and read with more comprehension, if you pause every once in a while to give your eyes some relief. Every ¼ second or so, your brain takes a microsecond pause to get a clear image of what you are learning. This pause is so rapid that most of us never notice it. But at each stop, your eyes try to bring words into focus. Scientists call these brief breaks fixations or visual gulps.

Whenever you try to read word by word, it limits your eyes to about four words per second, or a maximum of 240 words per minute.

Some basic visual stimulation exercises can help extend your eyes' area of perfect focus. That, in turn, will increase the amount of new learning that you can process in a single ¼-second visual fixation. Focus on the white space just above each line of letters. As you read, let your vision glide along the white space above words. That way, you gulp each line, rather than read word by word and inadvertently stop at every space between the words.

The letters on the opposite page are for practice. As you scan down each row, allow your eyes to pause just above the center letter for about a second as you notice the letters on either side without saying them in your mind. Then, move down to the middle letter of the next row. If you're patient with this exercise, you will automatically stretch your peripheral vision.

Z	A	M
Q	B	X
R	C	V
V	D	P
X	E	T
S	F	K
A	G	P

Q	Z	A	M	X
A	Q	B	X	S
V	R	C	V	N
Z	V	D	P	E
U	X	E	T	I
O	S	F	K	A
T	A	G	P	B

Q	Z	ABC	M	X
A	Q	BCD	X	S
V	R	CDE	V	N
Z	V	DEF	P	E
U	X	EFG	T	I
O	S	FGH	K	A
T	A	GHI	P	B

Learn Twice as Much in Half the Time

Sensory energy depends on a keen sense of interest and involvement. Yes, it's vital to stretch yourself to explore new kinds of learning and expand your horizons. At the same time, new information in a field that you care most about or find the most interesting is the easiest to learn.

Beginning with the next book or article you read, the following techniques may help to double your learning power, including your reading speed and comprehension.

Get the context and connection. You can't be forced to learn. Of course, with brute-force memorization, you can absorb a list of facts. But if you want to be involved and attentive, you have to see the benefit in reading. Link the subject of the text to one of the big dreams that you posted on your LifeMap (see Sensory-Energy Switch #3 for instructions on creating your LifeMap). What you read must be valuable in the bigger picture of your life or work. It can help you streamline your daily efforts and handle stress, get better at relaxing, build new insights for your advancement on the job, escape to another time and place in history or fiction, or just plain have some fun. If it doesn't seem interesting to you, why read it?

Choose your best learning position. Whenever you learn or read, your physical position has a lot to do with your attentiveness and effectiveness. Loosen your posture. Open your chest and neck position so that it's easier to maintain a smooth, rhythmic breathing pattern and draw in more oxygen to your brain and senses. Turn up the lights. Eat a snack. Adjust the angle of the book so your hands and arms are comfortable and the lighting on the page is best.

Pre-read using creative observation. For expanded, accelerated learning, you need to use as many of your senses as possible. Before reading the next book or article, scan it quickly. Begin with the title and author. What is the context? What is the sequence or outline? Are there

READING IS TO THE MIND

WHAT EXERCISE IS TO THE BODY.

—Sir Richard Steel, *The Tatler*, 1710

references? Is this philosophical, practical, or both? Could the subject be meaningful or important to you and your family? Skim through sample sections of the material.

If you're not excited about the content of what you'll be reading, set it aside or skip it. Believe me, we're all getting information overload. It's liberating to find what matters most to you. That's what you want to read or learn.

Read faster, and you'll read better. You've had a chance, in this chapter, to practice focusing your eyes above the words in each line. That's what you want to do every time you read. You don't need to think about speed. When your eye is no longer stopping in the break between each word, speed will come automatically. But the first thing that you'll notice is that all of your senses will be more absorbed in what you're reading.

Use a hand aid. At first, your hand can be a pacer for your eyes. Before flowing down the page, it's valuable to be able to scan at twice your normal speed from left to right under each line. By doing this, you can double your reading speed with equal or greater concentration. Move your index fingertip under the lines as you read. Your finger helps anchor your eyes to the page and frees you from the needless, slow-down habit of silently repeating every word you read. Move your right index fingertip (or your left, if you are left-handed) from the left margin to the right margin under each line as quickly as possible while still understanding the sentences.

This uses tactile feedback to provide a powerful link between your gaze and full attention and the page. Move your fingertip as smoothly and fast as your eyes can keep up. This alone can at least double your reading speed.

On narrow columns of writing, such as in the newspaper, you may be able to read easily and more quickly by bringing your finger down the center of the column while your eyes take in each line.

Ask reflective questions. When you question your own thoughts and what you read, you free yourself from word-by-word progress. Ask yourself, "What could this idea mean in my life? Can I apply this right now? Where is the author heading? Does the author's argument make sense?" Questions like these help free your mind to connect the meanings and applications of what you read.

Read vertically. Once you can pick up your reading speed by quickly moving your fingertip from left to right under each line, try tracing your fingertip under every other line, then every third line. Your brain can readily learn to accept words and phrases out of the usual order. With practice, in many types of reading, your mind can make instant sense out of sentences and entire paragraphs, rather than being dependent on reading every individual word in sequence.

Take frequent pauses and breaks. Nonstop learning creates rapidly diminishing returns. Neuropsychologists have found that in order for your brain to effectively file away and recall what it has learned, it needs to get at least several minutes of mental rest. Every 10 to 20 minutes, take a strategic pause.

If you read for several hours, you need to take a longer break. Try a quick catnap. Or do some radical change-of-mind activity. Think about something humorous or do a crossword puzzle after each concentrated learning experience.

Sleep Deeper

While the world's sleep debt mounts to trillions and trillions of hours, scientists are conducting extensive studies to rescue a highly stressed population from the high cost of sleeplessness. In a National Sleep Foundation poll, 56 percent of adults reported having insomnia at least a few nights every week. That number was more than double the incidence of insomnia reported 8 years before.

There's growing evidence that the majority of adults are getting grouchier and more error-prone because we're suffering from chronic partial sleep deprivation. We don't get enough sleep or, more often, we sleep poorly night after night.

Apart from the tension and irritability that accrues when we're weary and sleep deprived, we're also depleted of sensory energy. When we're just struggling to stay awake, there's little energy left over for enjoying the day. Our eyes get tired. Unexpected events are unwanted distractions rather than pleasant diversions. Our awareness diminishes as we focus on getting things out of the way.

Sight, touch, and hearing are dulled by sleepiness. When we're fighting to stay awake and get through the day, we don't have patience or concentration to enjoy the sights and sounds that might bring a moment's relaxation or pleasure.

Reading becomes a chore if we're struggling to keep our eyes open. Even common sensory pleasures like a patch of warm sunlight or a tasty meal can be more threatening than enjoyable. What if the sun makes you so drowsy you can't pay attention? What if the food makes you even groggier than you were before?

"One thing is absolutely certain in America: The quality and quantity of sleep obtained is substantially less than what is needed," says William Dement, M.D., Ph.D., chairman of the sleep-disorders clinic at the Stanford University School of Medicine. "A substantial number of Americans, perhaps the majority, are functionally handicapped by sleep deprivation on any given day."

If you count yourself among the sleep deprived, you're probably eager for a change, though you may doubt whether you can ever catch up. Despite the obstacles, however, catching up on your sleep may be easier than you imagine.

Getting More from Lights Out

Until recently, sleep has been the dark one-third of our lives, like the far side of the moon, a persistent mystery entangled with misconceptions and wonder. Sometimes, you eagerly fall asleep. Other times, you resist going to bed. And sometimes, sleep eludes you, no matter how hard you chase it. You lie awake, tossing and turning, frustrated, muscles tight, mind racing. Perhaps you finally get an hour or two of fitful, troubled rest, but upon awakening you feel robbed.

SLEEP IS THE ONLY MEDICINE

OF NATURE THAT GIVES EASE
AND RENEWS THE SPIRIT.

—Sophocles (ca. 495–406 B.C.), *Philoctetes*

We all covet great sleep. It's a natural, deep, refreshing experience that depends in part on knowing how to let go of each day. But what happens when the lights go out and you finally enter a state of unconsciousness where your brain and body go on automatic pilot?

Scientists used to regard sleep as a period of rest that was required by your brain and other organs to recover from the wear and tear of daily life. But extensive studies have revealed that a lot of activity continues when you're in a state of deep sleep. Your brain does not rest, at least, not all areas of your brain. In some regions, there's actually an increase of electrical activity, oxygen consumption, and energy expenditure during sleep.

Apparently, one purpose of this extra brain activity is to reinforce memories. In effect, the brain activity helps renew your brain and fortify your mental effectiveness. While you sleep, your brain is doing some late-night cramming for the next day.

But how will you feel when you wake up in the morning? Will your senses be fully alerted and revitalized by the quality of your rest?

Surprisingly, scientists know some clear, proven ways to make a sensory shift to produce measurably deeper sleep and increased energy afterward. There are several practical, little-known ways to reduce tense tiredness and promote deeper, more revitalizing sleep.

Zap the Tube

Millions of Americans fall asleep each night with the television on. The show is still airing, but finally exhaustion takes over and they nod off during a commercial break.

This has proven to be among the least relaxing ways to fall asleep. We carry our tensions to sleep with us, and it shows.

To sleep more soundly and contentedly, I think it's necessary to end the day by taking a few minutes to rebalance your perspective. For my grandfather Downing, this meant going outdoors, onto the porch roof, to peer through a telescope at the stars. To this day, I have not come across anything better to do before falling asleep. But there are many alternatives to stargazing that are just as rewarding to your sense of perspective.

Yes, they may take a minute or two, but we all need an effective way to let go of the day's tensions and worries before bedtime. Step outside and breathe some fresh air. Or just peer out a window to catch a glimpse of the stars. You might spend a moment looking at photos of loved ones, if you have them on your bureau or bed-side table. Or jot down some notes in your NoteStream diary.

Whichever way you prefer, this process of taking a break and restoring perspective will set your mind at liberty to prepare for rest.

Create a Timeless Sleep Space

Another key to good sleep is to hide your clock. Make sure that the face or the digital numbers aren't staring at you as you lie in bed. Turn the clock in the other direction. If you can see the time, there's a great chance that you'll repeatedly awaken during the night. You may not awaken fully, and in the morning, you may not remember being awake at all. But sleep researchers have noted that when there's a clock to be seen, people are more likely to keep checking the time. We simply sleep

SLEEP IS INTERWOVEN WITH EVERY FACET OF DAILY LIFE.
IT AFFECTS OUR HEALTH AND WELL-BEING, . . .
OUR ENERGY AND EMOTIONS, OUR MARRIAGES
AND JOBS, OUR VERY SANITY AND HAPPINESS.

—Peter Hauri, Ph.D., director, insomnia program, Mayo Clinic

better without time pressure. "The bedroom should be a time-free environment," says Peter Hauri, Ph.D., director of the insomnia program
at the Mayo Clinic.

Just as important, arrange for a gentle awakening that skirts the issue
of time. Of course, you'll probably need an alarm clock to help you
wake up. Go ahead and set it, but set it to wake you with music instead
of with the alarm buzzer. If you just set the alarm clock to go off with
a loud bleat or blast, you're starting the day with the message "Get up
now or you'll be late!" As I noted in Calm–Energy Switch #1, leaping
up to shut off an alarm clock is an abrupt jolt to your entire being. You
trigger a racing heartbeat, muscle tension, and stressful "emergency"
symptoms.

Test some alternatives that play down the time factor and ease you into
the day. Positive, energizing music set to come on with a timer and with
the volume just loud enough that you'll notice it and awaken is a far
better choice than the bleep–bleep–bleep of an alarm.

If possible, wake up at least a minute or two earlier than usual to lie
in bed, blink your eyes, move your arms and legs, and allow your body
to gradually adjust to being wide awake. (The wake–up movements in
Calm–Energy Switch #1 will help activate sensory energy as well as calm
energy.) How you spend these waking minutes can have a significant influence on your energy and performance all day long.

Raise Your Temperature Before You Go to Sleep

Doing at least 5 minutes of moderate exercise within 3 to 5 hours of bedtime can measurably deepen your slumber. Physical inactivity ranks among the prime causes of insomnia, and studies link physical fitness with improved sleep quality. But it's not just the exercise itself that's beneficial, it's the rise in body temperature that comes with exercise.

"If you can increase your body temperature 3 to 5 hours before going to bed, the temperature then will drop most as you are ready to go to sleep," explains Dr. Hauri. "The biological 'trough' deepens, and sleep becomes deeper, with fewer awakenings."

"People who take a hot bath or shower within 3 hours of bedtime get a similar benefit," according to James A. Horne, Ph.D., a sleep scientist at Loughborough University of Technology in England.

A brisk walk and a hot shower a few hours before bedtime sounds perfect, doesn't it? And that combination may be the perfect prescription for sleeping better.

Don't Mix Work and Sleep

Your sleep environment—that is, your bedroom—should be dedicated to sleep. It is not the place to think and talk about problems. Work stress, family turmoil, personal issues, financial planning are probably all things you have to contend with. But if your bedroom becomes the forum where you try to deal with those issues, you jam up the environment and prevent deepest rest.

Make it a household rule that your bedroom is a comfortable, relaxing haven. It's the place to have a warm, positive sexual relationship and it's the place to sleep, nothing else.

To follow this rule, some bedroom cleaning may be necessary. Do you have a computer in the room? Move it somewhere else. Is your briefcase in the room? Find another place for it at night. Do you leave mail, opened or unopened, on top of the dresser? Drop it in the study, the living room, anywhere but the bedroom. These are tangible reminders of all your obligations and pressures, and you don't want these to be the last things that you see before lights-out and the first things that you wake up to in the morning.

Instead of having all these reminders around, just keep a few blank notecards by your bed, suggest researchers. If you find that you wake up in the night stewing about problems or thinking of new ideas, scribble things down as quickly as you can. Then you won't have the additional worry of wondering whether you'll remember these things in the morning. You can literally put the thoughts aside, knowing that you can deal with them when you're fully awake.

There are also intangible but controllable factors that affect sleep. Make other rules such as no heated discussions in the bedroom, no brainstorming, no serious snacking, no worrying.

Researchers have found that all of these factors, tangible and intangible, can have a damaging effect on sleep patterns. They accustom your body to a "learned association with sleeplessness." Instead of getting you primed for sleep, the stressful reminders of life loom up even larger. Those reminders prime you for staying awake.

Use Sleep Scents

Here is a very simple consideration that, for some individuals, has proven valuable for promoting deepened rest. Scientists have long known that pleasing fragrances prompt us to take slower, deeper breaths and become more relaxed and refreshed. Every breath that you take passes currents of air molecules over the olfactory sites in your nose. Odors flood the nerve receptors in your nasal cavities, where the im-

You can turn off the light at bedtime, but great sleep does not come automatically. It takes personalized attention and planning.

You need the rest and rejuvenation that good rest brings. Sleep is what renews and expands your sensory energy. Yet many of those who fall asleep quickly and easily unknowingly hold on to excessive muscle tension all night long. That may be what's happening if you end up feeling more tired in the morning than you think you should be.

Here's How

Here's a 30-second remedy to help you wind down before you drift off to sleep.

1. Take several deep, pleasant breaths. With each breath, concentrate on tightening and then relaxing the muscles in your face, jaw, tongue, and neck.

pulses from five million nerve cells fire directly through the olfactory area of your brain to the cerebral cortex and limbic system. Certain scents seem to activate specific chemical messengers, or neurotransmitters, in your brain. Researchers have identified two scents that seem to help promote deeper, more restful sleep. Those fragrances are vanilla almond and apple spice.

I recommend these scents in their natural form since the effects of artificial scents are unknown and may even be detrimental to sleep. Try putting potpourri with either of these scents on your nightstand to see if it makes a difference in the quality of your rest.

2. Focusing on one body area at a time, extend this tense-and-release process across your chest and shoulders.

3. Repeat the tense-and-release process, moving down your back and abdomen.

4. Finally, tense and release your fingertips and toes.

With practice, you can actually use the tense-and-release process to drain all of the tension from your body.

It can also be helpful to accompany this physical release with mental suggestions that help you to give up feelings of tension and control. For some people, soothing music is an inducement to sleep. Others find help in bedtime prayers or positive affirmations. Or recall your fondest memories of soothing, wonderful sleep, perhaps from your childhood years or your favorite vacation. The objective is to do anything that you find to be helpful for putting the day to rest and deepening your pleasant drift into slumber.

Eat for Deeper Rest

The link between what you eat and the quality of your nightly rest has grown much clearer in the past decade. For obvious reasons, it's generally a good idea to avoid coffee, tea, and other caffeinated beverages within 4 to 5 hours of bedtime.

But don't go to bed hungry. If you just eat an early supper but skip having a mid-evening snack, you may end up experiencing a sharp drop in blood sugar in the middle of the night that can interfere with your sleep. That's the reason that I recommend delaying dessert after the evening meal and eating a light snack at mid-evening. The timing depends on your schedule, but for many people that means having a snack between 8:00 and 9:00 P.M.

For deepest sleep, you may want to test the link between what you eat and the quality of your nightly rest. Some studies at the Massachussetts Institute of Technology in Cambridge and a number of other institutions have suggested that you may sleep more deeply if you choose high-carbohydrate, low-fat, and low-protein foods. My own experience, for example, is to generally pass up dairy products when I snack. I find that they are relatively high in alertness-promoting protein. (See Energy Bites: Foods That Stoke Your Energy Furnace for some of my family's favorite evening snacks.)

Finally, if you choose to drink alcohol in the evening, do it early— generally, at least 4 hours prior to bedtime. Although alcohol makes some people drowsy, it actually distorts the normal brainwave pattern of sleep and prompts more frequent awakenings.

Start Your Day at the Same Time Every Morning

One widely celebrated American habit is sleeping in on weekends. Unfortunately, when you do that, your body's biological clock gets confused. There's even a name for this disruption pattern: It's known as free running.

You may think that free running is a good way to catch up on sleep that you've been missing during the week. Unfortunately, your body's sleep accountant doesn't operate on the basis of simple addition and subtraction. Free running tends to lower your energy rather than raise it.

In addition, there's a cumulative effect to free running. While you're likely to feel worn out and less alert after too much sleep, you may also have more difficulty falling asleep the next night.

"The worst thing in the world you can do [for your energy and rest] is sleep in on Sunday morning," says Charles Winget, Ph.D., a NASA scientist from Houston who is an authority on sleep cycles. "Essentially, you're becoming jet-lagged. You might as well fly from California to New York."

Even if your night's sleep has been briefer than usual, it makes sense to get up at about the same time that you usually do, he points out. Regular morning hours help synchronize your body's biological rhythms.

If you do choose to sleep in, it's a good idea to limit your extra time so you're not staying in bed more than an additional hour or so. Open the curtains to let in daylight as soon as you awaken. Then, take a walk outdoors or sit near a bright window. All of these actions help stabilize your sleep-wake rhythm and immediately boost sensory energy.

Part 5

Heartfelt
Energy

In recent years, leading-edge science has revealed to us many of the astonishing ways that the human heart can generate tremendous energy.

"The seat of the soul is to be sought in the heart," said Aristotle in the 4th century B.C. In Aristotle's day, as in ours, the heart was thought to have many more attributes than the mundane task of pumping blood. Phrases such as "learning by heart" or "good at heart" imply that the heart has a kind of majestic presence in all of our deepest thoughts and most compelling feelings.

Now, scientists know that the heart's energy is more than an imaginary construct of language. Scientific experiments show that the heart's energy, in the form of electromagnetic signals, is transmitted to every cell of the body and emanates outward.

In the 1990s, scientists in the emerging field of neurocardiology discovered a "brain" in the heart. Comprised of more than 40,000 neurons of various types, along with a complex network of messenger chemicals, proteins, and support cells, it acts independently of the head. This "heart brain," called a baroreceptor network, is as large as many key areas of the thinking brain and is sufficiently sophisticated to rate as a brain in its own right.

The Field of Binding Energy

The body, heart, and mind work on electrical energy. Research shows that the body's trillions of cells are strongly influenced by the heart, which generates energy and is, in turn, energized by huge electrical fields that engage us with life.

Studies show that the heart's electromagnetic field is by far the most powerful produced by the body. In fact, it is approximately 5,000 times greater than the field produced by the brain. According to research published in the *American Journal of Cardiology*, the electrical changes transmitted by the human heart can be felt and measured from 5 feet away. The heart's electromagnetic field not only permeates every cell in the body but also radiates outward and, in the most recent research, can be measured from 10 feet away with highly sensitive detectors known as magnetometers.

Another intriguing discovery is that heartbeats aren't just mechanical pump pulses; they have an intelligent "energy language" that influences how you perceive and relate to the world. Each and every heartbeat is linked to your thinking brain and to the parts of your nervous system that continually influence your perception and wareness.

Reaping the Benefits

Heartfelt energy will give you:

- Intrinsic motivation, the drive to contribute your best
- More trusting relationships with increased respect and value for yourself and others
- The courage to be more authentic and honest
- Increased focus on the positive things in life
- Confidence to speak up and stand out from the crowd
- Expanded empathy, the ability to relate better to others
- Clarified perspective and improved ability to keep your priorities straight
- Stronger commitments to doing more of what you love and more of what it takes to make the right things happen
- A deepened sense of contentment
- Increased ability to shape a unique imprint on the world through your life and work

A Presence within You

In helping to determine the way that you act and feel, your heart is a living presence. "The best and most beautiful things in the world cannot be seen or even touched," wrote Helen Keller. "They must be felt with the heart."

It's this aspect of the heart that comprises the fourth and final dimension in our advancement toward being 100 percent alive. It's heartfelt energy that informs your thoughts and actions, deepens your spirit and emotion, and brings you closest to others or to life's meaning.

It was the Nobel laureate Albert Schweitzer, M.D., who, speaking of the heart's role in higher qualities of life and work, cautioned that, "Your soul suffers if you live superficially." You are only as robust as that which you feel deep down and that for which you stand. Heartfelt energy takes you on a journey that does not necessarily lead to distant places but does, inevitably, lead you into places from which you have distanced yourself.

Far too many of us accept halfhearted life as our normal daily state of existence. We lose touch with the strong pulse of life within us.

Heartfelt energy helps unlock the depths of who you are and what you may yet become or achieve. Through heartfelt energy, you most significantly touch the lives of others and create an imprint on those lives. This energy is a wellspring of meaningful living, a powerful and significant source of the will to contribute to life in a society that increasingly seems cynical, scattered, and frantic.

A Driving Force

Heartfelt energy activates your deepest drive for a meaningful life and for significant relationships at work and at home. It also engages you in a profound and lasting search for your true voice and calling.

Heartfelt energy is also a sign of character. When heartfelt energy is absent in someone, you sense in them a shallowness or emptiness, despite any outer semblance of fitness or success.

When someone shows courage or commitment, on the other hand, you may quickly sense that it arises from heartfelt energy. This is a driving force of character that shapes each of us as an individual. When you have heartfelt energy, you can live your values and vision, rather than just talking about them.

You also have better health. We now know that this energy is linked to faster healing, strengthened immune function, and longevity.

Heartfelt energy moves you to care and to love, to share with others, and to learn all that you can from them, rather than pretending that you already know it all. It prompts a heightened degree of empathy and provides the vital energy to be more intimate and trusting with others.

Learning and Living by Heart

In terms of your creativity and ingenuity, it turns out that your heart not only is open to new possibilities but also actively and energetically scans for them. When people do their jobs with enthusiasm, we say that they "put their hearts into their work." Heartfelt energy has also been shown to be a necessary component of career success.

Jodi Taylor, vice president of the Center for Creative Leadership in Colorado Springs, headed an extensive project from 1995 to 1998 that examined the critical variables for success. The only statistically significant factor differentiating top leaders from the worst was caring.

The opposite of heartfelt energy is surface energy or political energy. It's not difficult to detect the difference. Surface energy includes Hollywood smiles, schmoozing words, and self-centeredness. When someone pretends to care, feigns honesty, or fakes commitment, that's surface energy. If you ever feel empty, distant, disillusioned, or disconnected, it may be because there's too much surface energy and not enough heartfelt energy in your life.

Without heartfelt energy, life exists out there, not in here. When you have heartfelt energy, relationships change for the better. This kind of energy is what helps to sustain you as you search for and then deepen a sense of higher purpose and meaning in your life and work.

Engage People Eye to Eye

When my daughter Shanna was 5, she learned to play Ping-Pong. Or should I say that we both learned?

We had spent part of one afternoon swimming at a nearby pool. Chelsea, my 8-year-old daughter, and her friend Meredith headed toward the indoor recreation area and began to play Ping-Pong. Shanna followed them inside and watched for a while. Pretty soon, they asked her to leave, complaining that she was pestering them and that she was too little to play. That's when she asked me to come in and watch with her. I did.

When the older girls finished, Shanna said, "Can we play, Daddy?"

"Sure."

I spent a few minutes trying to explain the basic objectives of the game. Shanna's head was barely above the edge of the table. I tried to imagine that view.

Shanna had the ball. She bounced it off the floor. Then, she bounced it on a nearby chair. When she tried to hit it with the paddle, she swung much too hard.

When she finally hit the ball, it ricocheted off a chair, rebounded against the wall, and zoomed straight between my legs. Shanna shrieked with laughter.

"No, Shanna, here's the way you do it," I said, demonstrating a proper serve. She swung, missed, chased after the bouncing ball, and then, spinning around, hit it backward between her legs. I ducked, swinging and missing, as it whistled past my shoulder and rebounded off the window beside me. More laughter.

"No, no, Shanna, that's not how you are supposed to do it."

"Who says?"

"Well, a rule book."

"But who was the person who said it?"

"I don't know."

"Did they have fun playing it?"

"They probably did."

"But what if it's more fun another way?" She looked at me expectantly.

I hesitated. There I was, all prepared to follow an instructional checklist. I was making this game into a chore, attempting to train a little girl in the art of Ping-Pong while she only wanted to have fun and try something new.

And that's when I stopped myself. Maybe I should leave the teaching to my 5-year-old. After all, she was the one having a great time, which was the purpose of the game. And while she was doing that, I was feeling concerned about the "proper" way to teach her traditional Ping-Pong, a game that—truth be told—I'd never even liked very much.

Looking back now, I'm very aware of that moment. It was as if her heartfelt energy caught up with me, engaging me with this young child and the possibilities of play. She taught me by catching my eye and my attention. I couldn't keep my intellect on track with preconceived notions or old mind-sets.

NOT BY CONSTRAINT OR SEVERITY

SHALL **YOU HAVE ACCESS TO THE WISDOM**, BUT BY

ABANDONMENT, AND CHILDLIKE MIRTHFULNESS.

—Henry David Thoreau, *Journal*, June 23, 1840

At that moment, I must have looked puzzled or stumped, because she announced, "Okay, then these are the new rules, Daddy. . . ."

She swatted the ball hard, and again it ricocheted off the picture window beside us. But this time, instead of hesitating to correct her form or disapprove, I jumped sideways and took a mighty swing.

I missed. She squealed with delight. And then I was laughing too. So were all of the adults and children nearby. With each new volley, it was contagious fun, probably way more fun than the founder of the official Ping-Pong rule book ever had in playing the game.

"Let's call this Pong-Ping, Daddy."

Okay, I thought.

It was much more spontaneous and fun than the old game of Ping-Pong. Unexpected, unexplained, it just emerged from the dynamics between Shanna and me. But I felt far more free to experiment with this new game and, indeed, far more human and alive.

Let It Shine

"The light that shines in the eyes is the light of the heart," said the 14th-century scholar and poet Rumi.

Based on scientific evidence and my own experience, I believe that he was right. And yet, when I work with leaders and organizations around the world, I see more and more people with no light in their eyes. It is evident that their hearts are not in their work. They are going through the motions, holding down jobs. They have lost or are losing their heartfelt energy.

In his book *The Language of the Heart*, James J. Lynch, Ph.D., codirector of the psychophysiology laboratory and clinic at the University of Maryland School of Medicine in Baltimore, explores the eye-to-eye valuing that one person gets from another. He describes the surge of energy that you experience each time you "glimpse the infinite universe behind another person's eyes."

It may seem a bit narcissistic to look yourself in the eye, but I think that it's worth doing once in a while. When you look at yourself in the mirror, what do you see in your eyes, reflected beneath the surface? If you had to say what's hidden in the depths of your gaze, what would it be? What do you find?

This simple exercise is worth doing because heartfelt energy is expressed to a significant degree through your eyes. In essence, you have to be able to look clearly into your own eyes before you can relate to others eye to eye.

A Look of Kindness

In America, it's common courtesy to look directly at another person in greeting. But looking at them sincerely and with kindness goes one step further, and it's an important step because it generates an energetic interchange of positive feelings between the two of you, even without a single word being spoken.

In its simplest form, this look is an expression of heartfelt energy. It's as unmistakable as a look of frustration, anger, disinterest, arrogance, or any other negative glance that speaks volumes. But when you give someone a genuine and kind glance of acknowledgment, you instantly convey a vital message, providing and communicating the positive, reinforcing energy that helps make other people feel recognized, respected, and valued.

"These looks are far beyond words: Eyes speak more profoundly than language the tenor of relatedness," writes Ruthellen Josselson, Ph.D., professor of psychology at Towson State University in Baltimore. "They express, surely and absolutely, how much and in what way we matter to the Other. Words may lie; eyes cannot."

It doesn't take much searching to witness the power of such eye contact. Think of the look in the eyes of someone arriving in an airport or a bus terminal and being warmly greeted by a family member. Or picture the lingering looks of those who are bidding each other goodbye. No words need to be spoken. The eyes convey the feeling of heartfelt energy.

Good Visibility

Think of how it feels to work hard at home or in a workplace of any kind where no one else seems to notice, much less care, that you are there making an effort. For every one of us, this feels devaluing, whether the other people mean it to feel this way or not.

In truth, we each need to be seen—to be acknowledged, even in a glance—by others in order to be made visible in the world. We cannot do this wholly on our own. Others must help. You're one of the people who can help those around you. Here's how.

Stay present. When you spend time with people, you may find yourself subconsciously exiting from conversations. This is rarely intentional, of course. But others know it, and when it happens, it can undermine your relationships and lead to unnecessary complications. Being in and out during a conversation is disrespectful and tiring, first to the other person and ultimately to you. When you're there, be there.

By the way, don't think that you can mask these subconscious exits. None of us can. Other people almost always see and feel it happening.

Leave when you have to. This is a corollary to staying present. Some people exit a conversation by switching on the TV. Others take business calls in the middle of a conversation. Yes, there may be a show that you want to watch. There may be a call that you have to make or take. But it's only fair to make a clean exit. Excuse yourself with an honest and appropriate explanation of what you want to do or have to do, and then go do it.

In the long run, and often in the short-run too, clarity pays. It's a lot fairer to the other person than being half-present or mentally exiting and reentering during a conversation.

Be emotionally honest. Beating around the bush, being vague, and sending other people mixed messages about what you truly mean are some of the quickest ways to block heartfelt energy. To the extent that you can use well-chosen words to say what you truly feel and believe, you find out who you are deep down. And the better you know yourself, the more clearly you can look someone else in the eye.

If you try to find words to genuinely express your feelings, not just the cheerful and uplifting feelings but the difficult and challenging ones as well, you allow others to see more of the real person you are. That makes it a lot easier to build trust and look them in the eye with honesty and clarity, knowing that you don't have anything to hide.

Plant your feet. The most exceptional people seem to always know accurately and instinctively where they stand at each moment. I call this constancy.

Constancy is different from consistency, which is a predictable, regular series of events. To me, constancy is the steady emanation of who you are. A lighthouse is emblematic of this quality. When I was a boy, my grandfather Downing would describe to me how the lighthouses of Scotland enabled sailors to find their way around the treacherous coastal waters to safe harbors. "Don't dim your light," he said to me. "And always look for the light in others."

Fight numbness. When certain things distract, frustrate, or irritate you, numbness can set in. Whenever you use your intellect to rationalize negative emotions, you are likely to feel drained. You get stuck in blame, defensiveness, hurt, regret, anger, remorse, and guilt. As time goes on, such emotions impair your senses and undermine your vitality. You feel less alive.

This is a warning sign, I believe. Your light of constancy is dimming, and if you let numbness take over, the light can go out of your eyes. When that happens, your first eye contact becomes wary, defensive, and suspicious rather than eager, open, and expressive. As this slowly drains your heartfelt energy, you become vulnerable to additional energy losses and emotional strains.

Do Less Rescuing

While the beam from a lighthouse may help guide sailors, it doesn't rescue them on cold, dark, and stormy nights. That's a job that they, and others, must take on themselves.

How does this relate to heartfelt energy? It's essential to remember that you can't make everything all better for anyone else. Your presence can be a great energizer to that person, and you get heartfelt energy in return. Your interest can lead to better communication and a

ABOVE ALL,

EVERYONE MUST BE RESPECTED

AS AN INDIVIDUAL.

—Albert Einstein (1879–1955), U.S. physicist

close affinity, an energy benefit for both of you. But by trying to rescue someone when you don't really have the time, capability, or expertise, you may find yourself floundering in stormy and treacherous waters.

One of the fastest ways to drain heartfelt energy is to feel that you need to keep making everything all better or to fix other people and their problems. With rare exceptions, it simply can't happen, and it doesn't work. But most people keep trying to do it anyway, and then they wonder why they feel so tired and stuck.

For one thing, few of us have the power to solve other people's problems, even in our own families. Instead, by genuinely relating to people, listening deeply, and validating their feelings appropriately, you can entrust them to be their own problem solvers. Here are some practical ways to put this into action.

Notice what's unique and valuable about another person. Each time you interact with or think about someone else, start by remembering or noticing what makes that person an individual. This helps you relate to others from your heart instead of only from your head. Your eyes will tell them what they need to know, that you recognize them, respect them, and value their individuality.

Let each person feel what they are feeling. Every moment, in situations of all kinds, people try to generate and express their heartfelt energy through feelings. If you respond, "But you shouldn't feel that way," you rob them of the essential vitality of their emotions. Looking away, shaking your head, or closing your eyes expresses the same thing. It feels like you're judging them. Don't. Instead, acknowledge their emotions, even when this may make you feel uncomfortable.

Avoid needless verbal battles. When someone else has feelings that include fear, anger, or resentment, it is easier than most of us realize to get caught up in their emotions and end up feeling argumentative and down. "Why is she blaming me? Why should I listen to this tirade?" you may think. At these moments, your eyes may be saying, "Don't say that" or "I don't want to hear that," reactions that could prolong or even increase the negative feelings rather than letting them play themselves out.

Try to keep the kindly light in your eyes. Just by listening and expressing genuine caring, without agreement—by responding, "That must be hard" or "I can tell that you're feeling stressed out right now"—you can let them know they're heard and encourage them to take responsibility for moving forward in a better way. Even when no words can help the other person fix what's wrong, the heartfelt energy expressed in your eyes is a strong and constant reassurance of this other person's fundamental and unique worthiness. This can make another feel as valued as a reassuring voice can.

Share the Ride

In close relationships, the heartfelt energy in eye-to-eye connections helps you stay in sync. In an intimate relationship, two lives eventually develop a connection that becomes tied into biological cycles. Researchers have discovered that couples who have close relationships show close correlations in their individual 24-hour circadian rhythms and 90- to 180-minute ultradian rhythms. Their overall activity patterns, appetites, need for diversion, and sexual rhythms all occur in synchrony.

One way to key in to your partner's rhythms and help establish and maintain feelings of closeness and intimacy is with frequent eye contact that expresses your heartfelt energy. There are many benefits when your wavelike biological rhythms are in close harmony, and there are correspondingly more conflicts and frustrations when you are on opposite waves.

In couples, unsynchronized heartfelt-energy cycles may also produce some frustrating sexual dilemmas. What happens when one of you is sexually aroused and sensually energetic, and the other one isn't? How do you share intimacy when one of you is in the mood for comforting, nonsexual cuddling, while the other is sexually aroused?

The more you can align your daily energy cycles with those of your partner, the greater your chances for lifelong, mutually satisfying closeness. Couples with exceptionally intimate and lasting relationships tend to unconsciously integrate their own individual ultradian and circadian rhythms. Couples who complain of feeling halfhearted or of losing heartfelt or sexual energy frequently report conflict and imbalance across these areas.

Any couple who have shared romantic glances over a candlelit dinner or who have glared at each other over the financial battlefield of an open checkbook know how much power, both positive and negative, can be carried in a single glance. When the balance of your thoughts and feelings are in close harmony, your eyes are wonderful communicators. You may not know what your partner is thinking, but with one look, you can tell instantly that he or she wants and needs something. In these moments, the heart and eyes speak volumes.

Seeing Eye to Eye

I'm sure that many of us have an image, buried somewhere deep in our idyllic view of the American landscape, of a contented couple seated on a porch swing, holding hands as they rock to and fro, talking softly and sharing warm glances as they watch the red sun dip below the horizon. All of the elements of heartfelt energy and synchrony are embodied by that bucolic picture—the rhythm and harmony of rocking to and fro, the comfort and homey feeling of the house in the landscape, and the presence of nature's force, emanating from the setting sun. And in this ideal setting, the glances shared by the couple are warm and loving.

Perhaps all would be well with your relationship if every evening were like this. More likely, you are indoors, the phone is ringing, the TV is on, you're rushing through housework, and someone has to think about dinner. But even if that's so, it's all the more reason why you have to make sure that your home and your relationships provide the heartfelt energy that each of us requires.

Here are several of the ways to increase heartfelt connections in your closest personal relationships.

Relate to each other eye to eye. When you talk, make genuine eye contact whenever possible. This helps ensure that each person feels visible and valued.

Don't leave or arrive without making eye contact. Whenever you say goodbye, look into the eyes of the other people in your household, taking time to see each individual at a time. This eye-to-eye validation keeps reaffirming your respect for others at the same time that it keeps boosting heartfelt energy.

Link touch to sight. Give a touch on the arm, a squeeze of the hand, or a hug to a family member.

Catch a glance when you walk. Going for a shared early-morning or evening stroll gives you a welcome chance for fresh air and open conversation. You will significantly increase heartfelt energy if you can pause for a moment, look at each other, enjoy the moment together. Catch your partner's eye when there's a moment of humor or enjoyment, and the heartfelt energy can brighten your whole day or evening.

In each of these simple actions, powerful verbal and nonverbal cues help to synchronize your heartfelt-energy rhythms. No matter how long you've been apart from each other, these are the important looks that can renew intimacy and create a closer bond between you and your partner.

Ask Openly and Listen Deeply

D oes everyone see what I see when I look at the world?"

The question came from a young boy at an inner-city Boys Club. Near the end of my tour of duty in the U.S. Marine Corps during the Vietnam War, I had a chance to do some volunteer work at the Boys Clubs of Los Angeles and San Diego, teaching martial arts classes.

The boy who asked the question did not know his own father. He would often stay after class, along with a number of the other kids, just to talk. They knew firsthand how difficult life can be, and they had a keen ability to ask open and honest questions, the kind that so many adults ignore or avoid.

Before I could answer him, I had my own question for this boy. "What is it that you see?"

He said, "I see me in your eyes."

I first thought he meant that he saw his own reflection in my eyes, the mirror of his own image. But no, he said, it wasn't that. He said that I was his friend. He saw his own life in my eyes.

So I was glad that he asked his question and that I had asked mine. I had found out something that I would not have discovered otherwise: that each of us, while seeing the world in our own way, hopes to have life reflected back to us from others.

A Telltale Response

According to researchers, whenever a person feels that they have been genuinely valued or deeply heard by someone else, they experience a moistening of the eyes. It's not enough for tears. But in bright light, you can clearly see their eyes moisten in response to heartfelt energy.

Researchers have also estimated that in more than 95 percent of daily interactions, there is no moistening of the eyes. One of the main reasons is that these are the conversations in which we do not feel valued or heard. Heartfelt energy, I believe, is missing.

But I also believe that you can introduce this valuable element in almost any interchange between two people. As that young boy did with me, you can change the landscape of the dialogue.

"While we speak with words, we speak also with our flesh and blood," says James J. Lynch, Ph.D., author of *The Language of the Heart* and codirector of the psychophysiology laboratory and clinic at the University of Maryland School of Medicine in Baltimore. "Study after study reveals that human dialogue not only affects our hearts significantly but can even alter the biochemistry of individual tissues at the furthest extremities of the body."

What's the Message?

Few things shape our lives as much as the communication that we share with others. The poet William Stafford wrote:

. . . It is important for awake people to be awake,
Or a breaking line may discourage them back to sleep;
The signals we give—yes or no, or maybe—
Should be clear; the darkness around us is deep.

Of course, it sounds like a contradiction to ask awake people to be awake. But what Stafford is saying is that the signals that you give can either encourage people to be awake or "discourage them back to sleep." When you pay attention, ask questions, and communicate heartfelt energy, the message is yes or perhaps no, when it needs to be, or even maybe. That's far different from trying not to face questions or avoiding answering altogether, which is what more and more people find themselves doing these days.

Our signals should be clear. I'm with Stafford on that. The darkness around us is very deep indeed, and we want people to know that we are listening. Signaling yes, no, or maybe helps confirm that we, too, are awake in life, not asleep in the rush and din of everyday living.

Asking and Listening

How can you learn if you don't ask? What enriches life most is the ability to explore the world and understand experience. That takes a willingness to ask challenging questions and engage in personal reflection.

According to Dr. Lynch, the human body is designed to benefit from a natural, heart-healthy rhythm between speaking and listening. Every time you speak, your blood pressure rises dramatically. To balance this soaring pressure, you need to listen genuinely and well. When you truly listen, your blood pressure drops below normal and provides you with a healthy recovery of energy and vigor.

Yet more and more people in today's rushed and noisy world seem to be talking loudly and listening hardly at all. And I've found that when

HEARING IS ONE OF THE FIVE SENSES. BUT
LISTENING IS AN ART. IT IS WHAT UNITES HUMAN BEINGS
IN ONE OF LIFE'S MOST SIGNIFICANT AND
MEANINGFUL INTERACTIONS: DIALOGUE.

—James J. Lynch, Ph.D., codirector, psychophysiology laboratory and clinic,
University of Maryland School of Medicine, Baltimore

people do seem to be listening, they're often doing it partially, in an act of theatrics. They're not really hearing. With this pattern, their blood pressures can stay too high, and they not only hurt their hearts but also lose heartfelt energy.

"What comes from the heart goes to the heart," said Samuel Coleridge, the 19th-century English philosopher and poet. Both asking and listening must make a direct connection to your heart. But how can you make that happen?

The answer, coming from those who have made a lifelong study of human interactions, is the name of this heartfelt-energy switch: "Ask openly and listen deeply."

The Asking Part

What does it mean to ask openly? First and foremost, it means not being afraid to ask. Whenever you withhold a question that you want to ask, you lose just a little more ground in your efforts to learn and grow, and your heartfelt energy wanes. To ask is to step forward or upward in life. It is often less important to know the answers than to be open to asking and pondering good questions.

Consider this: If you wonder what another person's motives or intentions are and you don't ask, you're just guessing. When researchers have asked people to guess what others are thinking and have then asked what those others are thinking, the guesses were right only about 10 percent of the time. That means that when you don't ask and you just trust your intuition, 90 percent of the time you're likely to be dead wrong in your assumption about another person's motives or intentions.

The trouble is that when you're vague in your understanding, when you're operating by guesswork and trying to read what people are thinking, you too often assume the worst. This is a natural instinct of the human brain. Think of the energy that is wasted on worry or anxiety if you guess or believe that someone is angry with you when they're really not. If someone close to you, a friend, colleague, or spouse, gives you a certain look, how do you interpret it? Is it disapproval? Impatience? Indifference? Distrust?

If you guess without asking, you can easily set off in an entirely wrong direction to mend a fence that hasn't been broken, to soothe feelings that have never been hurt, to patch up an argument that never occurred. Remember, 90 percent of the time when you try to interpret that look, whatever it is, you're wrong. The only way that you can possibly find out the truth of the situation is by asking.

The simple lesson is: Don't assume, ask. Seek to be as clear as possible about what you want to find out, and try to understand what others mean.

The Listening Part

Asking, of course, is only part of the story. Once you ask the honest, fearless question, you must also be fearless enough to listen very openly and curiously to what the other person has to say. And the moment that you begin to listen deeply, you can feel the heartfelt energy increasing and coming across. Few things feel more valuable and validating than to communicate with someone who listens deeply and well.

Often, it's not easy to disengage from the distractions in your mind. It may take a conscious act of will. If you need to, use the instant-calming sequence in Calm-Energy Switch #2.

Of course, this doesn't mean that you need to listen passively. Use clarifying phrases such as "What I hear you saying is. . . . Is that right?" Untangle whatever you're unclear about.

This simple act of genuine listening builds trust. And it's so much more direct. Your questions, your interest, your need to clarify will eliminate the fishing expedition that you often engage in when you take the indirect route.

Many people spend lots of time, energy, and effort trying to be heard. But because they never have an opportunity to answer questions directly and, when they do, they're not clearly heard, they end up posturing to get the attention that they want. Life becomes theatrics or a charade, which wastes everyone's time and energy. When you listen deeply, you demonstrate by example what it means to treat others as you would wish them to treat you. There's nothing more powerful to help drive away what Stafford calls "the darkness around us."

Questions about Life

For thousands of years, great thinkers and seekers have been willing to ask direct and heartfelt questions. And once they have asked those questions, they have been willing to pursue some very long journeys to search for the answers. In all of the great teaching and religious traditions, from Socrates and Aristotle to the preeminent thinkers and believers of today, the most meaningful quests have begun with questions like What is the purpose of life? Where do we find meaning? and What is the nature of good and evil?

Once you ask questions like these, you know how much heartfelt energy they can generate. Perhaps you remember intense discussions with like-minded or not-like-minded friends when the most urgent thing that you could imagine was to prove that you were right and they were wrong. Just beneath the surface energy of that debate, however, you were tapping into your deepest beliefs, your values, as shaped by your observation and experience; and your judgment, shaped by your sense of right and wrong.

Of course, I'm not suggesting that you want to dwell on such deep questions every hour of the day. But I do suggest that each of us has deeply felt values, experiences, and beliefs that we hold very dear. When we are asked about them or reflect on them, even briefly, we reconnect with a key source of our heartfelt energy. Such questions call forth the best of who we are and challenge us to live our lives more fully and with greater awareness.

Sooner or later, most of us face situations in life or work that deepen and expand heartfelt energy. We do it either by choice or when circumstances demand it, when we are confronted with the death of a loved one, the birth of a child, a serious illness, or the loss of a job that is important to our livelihood, ambitions, and sense of worth.

Tapping the Energy

Some questions energize you by revealing the deeper nature of your strength, courage, love, and creativity. These are fundamental questions that can awaken and increase heartfelt energy as you live your daily life. Depending on your relationship with the person you're asking, some of

TRY THIS NOW!

Who are the people whom you value the most? Whose opinions matter to you? Whose trust or respect do you most want to have? These are some of the people with whom you're most likely to share and feel the strongest heartfelt energy.

Before you answer those questions, it may help you to turn them around. Who are the people who respect and value you the most?

Here's How

Take out a piece of paper and write down several of the specific ways that you feel most valued by others. It may be eye-to-eye contact, words of support or concern, or the way they listen to you or encourage you to speak up. Your list may also include being held accountable for being your best or being asked what you feel rather than just what you think. Or it could be being recognized and rewarded for your efforts in some special ways.

Next, write down the names of four people who are vital to your success at work, in your community, or in your family life. Beside each name, write two specific ways that each of these individuals feels most valued or recognized by you. Are you valuing them from day to day the way that you most like to be valued? Do you know for certain that they feel valued in these ways?

To answer these questions, you need to ask these people directly. Only with this kind of genuine clarity can you truly relate to each person as an individual. It may seem risky to ask someone whether they truly feel valued by you, but it's a way to build trusting relationships by bypassing hidden assumptions and getting to the heart of the matter.

these questions may seem more compelling than others. But ask any of them, and you will be awakening new sources of heartfelt energy.

Who are you? No one is just a name, a profession, a position, or a set of relationships. Yet we often ask, "What do you do?" or "How do you know so-and-so?" or "Who are you married to (or dating)?" or "What do you plan to do?" Ask, "Who are you?" and you may begin to hear a voice with a life story. Beneath our joys and sorrows, our dreams and disappointments, is an essential nature that is whole and alive. People can easily say what they do or who they know or what their plans are, but that often doesn't touch their heartfelt energy. To do that, you need to hear something about their inner strengths and the unique experiences that have shaped who they are. And you need to find out what they're searching for that will be most meaningful to them.

What do you most love to do? This is a lot different from "What's your job?" or "Where are you working?" or "What do you plan to do?" Ask someone what they love to do, and you'll find out what that person's greatest sources of enjoyment are and get a glimpse into that individual's search to do more of those things. In our clearest moments, this is how we shape our dreams and guide our actions. Perhaps you'll discover when this person feels most content and alive. Yes, they may answer with a job description, if they have the perfect job and love it. More likely, you'll hear about long walks in the woods, a satisfying avocation, their joy in working with children, or their intellectual or spiritual pursuits. "I love to read" or "I love to fish" tells you far more about a person than their clothes, physical appearance, job description, or name does.

Who are the most exceptional people you have ever known? If you think about your own life and the mentors or teachers who have been most important to you, you'll realize the significance of this question. If you just want a conversation with someone, you can ask how they like their boss or how they're dealing with the neighbor who has unruly children and a barking dog. But it's unlikely that their heartfelt energy or yours is much connected to these relationships. When you ask, instead, about exceptional people, you may hear about family members, teachers, or friends. It could be someone they met only once or twice who, during those encounters, made a profound impression. Or it could be someone who shaped them as a person or a leader. You'll hear about people who were emotionally honest, who refused to live a lie or simply go through the motions for efficiency or a paycheck. They had the heart to break new ground, question old mind-sets, and extend a caring hand or a kind word.

What is one of the greatest challenges that you have faced and overcome? When I ask business leaders this question, few of them describe their successes. How people face setbacks and learn from them is often the most telling factor in shaping who they are and what they become. When you ask this question of others or yourself, you quickly learn something about their depth of heart and character.

What is the greatest form of respect and recognition that you have ever received? If you expect someone to reply to this question by describing a promotion or honor that they received at work, you may be surprised. In one nationwide survey of executives and office workers, 90 percent of the respondents said they had never felt genuinely recognized or respected at work. So the answer to this question is more likely to reflect the rewards that they have received from pursuits and interests outside of work or from moments of respect and recognition in their personal relationships.

What are your gifts to the world? Most of us believe that if we are given the chance, we can contribute to bettering the world. Needless to say, this is not a cocktail-party question. When you ask it, it must be with the utmost respect. In effect, you're asking another person to share their impression of how much of a difference they are making, on or off the job. It's also a question that taps deeply held assumptions about who we are and what we're doing here. The heartfelt energy that's generated can become a touchstone in your relationship with the other person. Often, it requires equal sharing on your part. How would you answer the questions What are you meant to do here? and What are you trying to do with your life?

If your house were catching fire and your loves ones were safe, what two or three things would you save—and why? This question prompts people to slow down and do some soul-searching. It helps keep our perspectives clearer.

Can you live today as if it were the last day of your life? We never know when or how we will die. Fourteen years ago, I lost five members of my extended family—two adults and three children—in a commercial airline crash. The suddenness and finality was an urgent reminder that life is fleeting. I realized how easy it is to take people for granted, even those we most care about or love. If we wish to not look back over our lives with regret, we will keep in mind and in our hearts that every effort we make and every contact we have with others leaves a mark. When you ask this question of yourself or anyone else, you are tapping into one important component of heartfelt energy, the urgency to define day by day who we are and what our lives mean to the world.

Get around Guesswork

By nature, the intellect is quick to make judgments and assumptions, especially when we're guessing or assuming the motives of others. As I've indicated, research indicates that our guesswork is usually wrong.

Few things constrict heartfelt energy faster than jumping to conclusions. When we don't ask for real answers, we may leap to conclusions, defend positions, or act all-knowing, without any basis for such attitudes.

In our overeager scrambles to reach conclusions, we can get trapped in an energy-draining maze of misunderstandings and relationship problems.

Here are some ways to avoid those pitfalls by asking questions that tend to generate heartfelt energy instead of draining it.

Don't look the other way or sweep things under the rug. Lots of us choose harmony over truth, and we almost always pay a price for it later. If there's a question or an issue that's left hanging, when you try to convince yourself that there's nothing to worry about or that it will probably all turn out fine, that's a good moment to double-check whether you're trying to ignore something that matters. Are there questions that need to be answered or things that you need to know more about? If so, trying to preserve the status quo is not the solution.

Too often, we work hard to pretend that problems don't exist; but at the same time, we may start to think that other people are against us. How can you even begin to assume that if you haven't asked and may not know for sure?

I'm certainly in favor of positive thinking. But when it's applied like frosting over real issues, we don't grow. Instead, we get trapped in life's theatrics and avoid meaningful questions and the straight talk that leads to real learning. Along the way, we end up trying to ignore many of the difficult, defining moments that produce the most intense heartfelt energy. The fact is that when applied with sensitivity and the proper timing, honesty saves time and builds respect. And it can help streamline your actions, along with helping others to do the same.

Share your views. Often, the best questions and the ones that are most productive of heartfelt energy begin with a statement about your own personal viewpoint. For example: "I could be wrong. Here's my view of this. . . . What's yours?" Or, "Here are my concerns. . . . What are yours?"

Recognize the other perspective. It pays to readily acknowledge the

WHEN WE LEARN NOT TO JUDGE OTHERS, . . .

WE CAN SIMULTANEOUSLY LEARN TO

BRING OUT THE BEST IN OURSELVES.

—Gerald Jampolsky, M.D., psychiatrist

other person's point of view. "You have a point there." Or, "I've never thought about it that way." Or, "I understand what you're saying." Notice that you're not necessarily agreeing and certainly not pretending to agree. These are just ways to acknowledge that you've heard the other person, you know what they're saying, and you can understand their point of view, whether or not you agree with it.

Hold the critiques. I suspect that so many of us are accustomed to giving advice or suggestions in the form of criticism that we aren't even aware that we sound more critical than helpful. If so, there's a risk that the majority of our interactions are having negative rather than positive effects.

"Flaw finding is the most dominant approach to giving feedback or criticism," says Stephanie Hughes, a sociologist at Boston University. "This helps explain why people experience criticism as a highly charged, negative emotional encounter and a personal attack."

To effectively give feedback and have it used constructively, you must be respected by the person who will be hearing the comments. If there's respect in the relationship and the other person values your advice, then the feedback may be helpful. But if not, there's a risk that your words may be heard as a flaw-finding critique.

Reveal your position. No one can automatically know your point of view unless you share it. And when you do, there's a gain in heartfelt energy, generated by the self-expression that leads to equal sharing in the relationship. Here are two of the emotionally honest statements that can prove very useful: (1) "This is what I experienced and felt . . ." and (2) "This is what I want or need: . . ."

Watch Your Words

"New scientific data reveal the links between the spoken word and the human heart," writes Dr. Lynch. These links, he goes on, show a relationship between the quality of dialogue and a number of health conditions, including hypertension, two major cardiovascular disorders, and migraine headaches. "Human dialogue is involved significantly in the development as well as the treatment of these diseases," he observes.

When we open our mouths to speak, adds Dr. Lynch, we are, in a sense, "attempting to bring the hearer inside our own world. Ordinarily, we tend to think of speech as words projected out, directed at, or aimed toward someone else. Yet a moment of reflection would reveal that quite the opposite is true of real speech. For when a person speaks, he or she is inviting others to come inside his or her world, into his or her reality—that is, into his or her body and ultimately into his or her mind's heart. Real speaking is communication in the most profound sense: It is an act of communion."

Genuine dialogue can occur only with feeling. It is far more of the heart than of the head. Feelings are what enrich good relationships and make us feel energized and alive when interacting with others.

Because of this, it's important to validate what you and others are feeling. If you don't, conversations too often go awry. Many people seem to have trouble understanding and responding to feelings. They have learned to be guarded or oblivious when feelings arise. But if you do that, it's easy to miss the heartfelt energy that is an essential part of good relationships. Here are some approaches that may help you be more comfortable when there's emotional content in your dialogue.

Go ahead, talk about feelings. It's not feelings themselves that lead to difficulties in life; it's how we acknowledge and handle them, or fail to do so. If someone can describe how they're feeling, it's a genuine and powerful attempt to communicate heartfelt energy. Whenever you acknowledge a feeling in yourself or others, you not only liberate heartfelt energy but also provide a clearer opportunity to respond more intelligently and empathetically in the next moment.

Accept that good people can feel bad from time to time. Everyone, including the "best" people, feels anger, gets frustrated, and stumbles or falls in their attempts to accomplish things. From time to time, we each feel alone, disappointed, overwhelmed, or confused. When we stop pretending every moment that we're just fine, we can better face the aloneness, difficulties, pressures, or confusion in ourselves as well as in others. In this way, we can be genuine about life's challenges, which boosts heartfelt energy and can make the challenges more manageable. It is also easier to own up to our own imperfections, stop bemoaning what we don't have and, instead, search more earnestly for what we do have, taking insightful and constructive actions to bring forth more of our strengths and talents.

Realize that your feelings are just as important as those of others. Many people try to minimize their own feelings because they have learned to assume that others' feelings are more important than theirs. Or they choose to hide feelings, not wanting to rock the boat. While that strategy may provide short-term relief, it often reappears as a long-term mistake. Other people's feelings are not more important; yours do matter. Unless you can acknowledge what you feel, you're likely to build resentment, and that can steadily erode your relationships.

Reframe problem talk into constructive focus. Reframing means taking the essence of what another person says and transforming it, in your response, into something more constructive. If you can do that, you turn a conversation from a tug-of-war into a mutual search for understanding.

For instance, suppose the other person says, "I'm right and that's all there is to it."

You reframe, "I want to make sure I understand your view. It's clear that you feel very strongly about this. I'd also like to share my own view of the situation."

Or suppose the other person says, "This is all your fault!"

You reframe, "I agree that I contributed to the problem. In different ways, we both did. Rather than focus on who's to blame, I'd like to look at how we got here and what we can learn going forward."

It's obvious, of course, that one sentence is not going to be enough in many cases. But you can see where you might start. In both of these examples, reframing moves the conversation forward constructively. Had you simply answered "You're wrong" or "It's not my fault," rather than reframing, the dialogue would have quickly turned into a full-blown argument.

The 24-Hour Give-a-Break Plan

Can you go a full 24 hours without saying a single unkind word about anyone? It's an interesting challenge.

The old playground chant claims, "Sticks and stones may break my bones, but words will never hurt me." You may have said it yourself at one point in your young life. But even then, you probably knew in your heart that it wasn't true.

Words can hurt. We know it all too well.

They can also heal. It's likely that the words that you speak and hear measurably influence every cell in your body, according to Dr. Lynch's research. What you say and hear has energy to help or harm.

Gossip can be one of the most hurtful forms of dialogue. But I believe that there's a way to talk about people that is less likely to undermine or injure them.

Talk about others in specific and clear ways. Be as kind and fair as you would want others to be when saying things about you. That doesn't mean that you need to be totally complimentary. Just be truthful. Keep your comments in perspective. If what you're saying is what you would like to hear about yourself, you're probably on the right track. Your concern about that person as well as your accuracy about repeating their comments or observing their actions or character can be yet another way to express heartfelt energy.

Empathize

What makes a good person?

I think that most of us would say that good people are those who care. Or perhaps we would give the reply that children gave to Robert Coles, M.D., researcher and psychologist at Harvard University, when they told him, "They are good of heart."

Good people, at least the ones whom we can most easily recognize, are the ones with empathy. Not only do we admire them, we often stand in awe of their ability to care. As far as we know, such caring is not an innate birthright. It is learned. And the caring not only uses heartfelt energy but also builds it.

Of course, in a cynical environment, perceptions may differ. People who are low in heartfelt energy and high in surface energy are often the most cynical of all. No matter what someone does, no matter how kind or generous their actions may seem, the cynics among us will always assume that the person has a hidden motive and that the motive is based on selfishness.

Today, however, the cynics' views are coming into question. Extensive research by Elliot Sober, Ph.D., professor of research and philosophy at the University of Wisconsin, Madison, and David Sloan Wilson, Ph.D., professor of biology at the State University of New York at Binghamton, shows that unselfish behavior is a vital and true feature of both biological and human nature. Integrating a wide range of studies, they demonstrate how people have evolved the capacity to care for others not as an afterthought, as has often been suggested, but as a central goal in itself for meaningful living.

The Energy in Helping

Helping others is a primary source of heartfelt energy. Research indicates that people who do regular volunteer work have greater life expectancies than those who do not perform such actions.

Whenever you learn something of the challenges that others have faced in their lives, it is your empathy that then deepens and enriches your experience of their efforts and value in the world. When you fail to look deeply at what others have experienced and endured, you lose touch with their vibrancy. When you presume to know what makes people tick but don't really explore their desires, motives, and fears, you can't really appreciate the hidden character of their lives.

I'm not suggesting that you can take on the problems of the world or responsibility for another person's life and try to fix everything and make it right. Rather, I advocate developing the empathy to readily sense where others are and what they need—and to do this with a discerning heart and, at the right times, an open mind and open hand.

In order to have heartfelt energy, we each must allow ourselves to be touched by life, by experiences, and by unique, individual people. Empathy is the outreach from your own heart to the people around you. It must be more than an instinctive and often unpredictable or random response. It must be a conscious attitude. Unless you are moved by the experiences of the heart, then your heart is rarely moved by the experiences of life.

Learning Empathy

One day when my son, Chris, was 11, I noticed him struggling to figure out how to better relate to his new sister Chelsea, who was about 9 months old.

Until this little girl's birth, he had been the only child. It had been years since he'd had much practice being around small children. Now, here was an attention-getting infant who couldn't even talk yet, and he had to fathom how to be her big brother.

That particular day, he noticed a small bird on the grassy yard near the back door to our home. Chris, who has always had a deep love of the outdoors, went right outside and picked up the bird, cupping it gently in his hands. It was trembling. He was trying to feel what was wrong with it, wondering if its wing had been broken.

I happened to be watching, and as I looked on, I was impressed by the gentleness of Chris's attempt to feel the little animal's needs and by the searching curiosity in his eyes. Something was wrong with this bird, and while he wanted to care for it, he also wanted to understand.

Eventually, Chris glanced around at the nearby picture window. I could almost read his thoughts as he concluded that the bird had stunned itself by colliding with one of the windows. He sensed that that was all that was wrong. Chris set the bird gently in the grass at the edge of the woods. He returned to the house. Minutes later, the bird flew away.

Soon afterward, he was holding little Chelsea in his arms. I could detect a change in how he held his little sister. Instead of trying to determine what she needed from her untranslatable movements and unintelligible sounds, he simply held her as he had held the bird, letting his feelings and senses help him understand. It seemed to come more easily to him now.

At the same time, he seemed more engaged with her, more comfortable in relating to her. At this point, she might have appeared to be little more than a helpless thing that needed careful handling. But the fact that he was now able to provide that with more empathy created a new bond between them.

Before the incident with the bird, Chris had been able to observe that Chelsea was helpless, and he was old enough to intellectually understand that she simply couldn't do a lot of things for herself. But when he'd held the bird in his hand, some *feeling* of helplessness was communicated to him that was stronger than objective understanding. I think he began to realize how a small, powerless creature can feel overwhelmed, curious, fearful, and in need. With that understanding of feeling, empathy was born. And Chris's story is a simple example of how empathy can be transferred from one life experience to another.

Getting Connected

It is the quality of your relationships, not just the number of friends that you have, that promotes heartfelt energy and health. People can feel profoundly alone even when surrounded by hundreds of acquaintances, if they aren't truly close to anyone.

The best way to have great friends is to be a great friend, and friendship begins with empathy. The great French author Honoré de Balzac wrote, "Listening to people talking, I could enter into their lives, feel their tattered clothes on my back, walk with my feet in their shoes; their desires, their needs, all passed into my soul, or my soul passed into theirs. It was the dream of a man awake."

In Latin, the word *emotion* means "the spirit that moves us." I don't believe that anything significant has ever been accomplished in human history without feeling. Always in life, there is a depth to each person that few others ever know—only those with empathy and close understanding.

Through feelings of empathy and compassion, you help yourself learn and grow, and you also enable others to begin to feel safe enough to talk about what is really going on in their lives. Then, they can tell their stories without fear of being judged, criticized, or abandoned. Once you begin to empathize with them, you can extend compassion and support to them, rather than remaining distant or unaffected.

When you learn to perceive other people's feelings beneath their words, you're likely to find that your feelings are more clearly understood as well. More often than not, empathy and compassion are returned to you in kind.

Where Empathy Begins

In *Mandela: An Illustrated Autobiography*, the South African leader writes of his 27 years as a political prisoner, "It was during those long and lonely years that my hunger for the freedom of my people became a hunger for the freedom of all people, white and black. I knew as well as I knew anything that the oppressor must be liberated just as surely as the oppressed. The oppressor and oppressed alike are robbed of their freedom."

In empathizing with his oppressor, Nelson Mandela took a leap that many of us may be incapable of accomplishing. He saw those who had taken him from his friends and family, imprisoned him, and tortured him in terms of *their* captivity. Somehow, he was able to understand their dilemma and empathize with it.

More often, in our everyday lives, empathy is not so difficult to achieve. We feel it spontaneously.

Consider the following story. A kindergarten teacher asks her students, "How many of you had breakfast this morning?"

Nearly half of the students raise their hands.

"What was the reason that you didn't eat breakfast?" the teacher asks those who didn't raise their hands.

Some children say that they got up too late and had no time to eat. A few say that no one in their families ate breakfast. One says that there was nothing good for breakfast, and another student agrees.

Then, the teacher comes to one girl who has not yet said anything. "And you, Martha?"

"It wasn't my turn."

"What do you mean?" asks the teacher.

Martha explains that there are eight children in her family and not enough food to go around. "We take turns," she says. "It wasn't my turn today."

What do you feel when you read this story?

Threads of emotion connect you with each experience that you have. You don't have to ponder where these feelings come from or analyze them to know that they exist. Feeling for this girl and empathy for her situation is far less demanding than figuring out a mathematical problem or understanding a foreign language. The feelings are spontaneous.

But then what? When you are engaged with the feelings of life in yourself and others, heartfelt energy has the power to move you, to inspire and activate your involvement. You may be intrigued or alarmed by statistical facts such as the number of children in America who go without breakfast every morning. But people who have the commitment and determination to actually launch a breakfast-for-kids program are likely to be inspired and driven by their empathy for children like Martha.

True, there are times when you may decide that the greatest kindness to another is to hold them responsible and accountable, when you may encourage them to stand fast or step up to the line and face a difficult situation. But that doesn't mean that you feel any less empathy for them.

You can't turn away from empathy. When you ignore human feelings, you inevitably ignore the human being who's experiencing them. That strategy is likely to result in a friend who turns away from you, a coworker who stops bringing energy to the problems that you have to solve, or a family member who no longer shows enthusiasm for new plans and ideas.

In terms of human energy, it can be mildly to severely debilitating to deny what you spontaneously feel or to suppress the impulses that draw you toward other people. The expression of empathy is a release of heartfelt energy, and you'll feel a measurable amount of energy in return.

With empathy, there is a much greater chance that you will focus on the positive things in life rather than on the negative and that you will look deeper than before to respect and value others. This doesn't mean that you approve of everything that you see. It means that your measuring, judging opinions have less of a dominating hold on you.

Getting the Benefits

Empathy and compassion are valuable for the gift that they give to others. These constructive forms of heartfelt energy are also, quite literally, health-enhancing and life-sustaining for those who give them.

According to a study published in the *Journal of Advancement in Medicine*, heart-centered, sincere, positive feelings boost the immune system. On the other hand, immunity may remain suppressed for up to 6 hours following each negative emotional experience.

The human connectedness that is derived from a positive and supportive social network helps you resist disease, enjoy life, and live longer. In fact, the existence of friendships is a good predictor of health and longevity. At the University of New Mexico School of Medicine in Albuquerque, more than 250 elderly individuals participated in a study that evaluated the intimacy and intensity of their relationships. Researchers concluded that people who had strong, open friendships also possessed a number of physical characteristics linked with reduced rates of disease. For example, those in the healthier, more intimate and friendly group had lower blood cholesterol levels and lower uric acid levels than those in other groups.

Sometimes, it takes such little effort to create positive feelings that it's a wonder that people don't take advantage of the opportunities all the time. Take the neighborhood lemonade stand, for instance. I still remember the sign that I put up as a 4-year-old: "Limmenaid 10 sents."

When I was a kid, I tried to make money every way that I could. That lemonade stand was only one method. I also delivered newspapers. I parked and washed cars. I painted fences and mowed lawns. I shoveled snow. My best customers were purchasers on many fronts. They went out of their way to "need" my services.

I remember what this meant to me. In all the years since, I have tried to help children find work. That's not hard to do, of course, especially when you travel. In Tibet, I hired two small boys who begged to "guard" my rented Land Cruiser while I climbed a nearby mountain. They did a great job. The Land Cruiser was still there when I got back. They beamed with pride as I thanked each of them and paid them for helping.

Beginning at a very young age, there is something special that happens inside you when you are entrusted by others to do something that makes you feel valued and proud. And there's something that happens inside you when you pass along some of the heritage of empathy that you've been given. That "something" is heartfelt energy.

Don't get me wrong. It's easy to rush by the kids who want to sell you lemonade, wash your car, or watch your Land Cruiser for a couple of hours. If you shake your head and say no to them, it won't feel like you've denied much—and you may have saved yourself some money and possibly some hassle. But there's a cost after all, the cost of repressing and denying the natural empathy that is part of your makeup.

Maybe you don't believe in paying those eager kids. Maybe it doesn't mean anything to you. That's fine. It isn't really about the money, anyway. It's about the sense of personal responsibility and entrustment. But if it does mean something to you and you don't do it, you may be sacrificing some of the energy that is your lifeblood.

Think Small

The poet William Wordsworth wrote:

Practice small acts of generosity.
The best portions of a good life . . .
Are the little, nameless, unremembered acts
Of kindness and love.

When I was a boy, whenever we would empty our closets and give away the spare clothes to Goodwill or the Salvation Army, my mother suggested that we add one extra item to the pile. Include at least one pair of good, warm socks, she said. This is a piece of clothing that is always appreciated, yet we take it for granted and rarely think to give it to others in need. At the moment that we included the socks, we learned that giving is more than emptying out closets. My mother's words reminded us that we weren't throwing away clothes. Instead, we were helping to meet the needs of other human beings, so we had to be mindful of what they really needed.

The release of heartfelt energy does not require great gestures. Whether you're buying lemonade from a child on the street corner or doing some small housekeeping chore for your spouse, you're expressing that energy in hundreds of often-unseen ways.

The "small acts of generosity" lauded by Wordsworth come in many forms. Pick up a piece of broken glass from the sidewalk and throw it away; no one will step on it. Put money in a parking meter for someone you don't know; you'll save them getting a ticket. Stop for a moment to smile at a toddler; the child may remember it all day. Share a word with the person at the checkout counter or front desk; you'll remind them that you appreciate what they're doing for you.

You don't need to do these things because it's a law or duty. The only reason to take these actions is because your heartfelt energy prompts you to do it. It is the most practical way of all to find new energy when you feel depleted.

Notes of Appreciation

There is increasing scientific evidence that gratitude and appreciation, when they are genuine and specific, not only increase heartfelt energy but also ignite it in others. This is particularly important between spouses or partners who live together, sharing many common day-to-day, emotional contacts.

Even when things are tough, you gain heartfelt energy when you find something to be grateful for and express your gratitude genuinely and

I CAN LIVE FOR A MONTH

ON **ONE GOOD COMPLIMENT**.

—Mark Twain (1835–1910), U.S. author and humorist

specifically. In fact, there are specific actions that you can take to show your appreciation and express it openly.

Use validation. This can come in the form of any comment, compliment, or appreciative remark that lets another person know that you understand them. "Validation is simply putting yourself in your partner's shoes and imagining his or her emotional state," explains John M. Gottman, Ph.D., professor of psychology at the University of Washington in Seattle and a leading researcher on what makes relationships work. "It's then a simple matter to let your mate know that you understand those feelings and consider them valid, even if you don't share them. Validation is an amazingly effective technique. It's as if you opened a door to welcome your partner."

Validation can take many forms, such as acknowledging responsibility (admitting, "Yes, I know this upsets you" or "It feels like I really made you angry"), apologizing (saying, "I'm sorry; I was wrong"), or expressing compliments (assuring, "I admire what you did" or "You have a talent for . . ."). Such validation can have a remarkably positive effect on the rest of the conversation, Dr. Gottman points out.

Express appreciation. How many times has your day been brightened by one small, unexpected gesture of appreciation or caring? Appreciation is not necessarily a grand gesture like buying a car, a piece of jewelry, or a refrigerator. Try loving glances, kind words, and a gentle touch on the arm.

Many women readily say that the little things matter much more than the big gestures that men sometimes feel obliged to make. What about sitting close together when you're watching television? Or what about checking with each other first before making plans? Do you occasionally buy flowers? Do you write thank-you notes? Between partners, these are often the most significant and expressive signs of appreciation.

"The casual details of everyday life are what allow long-term relationships to survive," observes William Nagler, M.D., psychiatrist at the University of California, Los Angeles, School of Medicine, who specializes in effective relationship communication.

Complete some sentences. No one likes to have their sentences finished for them. But in the right atmosphere, there's one kind of sentence completion that can actually help forge empathy within a relationship and restore heartfelt energy that may be waning. Spend a few minutes taking turns completing the following sentences with your partner or spouse.

- I feel valued when you. . . .
- I feel most respected when you. . . .
- I appreciate you the most because. . . .
- Here's the specific kind of respect, caring, and appreciation that I want and deserve. . . .

Remember to say please and thank you. I don't think that I'm the only one who has noticed that manners are falling by the wayside. This collapse of courtesy is leading to a loss of caring and cooperation. An overwhelming majority of Americans—89 percent in a recent nationwide poll—believe that incivility is a serious problem and is getting worse. Feel what happens each time you say please and thank you. Go against the tide and take action to bring courtesy back to your neighborhood.

Open the Lines of Communication

Some of the elements once thought to be vital to relationship success—love, similar backgrounds, coming from well-adjusted families—are secondary to how well a couple communicates and even argues, says Howard J. Markman, Ph.D., director of the Center for Marital and Family Studies in Denver, who, along with his colleagues, has spent nearly 2 decades studying what makes successful marriages work.

In a study of 325 married male executives, researchers found a strong correlation between the men's expressiveness and marital happiness. Expressiveness was defined as the man's taking an active interest in his wife, talking with her about herself and her concerns, and expressing affection toward her. Eighty percent of the marriages in which the husband saw expressiveness as an important part of the relationship were happy. This was in sharp contrast to the marriages in which the husband said that he did not value expressiveness. Nearly an equal percentage of those couples described themselves as being unhappy.

Based on long-term research, here are important pieces of day-in, day-out advice for men and women.

For men: Try not to avoid conflict. Sidestepping a problem or complaint won't make it disappear. You may feel uncomfortable when your wife vents her feelings, but in fact, by venting her feelings she's able to help keep your relationship healthy and secure.

For women: Confront him clearly but gently. For many reasons, in most relationships it's up to the woman to raise most of the important issues. But an outburst is not necessary, and it's likely to make your partner resist and withdraw. Can you be flexible enough to present the issues in a calm, clear, and gentle way? Be pleasantly persistent if he seems driven to keep changing the subject. Let him know that you are not attacking him and that you need him to join you in facing issues and conflicts in your relationship.

When Someone Stonewalls

As long as partners can communicate, heartfelt energy is alive in the relationship. But what happens when one spouse suddenly stops communicating and becomes silent? This withdrawal is known as stonewalling, and it can drain as much energy from a relationship as all the arguments on record.

Often, it's the man who stonewalls. He does so when he hears or anticipates criticism or senses that his wife is bringing up a difficult issue. When he feels threatened or overwhelmed, he withdraws. It's as if a wall went up. He avoids eye contact, barely moves his face, keeps his neck rigid, and even neglects to utter such simple acknowledgments as "Yes, I see" or "Uh-huh."

According to researchers, many women think out loud, sharing their struggles with their listeners and to some extent discovering what they want to say through the process of talking. But many men tend to process information differently. They tend to first silently mull over or think about what they've just heard or experienced.

Even though it's not fair, when a man stonewalls it often seems to be up to his wife to take control of what happens next. Dr. Gottman and other researchers have discovered that, in happy marriages, the wife usually interrupts the argument cycle. She ignores a negative comment or says something positive in the face of stonewalling behavior.

One of the challenges for women is to correctly interpret and support a man when he isn't talking. Women need to understand that often a man's silence means, "I don't know what to say yet, but I am thinking about it." Instead, women think that his silence means, "I am not responding to you because I don't care about you and I'm going to ignore you. What you have said to me is not important and therefore I am not responding."

Confide in Those You Trust

During challenging times, you especially need heartfelt energy. To keep this energy going strong, you must be honest with yourself and relate well to others. Without open, honest conversations, you can't come to know others well enough to trust them or count on them.

According to researchers, one of the most effective and meaningful ways to raise heartfelt energy and improve mind-body health can come from increasing your willingness to express your mistakes, confide your secrets, and reveal your hopes and fears. These expressions can take the form of either writing privately in a journal or confiding in a loved one, close friend, or trained counselor.

When the National Opinion Research Center asked the question "Looking over the last 6 months, who are the people with whom you discussed matters that are important to you?" those who described themselves as very happy were most likely to be people who could name at least five friends or relatives as confidants.

Researchers have discovered that suppressing deep guilt and misery, either consciously or subconsciously, requires such arduous physical effort that it takes a toll on your health. However, those who confide their troubles in a private diary, writing for as little as 5 to 15 minutes a day for 3 days, often experience marked improvements in their energy levels, attitudes, and immune function.

The Write Stuff

It may seem unlikely that writing things down could boost your heartfelt energy as well as confiding in another person can. But the very act of expressing your thoughts and feelings on paper seems to have the power to release all kinds of emotions.

"The benefits of writing lie in the act of letting go and expressing those deepest thoughts and feelings surrounding a personal upheaval," say psychologists Martha E. Francis, Ph.D., and James W. Pennebaker, Ph.D., of Southern Methodist University in Dallas. Based on their observations, they conclude that privacy is an essential component of writing to release heartfelt energy. "We encourage individuals to write for themselves as opposed to writing for someone else. . . . And people who write about personally upsetting experiences report that it is important for their essays to be kept anonymous and confidential."

In fact, it may even be best to destroy what you have written. Planning to share your thoughts and feelings with someone else can affect your mind-set while you write. "From a health perspective, you'll be better off simply making yourself the audience," says Dr. Pennebaker.

When writing, focus on the issues with which you are currently living, and explore both the objective experience (what is happening) and your feelings about it. Really let go, advises Dr. Pennebaker. What do you feel about it? Why do you feel that way?

Don't be concerned about temporarily feeling worse. "As we have found in all of our studies," observes Dr. Pennebaker, "you may feel sad or depressed immediately after writing. These negative feelings usually dissipate within an hour or so. In rare cases, they may last a day or two." But Dr. Pennebaker reports that the overwhelming majority of the volunteers who participated in the research reported feelings of relief, happiness, and contentment soon after the studies were concluded.

In many ways, the writing process can free you to express closely held emotions, allowing you to articulate these feelings at appropriate times with people you can trust. Even though the act of writing is personal and private, it may ultimately allow a greater sense of connectedness and renewed energy.

Discover Your Passion

What inspires the greatest enthusiasm in you? Can you turn a simple task or boring effort into an amazing and invigorating project that makes a difference and feels great? It isn't always possible, but more often than most of us realize, it can be done.

And there's a good reason to try. When you're doing things that inspire your passion, you don't need to worry about having enough energy. Heartfelt energy is ready and waiting, and as soon as you start to do things that you love, it comes bubbling to the surface.

But maybe it's not so easy to say what inspires your passion. Many of us had great dreams that cast magical spells on us during childhood. But there are few people who have seen most of their dreams come true. More often, we end up doing less and less of what we aspire to do, the things that we feel most passionate about, as adult life creeps up on us and we make choices that seem practical, rational, and sound.

So the first challenge may be this: Think of the times when you've felt most excited about things that were happening in your life. Think of the times when you had the following thoughts.

- Life is a blast.
- I'm thrilled to be doing this.
- I'm amazed at how much fun learning can be.
- I feel exhilarated and deeply enthusiastic.
- I feel deeply contented and satisfied.

The things that made you feel this way are some of the many sources of passion in your life. Have you been enjoying and developing any of them lately? If not, my question is "Why not?"

The Search Continues

In my experience, people do not discover their passions suddenly, out of the blue. Rather, we make continuous, ongoing discoveries about what we most love to learn and do.

In a sense, our passions begin teaching us even before we find them. But we have to be open to their influence. If we don't notice them, if we're numb, rushing headlong into the future, out of touch with our own hearts, we have to become more observant.

Take note whenever you feel the most excited and enthused with life or work. When you're talking and you see others' eyes light up, pay extra-close attention. It likely means that their passion is bubbling up, coming across, being communicated.

There are a number of fundamental ways to make discoveries about your most deeply compelling life interests, which is how some researchers refer to passions. Among them are:

AT ITS BEST, **LIFE IS PASSION**.

WITHOUT PASSION, WORK, LOVE, NOVELS,

ART, AND RELIGION ARE INEFFECTUAL.

—Honoré de Balzac, *La comédie humaine*, 1841

Your intuition. Be aware of the innate, persistent pull of the things that you get a kick out of doing.

Daily life. As you go through your day, note the contrast between things that you most enjoy doing and those that you don't like to do.

Life events. During difficult or challenging times, passions often come to the surface. Be aware of your reactions to birth, illness, marriage, divorce, changes in jobs, moves, or the death of a friend or loved one. Often, these are the occasions when life feels most fragile and precious and when we vow to spend more time doing what really matters to us.

Bolts out of the blue. Once in a while, life-changing events happen—near-death experiences, fortunate encounters with people who inspire or lead you, sudden awakenings. These and similar twists of fate can reveal deep passions within you and challenge you to pursue them.

Above all, keep in mind that passion and enthusiasm are natural parts of who you are. You don't need to wish for them; they're always within reach. You only need to give them a way to emerge and then thrive in your life and work. Sometimes, just writing a few morning notes, whether carefully thought out or scribbled in haste, is all you need to do to connect your inner heart with your outer actions and to better understand and appreciate the source of your passion.

Make LifeNotes

Whenever you put pen to paper, you make it easier to connect your heart—that is, your deep, sincere, authentic self—with your words.

A number of times in this book, I have suggested note-making methods that can help you tap into your personal sources of energy. I have another favorite way of doing this: creating what I call LifeNotes.

In order to utilize LifeNotes, you have to be willing to be emotionally honest with yourself. Other than that, all it takes is 2 to 3 minutes in the morning, plus paper and a pen. Here's what to do.

Get up 5 minutes earlier than usual, find your favorite well-lit spot, sit quietly, and listen deeply. Then, just write whatever you feel about what's going on in your life.

This is not a head exercise. If you try to outline your LifeNotes or put your thoughts in logical order, you risk turning this into an academic assignment. Instead, just seize this opportunity to openly reflect on your life and work. No matter how random or rough your thoughts, continue writing until you have something down on paper.

With emotionally honest writing such as this, you bypass what Michael Ray, Ph.D., professor of marketing and innovation at Stanford University, calls the voice of judgment. It won't take long before you feel the connection of heart and hand, without the mind acting as censor and inner critic. The key is to just write whatever you feel. It's an amazing thing: Your writing hand seems tied to your heart and finds it hard to lie.

Run-On Senses

Chances are that, if you just start writing and don't worry about form or grammar, a lot of what you express will be pet peeves and nagging frustrations. Great. Write them down.

Or you may find yourself intuitively exploring old resentments or new opportunities. Whatever comes up, it's real. And, according to researchers, it can offer a better way to navigate through the upcoming day or life in general. It's like the satisfaction you get from reading an honest, well-told story of someone's life. In this case, it's your own life story, honestly told, for your eyes only.

These notes are a good way to become more aware that your innermost thoughts and feelings have value. They are *your* truth, and never mind whether they're factually or technically accurate or truthful.

I've found, over time, that LifeNotes have enabled me to make more heartfelt and sincere presentations of how I see a situation or how I feel about a possibility that I'm facing in my work or life. And since these notes are for my eyes alone, they also help me realize more clearly that these are my thoughts, my feelings. I'm not at all surprised to discover that others may feel very differently about things and may hold their views just as passionately as I hold mine.

In light of this, I find myself disappointed less often. But also, I don't feel swayed or coerced into a changing view of my own feelings and enthusiasms. Because I know and trust my own feelings, I can instinctively value the differences between my own views and another person's, instead of resenting other viewpoints or feeling compelled to change them. We simply have different passions, you and I, and so it seems quite reasonable that your sense of truth and purpose does not need to be in line with my own.

Hitting the Right Notes

When you're jotting LifeNotes, make sure that you don't judge yourself. You never need to worry about what others may think, feel, or say if they knew what you were expressing. They'll never see these pages.

"We dream our lives in grand gestures," writes Kent Nerburn, a noted sculptor with a doctorate of philosophy in religion and art, "but we live our lives in small moments." Your LifeNotes give you the chance to get in touch with those small moments every morning, every day of the week.

LifeNotes are designed as a straightforward means of eliciting emotional honesty. You have plenty of wisdom. Let it come to the fore, and you can begin using it more effectively.

Here are some of the questions to ask yourself when you're writing.

- How did I listen to my passions and follow them yesterday?
- What can I do today?
- Who can help me increase my enthusiasm for and commitment to doing more of what I most love or may soon learn to love?
- How can I close the gap between where I am and where I most want to be?
- Today, will I do what I really want to do? Or am I just planning to do the same thing that I did yesterday?
- Is what I have what I really want, or have I settled for something less because it was easier or safer?

From time to time, you may have a creative breakthrough or some deep insight about yourself and others. Or you may get clearer about what questions to ask.

I encourage you to commit to trying LifeNotes for a minimum of a few minutes each morning, for 21 days, or 3 weeks. I believe that you'll be amazed at several things. First, you'll note the initial strength of your mental critic, the little voice in your head that says, "What a dumb idea. What a waste of time. Emotional honesty? Hah!" Second, you'll start to distinguish between your emotional buttons, the issues that make you incensed or off-balance almost instantly, and the deeper feelings or con-

WE MAY AFFIRM THAT ABSOLUTELY **NOTHING GREAT**
IN THE WORLD **HAS BEEN ACCOMPLISHED**
WITHOUT PASSION.

—Georg W. Hegel, *Philosophy of History*, 1832

cerns that are hidden beneath them. You'll start to understand your own unique emotional makeup, your strengths and vulnerabilities.

By the end of the very first week, I think that you'll start to feel a bit lighter and more energized when you finish writing. You'll recognize that you are, in fact, more prepared to be open, honest, and creative throughout the day.

Things to Touch On

If you have days or even weeks when nothing seems to spark your imagination or excite you, you may need a jump start to rediscover your heartfelt energy. One way to make that rediscovery is with affirmations that can help bring your enthusiasms into focus. Here are several practical things to consider.

Acknowledge that there's no one else like you. This sounds like common sense, but it's not common practice. One reason for this is that we live in a world that is trying, in hundreds of ways, to make us feel invisible, dispensable, and interchangeable rather than like one-of-a-kind individuals with untapped energy.

Sometimes, we're so quick to see what's wrong in ourselves, in other people, and in situations that it's almost as if we were trained to notice deficits. For a few minutes, just for practice, think of some greatness in one other person. Then think of some rare and invigorating qualities that you have. How can you build upon those qualities?

When you plan for what's next, begin with your heart instead of with your head. There's a growing body of evidence that the highest reasoning depends on emotional intelligence—the ability to sense and apply the feeling side of intellect—as well as on mental intelligence. What are your longest-held and most compelling life interests? These passions help define which kinds of activities make you feel most committed and, ultimately, most contented.

"Think of a deeply embedded life interest as a geothermal pool of superheated water," Harvard University researchers Timothy Butler and James Waldroop suggest. "It will rise to the surface in one place as a hot spring and in another as a geyser. But beneath the surface—at the core of the individual—the pool is constantly bubbling."

If you recognize and respect what bubbles up, you'll introduce more heartfelt energy into your decision making. If you try to make a decision and one course of action just feels wrong, don't try to explain it away. That feeling is bubbling up from somewhere. Maybe it comes from a fear that you want to conquer. Or maybe it's the instinctive knowledge that the course of action isn't in line with your goals and your values. Either way, your heartfelt energy is sending up a message, and you need to pay attention to whatever rises to the surface.

Ask "Why not?" rather than "Why?" There's no way that you can anticipate what a new experience will be like, so why not go for it? It could be something that challenges you to learn and grow. It could be an experience that you enjoy, even love. If you approach experiences with a willingness for the best to happen, you will find the courage to do more and doubt less. Each choice can help build up your spirit of confidence.

Don't delay. We live in a paradoxical full-speed-ahead society of skilled procrastinators. Don't postpone things. I'm not suggesting that you engage in frenetic motion or chronic rushing; I'm suggesting that you have an attitude and exuberance for life based on continued exploration. Each time you delay the pursuit of your passion, a bit more of your natural exuberance dies and it gets harder to do what you're passionate about. Listen to your heart, and move accordingly.

Move Ahead

Anything that blocks your strengths, talents, and passions can leave you feeling empty, frustrated, or just plain lost. You certainly want to remove those blockages to get rid of the things that stand in your way. The question is, how?

"Where your talents and the needs of the world cross, therein awaits your vocation," Aristotle said. One of the challenges of living a high-energy life is finding or creating the work that you were born to do. This can happen in a thousand small ways. Perhaps you can speak out and loosen your job descriptions, asking to do more of what you love to do and less of what you don't. Perhaps the key is offering to take greater responsibility for the results that you produce and the discoveries that you make along the way.

You were born with unique potential. But often, you probably just try to make do, go along, and get by. Deeper in your heart, a voice tells you that there's no getting away from the calling or prompting of your passion.

Fortunately, when you begin to obey that voice and more actively pursue your passions, you'll find more energy than you knew you had. That's your heartfelt energy.

How will you know? It's when you end up saying things like "I couldn't not do it" or "I couldn't be silent; I had to raise my voice and take a stand" or "I had to step forward; there was nothing else for me to do." Often, when you have these feelings, you just have to act on them. As you do, your actions shape what you become. You discover how to listen more closely to the inner voice that guides you to your heartfelt energy.

And, just as naturally, that inner voice will speak to others. When you realize your deepest sources of enthusiasm for life and become clearer about what your passions are, you'll find that you'll want to talk about them and share them openly and honestly. Yes, it takes some fearlessness to explore what the human heart feels and knows. But few efforts in life pay greater dividends in either energy or happiness.

Leave Your Imprint

T he story came in a news report, and once I'd heard it, I couldn't stop wondering about how it had happened and thinking about all of its ramifications and implications. It concerned a young public-school teacher. She had been teaching for 8 years. She was used to the routine, but eager for a challenge. She hoped to be given a class of gifted students.

On the first day of preparation week, prior to the start of classes, she opened her packet of registration materials. As in previous years, there was a one-page listing of the students in her class. And alongside each name, as was customary in this school, the school administrators had listed each student's IQ score in bold type.

The teacher blinked. All of the numbers were in a remarkably high range—from 130 to 155.

The teacher was delighted. She knew that the year would hold more challenges than ever before. For this class, she would have to prepare harder and more creatively. She would have to make sure that every stu-

MOST PEOPLE LIVE IN A VERY RESTRICTED CIRCLE OF THEIR POTENTIAL BEING. **WE ALL HAVE RESERVOIRS OF GENIUS** TO DRAW UPON, OF WHICH WE DO NOT DREAM.

—William James, *Energies*, 1899

dent received individual attention and got challenging assignments. She could help them excel; she knew it.

She also knew that this group would, in all likelihood, be far better mannered than any previous class that she had taught. She anticipated fewer discipline problems.

After scanning the rest of her registration packet, she set about getting ready for her students. Knowing that gifted children need to have class work tailored to their unique needs, the teacher gathered new resources and devised a wide range of opportunities for extra credit.

On the first day of class, according to the news story, she told the class, "It's wonderful to have the opportunity to work with students as gifted as each of you." The students met her expectations, even exceeded them. They were enthusiastic and attentive, snapped up the extra-credit projects, and plunged wholeheartedly into lively classroom discussions.

More parents got involved than ever before, and the teacher herself was continually challenged, searching for new and more inventive ways to bring out the genius in each individual. She gave genuine and specific recognition for each student's efforts, writing out personal notes of congratulation. She worked longer and harder than ever before in her career as a teacher, but the work was both fun and challenging. She was having the time of her life.

Judging from interviews with parents, students, and administrators, it was a remarkably successful year for this group of students. Many students noted extraordinary achievements, and they received numerous awards for successful work that went well beyond their grade level.

No one, least of all the teacher, was prepared for the revelation that came at the end of the school year. Appearing for her administrative review in June, the teacher was congratulated by the principal. It had obviously been an exemplary year. Their conversation after that, as she recalled it, went something like this.

"I knew this would be possible once you gave me the class of gifted students," she said.

"What do you mean?" asked the principal.

She reminded him of the stellar IQ score of each of the students in her class. And she thanked the principal for giving her the gifted class.

"Oh, no," the principal explained. "Those weren't IQ scores."

That year, the school had changed its policy. Attorneys had advised the administration that IQ scores should be kept completely private. So they had been omitted from the class list. It had all been explained in the registration packet. But the teacher realized that in her excitement about teaching the new class of gifted students, she hadn't bothered to carefully read all of the introductory materials that came with her class list.

If those weren't IQ scores, she asked, what were they?

"Locker numbers," replied the principal.

Trusting That There's Greatness in Others Helps Make It So

It's not hard to see why I thought this story was memorable. As an experiment in education, motivation, and human interactions, it would be hard to devise more elegant proof of the power of positive influence. Here is a teacher who, because of her belief about the genius in her students and a newly regenerated enthusiasm for herself, created the kind

(continued on page 418)

The Heart's Horizon

Heartfelt energy often travels by circuitous routes. You leave all kinds of messages. Only some of those messages are transmitted by words. Other messages are conveyed by the way you live, the example that you set with your own life. And there's yet a third kind of message—the feelings that others have when they're around you.

You can never tell who will read your written messages, nor do you know how many people will experience the more intangible messages that come from being in your presence or sharing your emotional life. Yet your words, feelings, and actions leave powerful threads of heartfelt energy that travel through time.

Whenever you face one of life's great challenges, it's easy to feel overburdened and overwhelmed by what seems to be expected of you. What's vital at such times is a clear sense of history and memory. I call this the heart's horizon. It can be one of the most vital ways to regain your perspective. Often, the heart's horizon is expanded by the thoughts, memories, or legacies that are passed on from generation to generation.

Here is a journal entry from Helen Downing, 8 years old. Her mother was sitting by her bed and recorded what she had to say. The date was December 7, 1934. The entry reads:

> I love to look up at the sky and sun and stars. When will I do that again?
> My favorite story is about Heidi. I dream about the Swiss mountains,
>   which I have never seen. I hope to go there sometime.
> I like laughing and holding flowers in my hands. I like feeling the wind in
>   my hair. I want to run and dance again. What will tomorrow bring
>   when I wake up in the world?

Helen, the child who spoke those words in 1934, was an aunt I never knew. My grandmother, the woman at her bedside, knew that Helen had spinal meningitis. In those days, there was not yet a cure for the disease. Helen was at the Mayo Clinic, where my grandfather, who was a surgeon, and a team of physicians and nurses worked for 6 days trying to save her life. She died on December 8, 1934, the day after this journal entry was written.

I have such a strong sense of that 8-year-old's imprint on the world, on my grandmother and grandfather, on my mother, and, even as I read and record these words, on me. Because of my grandmother's great love and care for that child, I learned the words spoken by that 8-year-old girl the day before she died. To me and to so many others in my family, this moment is part of the heart's horizon. It exists in our family's history as the moment when darkness moved in. But because life goes on and generation follows generation—and because all families have survived such tragedies—the message left by this little girl can speak to you as well as to me.

My grandmother's prayer, after the funeral, was "May I be in a measure worthy of her memory."

Throughout history, philosophers have said that it is only when the days of our lives are framed by our own mortality that we are truly alive. There's no way to plan or prepare for the moments that will leave an imprint on others, that will transmit our heartfelt energy into the future. Any moment could be the one that counts. That's why it's so important to make every moment feel more compelling and valuable.

of school year that leaves a lasting influence on the students, parents, school, community, and probably on other teachers as well.

What actually changed in her world to make this remarkable year possible? She simply believed in her heart that her students were gifted. She reinforced their belief in themselves with her own belief that they were, indeed, geniuses in their own unique ways and that they could accomplish remarkable things. She further reinforced her own belief, and theirs, by putting exceptional creative effort into her work. And not surprisingly, each of those students rewarded her efforts and their own by producing exceptional results.

It's this kind of interpersonal, human alchemy that so often has scientists of human behavior wondering just what they're dealing with. After all, IQ tests have been valued by educators for decades because their results are measurable, quantifiable. They are relatively fixed, or permanent. They seem to tell us a great deal—though, assuredly, not everything and perhaps not much—about the intellects of those who take the tests.

But as we are now discovering, IQ reflects at most a very small part of the full story of a person's strengths, talents, and successes in life and work. As this story so vividly illustrates, all the other qualities of intelligence, including curiosity, creativity, and a sense of self-worth, are profoundly affected by immeasurable influences such as a teacher's respect. If a teacher believes in a student, that student will often shine.

Not only that, but this story tells us that the teacher, too, is likely to perform better. The student's response inspires the teacher to be more involved, more creative, more inspiring, and more challenging in ways that lift that student to new heights.

What a testimony to heartfelt energy. There was enough in one teacher to feed an entire classroom of students and significantly change their performance for an entire year. And when you look at everything that went on in that creative dynamic, you don't get a simple formula.

But you do get a simple fact: If we use our heartfelt energy, we have the power to leave an imprint on other people's lives.

"On the surface," wrote philosopher Abraham Heschel in 1965, "I am an average person, but to my heart I am not an average person. To my heart, I am a great moment. The challenge I must face is how to give everything I have inside to fulfilling this moment."

Shaping Things to Come

Ideally, of course, we would learn another lesson from this teacher who was so wonderfully deluded by locker numbers. We would learn to look at everyone, including ourselves, as a one-of-a-kind genius.

What if we could do that? Let's say that we could treat each person as someone who could learn best and contribute the most only when enabled to discover, develop, and live their passions. What might be possible? Wouldn't that help bring out the hidden genius or greatness in every person we meet and, quite possibly, the genius in ourselves?

I have mentioned my grandparents a number of times in this book. It's absolutely clear to me how, along with my parents and a few key mentors in my life, they left their marks. I can feel the warmth of their good wishes for me, their love, and their conviction that, if they spoke carefully enough and showed me by example what was important to them, I would learn. They left their imprints on me in many ways. Here's one small example that comes to mind.

When I was about 10, I had been spending lots of time after school playing baseball. One day during practice, I quit early and headed home. On the way, I stopped at my grandparents' house.

My grandfather was puzzled that I had quit early, and he asked me why.

"I just don't like it," I replied.

I can still see the expression in my grandfather's eyes as he wondered

THE RUNG OF A LADDER WAS NEVER MEANT TO REST UPON, BUT ONLY TO SUPPORT YOU LONG ENOUGH TO ENABLE YOU TO **REACH FOR SOMETHING HIGHER**.

—Thomas Henry Huxley (1825–1895), English biologist and essayist

to himself whether he should force me to go back and keep practicing. I'd obviously had my fill of playing catch and swinging the bat. Of course, he could give me a lecture on the great importance of practice, practice, practice. But would that inspire me, or would it make me more defensive than he sensed I already was?

Instead, he motioned for me to follow him into the small, dusty storage building along the driveway to his house. Before I could ask what we were doing in there, he reached up to a high shelf and retrieved a dusty baseball glove. The glove looked odd—small, thick-fingered, and darkened with age. The only time I'd seen a glove like this was in sepia photographs of baseball history. It was the kind of glove that you'd expect to find in the Baseball Hall of Fame next to a picture of baseball founder Abner Doubleday, not tucked on a shelf in a darkened storage building.

My grandfather handed it to me. As I looked at the leathery relic, turning it this way and that in my hand, he explained that it had belonged to his brother, Will. As a young man growing up in the 1890s, Will had been an early enthusiast of the newly created game of baseball.

I was puzzled. Knowing that my grandfather had an innate dislike for quitters, I braced once again for the expected lecture on the value of perseverance and tenacity. Instead, he said nothing and simply watched me holding his brother's glove.

Taking out his handkerchief, my grandfather gently wiped away the dust from the glove. "Try it on," he said.

I slid my hand inside. My fingers were too small to fit snugly. Will, after all, had probably been twice my age when he wore this glove. Even though it was a loose fit, I could clearly feel something inside: the imprint of another young man's hand in the leather.

"It doesn't fit me," I said.

"That's because you'd have to make it your own first," my grandfather nodded. "You'd have to break it in."

My grandfather explained that Will's coach had instructed him with great care on how to break in the glove, and Will had followed the instructions to the letter. He'd soaked it, then worked it by hand and left it wrapped tightly around a baseball at night. Through innumerable practices and games, the finger pads and pocket of the glove had eventually been shaped to exactly fit his hand.

"You are touching Will's hand," my grandfather said.

Inside the glove, my fingers tingled. For a few moments, it was as if Will's hand, the hand that had created these indentations, were alive there, even in memory, after all those years. Just then, the glove was more than an old leather baseball mitt. It was the mark or very essence of another person's life in another time and place.

"Robert, you know that you don't have to keep playing baseball," said my grandfather. "There are many other pursuits in your life that you already seem to love more than this game. You must keep learning to know what you're most drawn to do and then to follow these things with energy and commitment. But before you say goodbye to baseball, I want you to carefully remember the shape of Will's hand. Whenever you touch something, you have the chance to shape it and make it your own."

With the afternoon light shining through the doorway, my grandfather turned away and walked from the storage building, leaving me with the old baseball glove of his younger brother who had died long ago.

Imprints

That was 40 years ago. I love to play catch with my children and friends, but I don't play baseball these days. I've gone on to many other things, and I have listened to my grandfather's advice in trying to find my way in life. But as I write these words, I remember the shape and feel of that glove.

Just as we have the power to shape things, we are shaped by them. I believe that this imprint is the deepest energy switch in the human heart.

It takes time to shape a glove. It takes time to shape a life or a passionate pursuit or a dream or a growing child. Everything that we shape takes time. But that time isn't made up of years; it's made up of small moments that eventually turn into years. In essence, what we are shaping and becoming is always within our reach.

I suppose that for many people, it's obvious—when they stop long enough to reflect on it—why we often don't spend the time to more wholeheartedly and clearly shape what we leave behind. We get too busy. We lose energy. We lose touch.

Whenever we lose sight of the unique imprint we are shaping, or failing to shape, that oversight can become the source of many disappointments. Years later, these are the regrets that many people feel most acutely. Deep satisfaction, the heartfelt energy that truly comes from the heart, can be expressed only when we are aware of our imprints as we are making them. Every day, not only sometime later on, we each need to know that our efforts have counted in specific ways.

Meaning is not something that you trip over, or snap in place like the pieces of a puzzle. It is something that we each must weave into our lives. The threads are within you. You can draw them together. And when you do, the pattern is unique—and lasting.

Part 6

Conclusion

Trust Your Skillpower

In one of my earlier books, I made the argument that the quality that we call willpower is often overrated. What we need to develop instead is something quite different. However strong or weak our willpower, we really need *skillpower* to reach our goals as quickly, easily, and smoothly as possible.

Willpower alone won't work. In fact, trying to exercise willpower all the time is a severe energy drainer. Whenever you're under pressure, your brain's natural instinct is to do more of the same, only harder, longer, and faster. You buckle down. You implore yourself to never waver. You struggle to reach your goals. All those reactions to pressure involve willpower, but as you've probably discovered, trying to exercise your willpower all the time can be demoralizing and exhausting.

In fact, the belief in willpower is a kind of magical thinking. What is willpower, after all? To some people, it's like a lucky rabbit's foot. Carry it around all the time, and maybe, just maybe, you'll be lucky enough to

APPROACH EVERY DAY IN YOUR LIFE
AS IF IT WERE YOUR LAST.

—Marcus Aurelius Antoninus (A.D. 121–180), Roman emperor

have all the energy that you need to get everything done. In other words, if you believe in willpower, you also believe that you'll find the energy somewhere, somehow, mysteriously, just at the moment when you need it. Tensions rise. Effort increases. But results?

More often than we assume, willpower is not required. Despite repeated attempts, all that these struggling efforts have frequently done is to make us feel exhausted, depleted, and worn down.

Now what? This is where skillpower comes in. No, you don't have to work harder. You don't have to push nonstop or add more strain to your life to feel energized. You can use 21st-century skills to excel at 21st-century life.

Why More Skill Than Will

You don't need to rely on repeated doses of willpower if you have the skills that you need. The 20 switches that turn on energy can be simply and readily learned, practiced, and repeated. Each one of those switches is supported by scientific insights from experts and specialists who have observed that specific outcomes are the results of specific actions.

Many of us have come to believe or at least hope that because something has been spoken out loud or has been written on an action list, it will actually happen on its own—puff, like magic.

In contrast, the energy switches in this book are actually what some scientists call mechanisms, which are the means by which a result is achieved or a purpose is accomplished. This goes beyond willpower, goal-setting, or planning. It's about how you actually make more of the right things happen.

Mechanisms are simple, specific, measurable changes in how you face life and work, in how you act, interact, create, move, listen, pause, and get things done. With these mechanisms, you close the distance between where you are and where you want to be.

Skills in Action

As you've seen in this book, you can readily increase the four different kinds of human energy that help make you feel 100 percent alive. But if you're going to use the critical energy switches, you need to practice them. Some of these skills may come almost automatically, and you can use them instinctively. But others require testing and practice. Otherwise, they may be lost or forgotten. That's why it's so important to trust your skillpower.

If some of these skills are completely new to you, they may not be automatic at first. In fact, when you're in circumstances that cause tension or distress, you may feel as if you've forgotten all the energy switches you ever learned. Instead, you may have an instinctive fight-or-flight reaction. That is, you either want to attack the problem furiously or you want to run away. Those are natural responses.

But they aren't the best responses. What I'm suggesting is that, one at a time, you put your trust in the energy switches that are described in this book. Test them. Every day, you face circumstances that call for energy switches. Not just situations that produce tension or stress but also those that produce fatigue, boredom, disinterest, and lapses of memory.

When you're in these situations, when you're feeling overwhelmed or stuck, I encourage you to test the energy switches.

Whenever you find yourself saying, "I don't have time to stop what I'm doing, even for a moment," consider the "energy win" from a brief break or pause.

For example, think about how you're feeling right now, at this exact moment. If you're fading, you can use Active-Energy Switch # 1: Plan Your Time-Outs to take a quick break and return to this book again with sharpened attention. Or perhaps the tension has been gathering in your back, neck, and shoulders, and you need Calm-Energy Switch #3: Hold Your Head High. Or you might be reading too slowly and losing energy because your mind is dragged down by the pace. Use Sensory-Energy Switch #4: Strengthen Your Sight Skills.

Next, shift your concentration from this book to some interaction, task, or event that's coming up. Think about something that you've been putting off, an expectation or obligation that you literally get tired just thinking about. Have you been blaming yourself for not getting it accomplished? Well, you can skip the guilt and just trust your skillpower. If the prospect of that task makes you tense and nervous and you don't feel like you ever have time for it, maybe you need Calm-Energy Switch #5: Find Breathing Space to discover how that task can be valuable, enjoyable, or amusing. Or call on Heartfelt-Energy Switch #2: Ask Openly and Listen Deeply. If your upcoming obligation involves communicating with other people, heartfelt-energy switches, such as Switch #1: Engage People Eye to Eye or Switch #3: Empathize, may be your best sources of renewed energy.

In other words, if you trust the switches that you've learned about and tested, you know you don't need to rely on old habits of tension or willpower. You have the skills to turn on the energy you need, when you

LET THE BODY THINK

OF ENERGY AS STREAMING, POURING

RUSHING AND SHINING INTO IT FROM

ALL SIDES.

—Plotinus (A.D. 205–270), Roman philosopher

need it. And when you trust the skills that you've learned, you can rely on them to help you achieve more of what you want. When that happens, skillpower takes the controls and willpower takes a backseat.

Predictable Outcomes

One of the reasons that I have asked you to try out the energy switches while reading this book is that I want you to demonstrate to yourself that they really work. You may be persuaded by the research. You may understand the logic behind why these switches are useful. But unless you actually try them out, you won't be able to convince yourself that they're truly effective.

I am reminded of the time the Nobel Prize–winning Danish physicist Niels Bohr, father of quantum mechanics, was asked whether he believed in the results of the unexpected things that he was discovering in an experiment. "But surely you don't believe it works," said a friend about a particular mechanism that Bohr had built and put to the test, one which was already producing remarkable, measurable results.

"True enough," replied Bohr. "But I understand that it works whether I believe in it or not."

The whole premise of the energy switches is that if you take the specific actions that I've described in this book and tailor them to your own needs and lifestyle, you'll get solid, predictable benefits that give you more of the vigor and stamina that you want and deserve.

And each of these specific outcomes creates more energy. More calm energy to infuse your life with greater contentment, creativity, mastery, and a sustained sense of well-being. More active energy to help you feel vibrantly alive. More sensory energy to engage with the richness of life and turn back the aging clock. More heartfelt energy to bring you closer to the people who matter the most to you and the efforts that can make the greatest difference.

Each of us has amazing and largely untapped reserves of calm, active, sensory, and heartfelt energy. But if you want to consistently unlock the sources of that energy, you can't rely on luck or willpower. You need to try the switches; develop the kinds of simple, practical, scientifically based, do-them-anywhere skills that I have described; and then trust those skills. If you keep exploring these newfound ways to bring out more of your best everyday, you will unlock untold reserves of energy. Few investments of time or effort pay greater dividends.

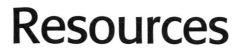

Resources

Foods That Stoke Your Energy Furnace

A key part of a high-energy lifestyle is choosing the right food at the right time. Usually, this means taking advantage of easy, great-tasting snack-size portions that my wife, Leslie, and I call Energy Bites.

The simple scientific truth is that when you eat a small amount of healthy, delicious food every few hours of the day, your metabolism revs up. Your brain, body, and senses make more energy. This not only helps to keep you slim and healthy, it also gives you a heightened sense of being alive and more fully engaged with life.

One of the keys here is knowing whether you want more calm energy or active energy. For calm energy, we've found that the best snacks are generally low in fat, low in protein, and high in complex carbohydrates and fiber. This provides lasting fuel for easygoing vigor and relaxed emotions. Complex carbohydrates include whole grains and legumes.

For active energy, our favorite snacks are low in fat, moderately high in protein, and high in complex carbohydrates and fiber. The extra bit of protein has been shown to healthfully shift brain chemistry toward

TELL ME WHAT YOU EAT,

AND I WILL TELL YOU WHAT YOU ARE.

—Anthelm Brillat-Savarin, French gastronome

alertness, according to scientists including Judith J. Wurtman, Ph.D., a nutritional researcher in the brain and cognitive-sciences department at the Massachusetts Institute of Technology.

While the nutritional composition of our snacks is important, we also take into consideration their convenience and taste. Energy Bites need to be easy to make (and, in many cases, easy to prepare in advance), easy to carry along, and easy to enjoy because they taste so good. Otherwise, why bother?

To plan your Energy Bites and regular meals, you may want to create a chart. I use one that has categories for the nine key times that I eat during each day.

1. Wake up (within the first half-hour or so after rising in the morning)
2. Breakfast
3. Mid-morning snack
4. Lunch
5. Mid-afternoon snack
6. Heading-home snack (in late afternoon or early evening, as the most intense work of the day winds down)
7. Walk-in-the-door snack (within the first half-hour or so after arriving home)
8. Light dinner
9. Mid-evening snack/delayed dessert

As a general rule, the snacks earlier in the day should be geared toward active energy, while those later in the day should emphasize calm

Gauge Your Snack Reaction

Each of us is unique in how we respond to Energy Bites. As you develop your own favorites, become aware of how you react to the following qualities of each snack.

Temperature. Do you feel increased calm energy or active energy when you eat or drink something that's ice cold? What about something that's pleasantly hot?

Timing. At different hours of the day, do you feel more energized or relaxed when you eat certain snacks?

Taste. Besides tasting good—which is always important—which snacks have the smells and flavors that provide you with an immediate pick-me-up? Stimulating scents and tastes identified in research include lemon, orange, and chocolate.

Likewise, do certain smells and flavors readily relax you? Scientists have found that vanilla and apple-cinnamon sometimes have this effect.

Spiciness. Remember the research noting that spices such as cayenne and jalapeño peppers and even ginger may increase metabolism and help burn excess calories? How do these seasonings affect you? Do they boost your alertness or simply taste good?

Protein content. As noted in Active-Energy Switch #2, some scientists believe that snacks that are higher in protein—usually with 3 grams or more—tend to promote increased alertness and vigor in a number of people. How does this kind of snack make you feel?

energy. This is a very individualized decision, however. You need to consider how demands for your attentiveness and involvement change with the flow of activities throughout the day and evening.

If you want to have extra active energy later in the day, you can easily increase the protein content of an Energy Bite by adding one of the following:

- A small glass of fat-free milk or low-fat soy milk
- A half-cup of low-fat yogurt or cottage cheese
- A few peanuts, almonds, or pumpkin seeds

Beyond the recipes in this section, some of my family's favorite Energy Bites include homemade caramel popcorn, banana splits made with low-fat frozen yogurt, fresh fruits, and all kinds of blender smoothies. For other ideas, refer to my previous book *Low-Fat Living* and Leslie's book *Low-Fat Living Cookbook*. (You can order both books directly from the publisher; visit the Web site at www.preventionbookshelf.com or call 1-800-848-4735).

At first, eating so often over the course of a day takes some getting used to. Many of us have learned to ignore our hunger; we inadvertently starve ourselves, thinking this is a good way to lose weight. While it doesn't take off pounds, it does leave us tense and tired.

People from all over the world contact Leslie and me to tell us how great they feel after making Energy Bites part of their active, high-energy lifestyles. Our advice to you is to have fun with these recipes and to make note of the immediate and lasting results.

Loaded Oatmeal Cookies

Prep time: 15 minutes

Cooking time: 10 to 12 minutes

These chewy whole-grain cookies are a great afternoon snack to help you slow down after a busy day. You can flavor them with a variety of goodies.

- 2 **cups whole-wheat pastry flour or unbleached flour**
- 2 **cups quick-cooking oats**
- 1 **teaspoon ground cinnamon**
- 1 **teaspoon baking soda**
- ¼ **teaspoon salt**
- 8 **tablespoons unsalted butter or margarine, softened**
- 1 **cup packed brown sugar**
- ¾ **cup sugar**
- 4 **egg whites**
- ¼ **cup fat-free milk**
- 1 **tablespoon vanilla extract**
- 1½ **cups mixed dried fruit, chopped nuts, and/or chocolate chips**

Preheat the oven to 350°F. Coat 2 baking sheets with cooking spray.

In a medium bowl, combine the flour, oats, cinnamon, baking soda, and salt.

Place the butter or margarine in another medium bowl. Using an electric mixer, beat until creamy. Add the brown sugar, sugar, egg whites, milk, and vanilla extract. Beat until smooth. Gradually stir in the flour mixture until well-combined. Stir in the dried fruit, nuts, or chocolate chips.

Drop the dough by rounded teaspoons onto the prepared baking sheets about 2" apart. Bake one sheet at a time for 10 to 12 minutes, or until the cookies are lightly browned on the edges. Remove to a rack and cool.

Makes 52

Per cookie: 85 calories, 2 g protein, 16 g carbohydrates, 2 g fat, 5 mg cholesterol, 1 g fiber, 43 mg sodium

Ricotta Cheesecake Cups

Prep time: 15 minutes

Cooking time: 45 minutes

Rich and creamy cheesecake can be a great energy booster when it's made with low-fat and fat-free cheeses. Bake these cakes in single-serving sizes so they're available for a quick and easy snack.

16	ounces low-fat ricotta cheese, softened
4	ounces Neufchâtel cheese, softened
4	ounces fat-free cream cheese, softened
½	cup sugar
1	vanilla bean, halved lengthwise
3	eggs

Preheat the oven to 325°F. Place paper liners in a 12-cup muffin pan. Fill a large baking pan with enough water to cover the bottom of the muffin pan but not come over the top. Place the baking pan in the oven to preheat.

In a large bowl, beat the ricotta with an electric mixer until creamy. Add the following ingredients in order, beating after each addition: the Neufchâtel, cream cheese, and sugar. Using a knife, scrape the seeds from the vanilla bean, then add the seeds to the cheese mixture (discard the remaining pod). Beat until smooth and creamy. Add the eggs. Beat until smooth and creamy.

Spoon the batter into the prepared muffin pan. Place the muffin pan in the baking pan of hot water. Bake for 45 minutes. Turn off the oven and open the door slightly. Let the cheesecake cups cool slowly in the oven for 15 minutes. Remove from the oven and cool in the pan on a rack. Cover lightly and refrigerate for at least 1 hour or overnight.

Makes 12

Per cheesecake: 124 calories, 10 g protein, 11 g carbohydrates, 5 g fat, 66 mg cholesterol, 0 g fiber, 165 mg sodium

Mixed-Berry Pie

Prep time: 10 minutes

Cooking time: About 1 hour

The combination of berries makes this calming snack a rich and satisfying treat.

- 5 **cups frozen mixed berries (blueberries, raspberries, strawberries, blackberries)**
- ¾ **cup sugar**
- 1 **teaspoon ground cinnamon**
- ¼ **cup Chambord liqueur**
- 6 **tablespoons arrowroot or cornstarch**
- 1 **tablespoon lemon juice**
- 1 **unbaked deep-dish pie crust**
- 1 **tablespoon packed brown sugar**

Line a baking sheet with foil. Place in the oven and preheat to 425°F.

In a large bowl, combine the berries, sugar, and cinnamon.

In a cup, combine the Chambourd, arrowroot or cornstarch, and lemon juice. Stir well and pour over the berries. Toss until well-combined.

Spoon the berry mixture into the pie crust. Sprinkle with the brown sugar.

Bake for 15 minutes. Reduce the heat to 350°F and bake for 40 to 45 minutes, or until the filling is bubbling. Remove to a rack and cool.

Makes 9 servings

Per serving: 239 calories, 1 g protein, 44 g carbohydrates, 6 g fat, 4 mg cholesterol, 3 g fiber, 64 mg sodium

Hints: For an extra-special touch, try serving the Mixed- Berry Pie à la mode, with vanilla frozen yogurt or low-fat ice cream, and top with chocolate syrup.

For a fat-free alternative, you can bake the filling in ramekins, instead of in the crust.

Lemon Lift Muffins

Prep time: 15 minutes

Cooking time: 20 minutes

These muffins are packed with high-energy ingredients. They are great for breakfast, as a mid-morning snack, or for an extra mid-afternoon boost.

1¼	cup whole-wheat pastry flour
¾	cup sugar
½	cup nonfat dry milk
¼	cup toasted pine nuts (optional)
3	tablespoons soy flour
½	teaspoon baking powder
½	teaspoon salt
⅛	teaspoon baking soda
6	ounces fat-free lemon yogurt
4	egg whites or 2 eggs
3	tablespoons unsalted butter, melted, or canola oil
2	teaspoons grated lemon peel

Preheat the oven to 350°F. Line a 12-cup muffin pan with paper liners or coat with cooking spray.

In a small bowl, combine the whole-wheat flour, sugar, dry milk, pine nuts (if using), soy flour, baking powder, salt, and baking soda.

In a medium bowl, whisk together the yogurt, egg whites or eggs, butter or oil, and lemon peel. Add the flour mixture and stir just until combined. Spoon the batter into the prepared muffin pan.

Bake for 20 minutes, or until the tops are lightly browned and a wooden pick inserted into the center of a muffin comes out almost clean. Cool in the pan on a rack for 5 minutes. Remove to the rack and cool completely.

Makes 12

Per muffin: 145 calories, 5 g protein, 25 g carbohydrates, 4 g fat, 8 mg cholesterol, 2 g fiber, 174 mg sodium

Hint: The nutritional value of pine nuts varies with the species of tree from which they come. Piñons, which grow in the southwestern United States, are in limited supply. A better choice is pignolis, which are imported from Spain and the Mediterranean region. Besides being more available than piñons, pignolis have more than double the protein but less fat and fewer calories.

The Skinny on Nuts and Seeds

Nuts and seeds are a main protein source for many cultures around the world. And they're very versatile. They add texture, flavor, and nutrients to baked goods, casseroles, salads, and desserts.

Although most nuts are quite high in fat, much of it is unsaturated. Eaten in small quantities, they are a wonderful addition to a healthy diet. They also contain a variety of essential nutrients, including calcium, B-complex vitamins, and vitamin E.

The following table compares the nutritional profiles of various types of nuts and seeds, per 100-gram serving.

Variety	Fat (g)	Protein (g)	Calories
Almonds	54.2	18.6	598
Cashews	45.7	17.2	561
Peanuts	48.4	26.3	568
Pecans	71.2	9.2	687
Pine nuts (pignolis)	47.4	31.1	552
Pine nuts (piñons)	60.5	13.0	635
Pistachios	53.7	19.3	594
Pumpkin seeds	46.7	29.0	553
Sesame seeds	53.4	18.2	582
Sunflower seeds	47.3	24.0	560
Walnuts (English)	64.0	14.8	651

Peanut Butter Bursts

Prep time: 25 minutes

Cooking time: 5 to 7 minutes

Try one of these treats when you need something sweet and satisfying. Carry them in your purse, briefcase, or backpack. They're great for a midday snack. One batch lasts for weeks when stored in a covered container in the refrigerator.

1	**cup natural peanut butter**
½	**cup honey**
½	**teaspoon vanilla extract**
¼	**cup sunflower seeds**
¼	**cup pumpkin seeds or finely chopped almonds**
2	**cups quick-cooking oats**
¼	**cup chopped dates or other chopped dried fruits**
¼	**cup wheat bran, wheat germ, or oat bran**
¼	**cup warm water**
4	**tablespoons sesame seeds**

Preheat the oven to 350°F.

In a large bowl, mix the peanut butter, honey, and vanilla. If needed, heat in the microwave oven to soften.

Place the sunflower seeds and pumpkin seeds or almonds on a baking sheet and toast for 5 to 7 minutes, or until lightly browned.

Add the toasted seeds; oats; dates or other fruits; wheat bran, wheat germ, or oat bran; and water to the peanut butter mixture. Stir until well-blended.

Roll the dough into 42 walnut-size balls. Roll each ball in the sesame seeds to coat. Place in a single layer on a baking sheet. Refrigerate for several hours. Store in a covered container.

Makes 42

Per burst: 77 calories, 3 g protein, 8 g carbohydrates, 4 g fat, 0 mg cholesterol, 1 g fiber, 1 mg sodium

Energy Bites: Foods That Stoke Your Energy Furnace

Fresh Cranberry Loaf

Prep time: 20 minutes

Cooking time: 1 hour

Fresh berries are readily available in autumn, but frozen work just as well. The bread is great for breakfast, a snack, or dessert.

2	cups fresh cranberries, halved
⅓	cup chopped pecans
1	teaspoon grated orange peel
2	tablespoons + 1 cup sugar
2	cups whole-wheat pastry flour or unbleached flour
1½	teaspoons baking powder
½	teaspoon salt (optional)
½	teaspoon baking soda
2	tablespoons unsalted butter, melted, or canola oil
2	egg whites or 1 egg, lightly beaten
⅓	cup orange juice
¼	cup fat-free milk

Preheat the oven to 350°F. Lightly coat a 9" × 5" loaf pan with cooking spray.

In a small bowl, combine the cranberries, pecans, orange peel, and 2 tablespoons of the sugar. Set aside. In a large bowl, mix the flour, baking powder, salt (if using), baking soda, and the remaining 1 cup sugar.

In another small bowl, mix the butter or oil, egg whites or egg, orange juice, and milk. Pour into the sugar mixture and stir just until well-mixed.

Stir in the cranberry mixture. Pour into the prepared pan and bake for 1 hour, or until a wooden pick inserted into the center comes out clean. Cool in the pan on a rack for 10 minutes. Remove to the rack and cool completely.

Makes 12 servings

Per serving: 197 calories, 4 g protein, 37 g carbohydrates, 5 g fat, 6 mg cholesterol, 4 g fiber, 127 mg sodium

Cinnamon Scones with Walnut Cream

Prep time: 25 minutes

Cooking time: 12 to 15 minutes

Scones are an English favorite, often snacked on with a relaxing cup of warm tea. Spread this low-fat, whole-grain version with Walnut Cream instead of the usual butter.

Cream

2	tablespoons walnuts
3	tablespoons (about 1 ounce) fat-free cream cheese, softened
1	teaspoon unsalted butter or margarine, softened
½	teaspoon sugar

Scones

1½	cups unbleached flour
1	cup whole-wheat pastry flour
¼	cup brown sugar
1	teaspoon baking powder
½	teaspoon baking soda
½	teaspoon salt
1	teaspoon + ¼ teaspoon ground cinnamon
3	tablespoons unsalted butter or margarine, well-chilled
¾–1	cup buttermilk
2	teaspoons sugar

To make the cream: In a food processor or blender, grind the walnuts. Add the cream cheese, butter or margarine, and sugar. Process until smooth and creamy. Place in a small dish. Cover and refrigerate until ready to serve with the scones.

To make the scones: Meanwhile, preheat the oven to 400°F. Line a baking sheet with parchment paper or coat with cooking spray.

In a large bowl, combine the unbleached flour, whole-wheat flour, brown sugar, baking powder, baking soda, salt, and 1 teaspoon of the cinnamon. Using a food processor, pastry blender, or two knives, cut in the butter or margarine until the mixture forms fine crumbs.

Make a well in the center of the flour mixture and pour in ¾ to 1 cup buttermilk, or just enough that the dough sticks together. Using a fork, stir just until combined. Turn the dough out onto a lightly floured surface and knead gently just until the dough holds together.

Roll the dough to about 1" thickness. Using a 2" biscuit cutter or the rim of a glass, cut the dough into rounds and place on the prepared sheet. Continue rolling and cutting until all the dough is used to make 10 scones. Be careful not to overwork the dough.

Combine the sugar and the remaining ¼ teaspoon cinnamon. Sprinkle on the top of each scone.

Bake for 12 to 15 minutes, or until the scones just begin to brown. Remove to a rack and cool.

Serve with the cream.

Makes 10

Per scone: 192 calories, 5 g protein, 31 g carbohydrates, 5 g fat, 12 mg cholesterol, 2 g fiber, 282 mg sodium

Hint: If you don't use buttermilk often, look for dried cultured buttermilk in the baking section (near the dry milk) of your grocery store. It has a long shelf life if kept in the refrigerator and is convenient to use. Just mix with water according to the package directions. You can make only as much as you need.

Orange–Poppy Seed Biscotti

Prep time: 15 minutes

Cooking time: 40 minutes

Try one of these twice-baked cookies with a morning cup of tea, coffee, or fat-free milk. The light orange flavor and the addition of some higher-protein ingredients make for a great morning or mid-afternoon pick-me-up.

1¾	cups whole-wheat pastry flour or unbleached flour
¼	cup soy flour
¼	cup fat-free dry milk
2	tablespoons poppy seeds
1½	teaspoons baking powder
⅛	teaspoon salt
3	tablespoons unsalted butter or margarine, softened
2	eggs
1	tablespoon grated orange peel
1	teaspoon vanilla extract
½	cup + 1 tablespoon sugar

Preheat the oven to 350°F. Coat a baking sheet with cooking spray.

In a large bowl, combine the whole-wheat or unbleached flour, soy flour, dry milk, poppy seeds, baking powder, and salt.

In a medium bowl, beat the butter or margarine with an electric mixer until creamy. Beat in the eggs, orange peel, vanilla, and ½ cup of the sugar. Add to the flour mixture and stir until well-combined.

Divide the dough in half and place each half on the prepared sheet. Shape into 2 logs, each about 10" × 4" and ¾" thick. Sprinkle with the remaining 1 tablespoon sugar.

Bake for 20 minutes. Cool on the baking sheet on a rack for 10 minutes.

Diagonally slice each log into ½" pieces. Place each piece cut-side down on the baking sheet.

Bake for 20 minutes longer, or until beginning to brown slightly. Remove to a rack and cool.

Makes 28

Per biscotti: 67 calories, 2 g protein, 10 g carbohydrates, 2 g fat, 19 mg cholesterol, 1 g fiber, 45 mg sodium

Blueberry-Cream Fruit Dip

Prep time: 5 minutes

This dip for fresh cut-up fruit is creamy and has a bit of protein from the cream cheese. It goes great with strawberries.

1   **banana**
1   **cup blueberries**
3   **ounces Neufchâtel cheese or low-fat cream cheese**
2   **tablespoons orange juice**
1   **teaspoon lemon juice**

In a blender, combine the banana, blueberries, Neufchâtel cheese or cream cheese, orange juice, and lemon juice. Blend into a smooth puree. Store in the refrigerator in a covered container for up to 3 days.

Makes 1½ cups

Per ¼-cup serving: 70 calories, 2 g protein, 9 g carbohydrates, 4 g fat, 11 mg cholesterol, 1 g fiber, 58 mg sodium

Multi-Grain Soft Pretzels

Prep time: 20 minutes

Cooking time: 12 to 15 minutes

Although these pretzels are made with yeast, they don't need to rise, so they're fast and easy to make. They're great for a calming whole-grain snack.

¾	**cup warm water (110°–115°F)**
1	**tablespoon active dry yeast**
2	**teaspoons sugar**
½	**cup whole-wheat flour**
¼	**cup mixed whole-grain flour (barley, oat, brown rice, oat bran, cornmeal, etc.)**
½	**teaspoon salt**
1¼–1½	**cups unbleached flour**
1	**egg, well-beaten**
1	**teaspoon coarse kosher salt**

Preheat the oven to 425°F. Coat a baking sheet with cooking spray.

In a large bowl, combine the water, yeast, and sugar. Set aside for 5 minutes, or until foamy. Add the whole-wheat flour, mixed whole-grain flour, salt, and 1¼ cups of the unbleached flour. Stir to mix.

Turn out onto a floured surface and knead for 10 minutes, or until smooth and elastic. If the dough seems too wet, knead in a little more of the unbleached flour.

Divide the dough into 12 pieces. Roll each piece into a 15" strip. Shape each strip into a pretzel. Place on the prepared baking sheet.

Brush each pretzel with the egg and sprinkle with the coarse salt. Bake for 12 to 15 minutes. Remove to a rack and cool.

Makes 12

Per pretzel: 85 calories, 3 g protein, 16 g carbohydrates, 1 g fat, 18 mg cholesterol, 2 g fiber, 297 mg sodium

Chocolate–Chocolate Chip Biscotti

Prep time: 15 minutes

Cooking time: 40 minutes

Sweet and crunchy, these low-fat chocolate treats are perfect for satisfying late-afternoon or evening cravings. They're a big hit with kids too.

2	cups whole-wheat pastry flour or unbleached flour
¼	cup unsweetened cocoa powder
1½	teaspoons baking powder
¼	teaspoon salt
2	tablespoons unsalted butter or margarine, softened
1½	cups sugar
3	eggs
2	teaspoons vanilla extract
½	cup chocolate chips

Preheat the oven to 350°F. Coat a baking sheet with cooking spray.

In a large bowl, combine the flour, cocoa, baking powder, and salt.

In a medium bowl, beat the butter or margarine with an electric mixer until creamy. Beat in the sugar, eggs, and vanilla.

Add to the flour mixture. Add the chocolate chips. Stir to combine.

Divide the dough in half and place each half on the prepared sheet. Shape into 2 rectangles, about 12" × 4" and ¾" thick. Bake for 20 minutes. Remove to a rack and cool for 10 minutes.

Diagonally slice each rectangle into ½" pieces. Place each piece cut-side down on the baking sheet. Bake for 20 minutes longer, or until beginning to brown slightly. Remove to a rack and cool.

Makes 36

Per biscotti: 79 calories, 2 g protein, 15 g carbohydrates, 2 g fat, 20 mg cholesterol, 1 g fiber, 43 mg sodium

Strawberry-Banana Boost

Prep time: 5 minutes

Shakes and smoothies make fast and easy snacks. They taste great, can be low in fat, and travel well in a Thermos. Try this icy-cold energy drink whenever you need a boost.

- 1 **banana**
- 2 **cups frozen strawberries**
- 8 **ounces fat-free or low-fat strawberry yogurt**
- 1 **cup fat-free milk or low-fat soy milk**

In a blender, combine the banana, strawberries, yogurt, and milk. Blend until smooth.

Makes 2 servings

Per serving: 268 calories, 11 g protein, 57 g carbohydrates, 1 g fat, 2 mg cholesterol, 5 g fiber, 137 mg sodium

Hints: Any fruit can be substituted for the strawberries. If the fruit isn't frozen, throw a few ice cubes into the blender.

For an extra protein boost, try adding a scoop of soy powder or other protein power and blend well.

Raspberry Chiller

Prep time: 5 minutes

This smoothy is perfect for the afternoon wind down. Loaded with fruit and fruit juice, it gives you a jump on meeting your daily fruit-and-veggie requirement. It's also a good source of fiber.

- 1 **banana**
- 2 **cups frozen raspberries**
- ¾ **cup apple juice**

In a blender, combine the banana, raspberries, and apple juice. Blend until smooth.

Makes 2 servings

Per serving: 354 calories, 2 g protein, 90 g carbohydrates, 1 g fat, 0 mg cholesterol, 13 g fiber, 6 mg sodium

Chocolate Power-Plus Shake

Prep time: 5 minutes

Sweet, flavorful, and filling, this shake is packed with ingredients that can help energize you.

- 1 **banana**
- 8 **ounces fat-free or low-fat coffee or vanilla yogurt**
- 1 **cup fat-free or low-fat chocolate frozen yogurt or ice cream**
- ½ **cup fat-free milk or soy milk**
- 1 **tablespoon natural peanut butter**

In a blender, combine the banana, yogurt, frozen yogurt or ice cream, milk, and peanut butter. Blend until smooth.

Makes 2 servings

Per serving: 341 calories, 12 g protein, 66 g carbohydrates, 4 g fat, 1 mg cholesterol, 3 g fiber, 137 mg sodium

Triple-Orange Pound Cake

Prep time: 20 minutes

Cooking time: 50 to 55 minutes

Try this cake as an afternoon snack, or serve it with low-fat frozen yogurt.

3½	**cups whole-wheat pastry flour or unbleached flour**
1½	**teaspoons baking powder**
¼	**teaspoon baking soda**
¼	**teaspoon salt**
6	**tablespoons unsalted butter or margarine, softened**
2	**cups sugar**
4	**eggs**
2	**egg whites**
½	**cup orange marmalade**
	Grated peel of 2 oranges
¾	**cup orange juice**
2	**teaspoons vanilla extract**
2	**tablespoons confectioners' sugar**

Preheat the oven to 350°F. Coat a 9-cup Bundt or tube pan with cooking spray. Sprinkle the pan with some flour and tap upside down to remove excess.

In a medium bowl, stir together the flour, baking powder, baking soda, and salt.

In a large bowl, beat the butter or margarine with an electric mixer until creamy. Beat in the sugar. Add the following ingredients in order, beating after each addition: the eggs, egg whites, marmalade, orange peel, orange juice, and vanilla. Add the flour mixture and beat on the lowest setting just until combined. Stir by hand to finish mixing. Pour batter into the prepared pan.

Bake for 50 to 55 minutes, or until a wooden pick inserted into the center comes out dry. Cool in the pan on a rack for 10 minutes. Remove to the rack and cool completely. Sift confectioners' sugar over the top.

Makes 18 servings

Per serving: 254 calories, 5 g protein, 48 g carbohydrates, 6 g fat, 58 mg cholesterol, 4 g fiber, 114 mg sodium

Raspberry-Banana Fruit Sauce

Prep time: 5 minutes

Here's one snack we don't mind the kids eating before dinner. We like to serve it when the whole family is hungry and the meal won't be ready for a while. The fruit and sauce curb our appetites without filling us up. Plus, it gives us (especially the kids) another serving of nutritious fruits. Leftovers keep in the refrigerator for several days. Just cut up some fresh fruit—apples, bananas, pears, pineapple, melon, kiwifruit, or even grapes—and with a wooden pick or fork, dip the pieces into the sauce.

1   **banana**
1   **cup raspberries**
2   **tablespoons orange juice**
1   **teaspoon lemon juice**
    Pinch of ground cinnamon

In a blender, combine the banana, raspberries, orange juice, lemon juice, and cinnamon. Blend into a smooth puree. Store in the refrigerator in a covered container.

Makes 1½ cups

Per ¼-cup serving: 30 calories, 0 g protein, 7 g carbohydrates, 0.5 g fat, 0 mg cholesterol, 2 g fiber, 0 mg sodium

Apricot-Almond Spread

Prep time: 10 minutes

This creamy spread can give you an energy boost whenever you need one. Spread it on your morning toast for a quick breakfast or on Cinnamon-and-Sugar Pita Crisps (page 456) for a sweet mid-morning or mid-afternoon snack. Our kids love it as an after-school, before-sports-practice treat.

15   **unsalted almonds, toasted**

½   **cup fat-free or 1% cottage cheese**

2   **ounces Neufchâtel cheese or low-fat cream cheese**

¼   **cup fat-free milk**

¼   **vanilla bean**

1   **teaspoon sugar**

8   **dried apricots, chopped**

In a food processor or blender, finely grind the almonds. Add the cottage cheese, Neufchâtel cheese or cream cheese, and milk. Using a knife, scrape the seeds from the vanilla bean, then add the seeds to the processor (discard the remaining pod). Add the sugar. Process until smooth and creamy. Add the apricots and blend well. Store in a covered container until ready to serve.

Makes 5 servings

Per serving: 113 calories, 7 g protein, 11 g carbohydrates, 6 g fat, 9 mg cholesterol, 2 g fiber, 126 mg sodium

Hints: To toast almonds, place them in a dry skillet over medium heat. Cook, shaking the pan often, for 2 minutes, or until lightly browned and fragrant.

For a quick and easy way to chop dried apricots or any sticky dried fruits, use kitchen shears to snip into small pieces.

Roasted Pepper and Olive Tapenade

Prep time: 15 minutes

Need a little something to take the edge off your pre-dinner hunger? This spread is easy to make and keeps well in the refrigerator for up to a week. Serve it on whole-grain crackers, or try it with the Savory Pita Crisps (page 457).

- 1 **clove garlic**
- 1 **tablespoon parsley**
- 1 **tablespoon fresh basil**
- 7 **dry-packed sun-dried tomatoes, soaked in boiling water for 5 minutes**
- ½ **cup pitted kalamata or black olives**
- ½ **cup jarred roasted red peppers, chopped**
- 2 **tablespoons capers, drained**
- 1 **teaspoon lemon juice**
- ½ **teaspoon grated lemon peel**
- ½ **teaspoon herbes de Provence or Italian seasoning**
  Ground black pepper

In a small food processor, combine the garlic, parsley, and basil. Process until finely chopped. Drain the tomatoes. Add to the processor and process until finely chopped. Add the olives and process until chopped but not pureed.

Transfer to a small bowl. Stir in the red peppers, capers, lemon juice, lemon peel, and herbs. Season with the black pepper to taste. Store in a covered container in the refrigerator.

Makes 1¼ cups

Per 1-tablespoon serving: 15 calories, 0 g protein, 3 g carbohydrates, 1 g fat, 0 mg cholesterol, 0 g fiber, 84 mg sodium

Cinnamon-and-Sugar Pita Crisps

Prep time: 5 minutes

Cooking time: 7 to 10 minutes

These crisps are sprinkled with cinnamon and sugar before baking. This gives them a sweet crunch that makes them the perfect complement to nut butters, jams, or cream cheese. They are versatile enough to eat at any time of day, depending on the type of spread you choose to pair them with.

2   **whole-wheat pitas**

2   **teaspoons sugar**

½   **teaspoon ground cinnamon**

Preheat the oven to 350°F. Coat a baking sheet with cooking spray.

Cut each pita into 6 triangles. Break each triangle into 2 chips. Place the triangles in a single layer on the prepared baking sheet. Coat with cooking spray.

In a small cup, combine the sugar and cinnamon. Sprinkle each chip with the mixture.

Bake for 7 to 10 minutes, or just until beginning to brown. Watch carefully; they burn easily. Store in an airtight container.

Makes 24

Per serving (4 chips): 16 calories, 1 g protein, 3 g carbohydrates, 0.5 g fat, 0 mg cholesterol, 0 g fiber, 28 mg sodium

Savory Pita Crisps

Prep time: 5 minutes

Cooking time: 7 to 10 minutes

Our family loves these Italian-tasting crisps topped with a flavored cream cheese like garlic or herb, slices of cheese, or Roasted Pepper and Olive Tapenade (page 455).

- 2 **whole-wheat pitas**
- 2 **teaspoons grated Parmesan cheese**
- ½ **teaspoon Italian seasoning**
- ¼ **teaspoon garlic powder**
- ¼ **teaspoon salt**
-    **Ground black pepper**

Preheat the oven to 350°F. Coat a baking sheet with cooking spray.

Cut each pita into 6 triangles. Break each triangle into 2 chips. Place the triangles in a single layer on the prepared baking sheet. Coat with cooking spray.

In a food processor or blender, combine the cheese, Italian seasoning, garlic powder, and salt. Add the pepper to taste. Process into a fine powder. Sprinkle each chip with the mixture.

Bake for 7 to 10 minutes, or just until beginning to brown. Watch carefully; they burn easily. Store in an airtight container.

Makes 24

Per serving (4 chips): 15 calories, 1 g protein, 3 g carbohydrates, 0.5 g fat, 0 mg cholesterol, 0 g fiber, 55 mg sodium

Chili-Lime Pita Crisps

Prep time: 5 minutes

Cooking time: 7 to 10 minutes

Similar to Mexican tortilla chips, these crisps are the perfect match for bean dips, salsa, or even flavorful cheeses.

2	**whole-wheat pitas**
1	**teaspoon nonfat dry milk**
1	**teaspoon chili powder**
1	**teaspoon grated lime peel**
¼	**teaspoon ground cumin**
¼	**teaspoon ground coriander**
¼	**teaspoon sugar**
	Salt
	Ground black pepper

Preheat the oven to 350°F. Coat a baking sheet with cooking spray.

Cut each pita into 6 triangles. Break each triangle into 2 chips. Place the triangles in a single layer on the prepared baking sheet. Coat with cooking spray.

In a food processor or blender, combine the dry milk, chili powder, lime peel, cumin, coriander, and sugar. Add the salt and pepper to taste. Process into a fine powder. Sprinkle each chip with the mixture.

Bake for 7 to 10 minutes, or just until beginning to brown. Watch carefully; they burn easily. Store in an airtight container.

Makes 24

Per serving (4 chips): 15 calories, 1 g protein, 3 g carbohydrates, 0.5 g fat, 0 mg cholesterol, 0 g fiber, 30 mg sodium

Quick Bean Dip

Prep time: 5 minutes

You can make this dip quickly, and it will keep for several hours unrefrigerated. So mix up a batch, spoon it into a covered container, and serve it with low-fat or baked tortilla chips. Or try it with the Chili-Lime Pita Crisps on the opposite page. Adjust the amount of spiciness by adding more or less jalapeño pepper.

1	**small onion, halved**
1	**clove garlic**
½–1	**jalapeño pepper, halved and seeded (wear plastic gloves when handling)**
1	**can (15 ounces) pinto beans, drained and rinsed**
3	**tablespoons orange juice**
1	**tablespoon olive oil**
1	**tablespoon tomato paste**
½	**teaspoon ground coriander**
½	**teaspoon ground cumin**
¼	**teaspoon white or red wine vinegar**
	Salt
	Ground black pepper

In a food processor, combine the onion, garlic, and jalapeño pepper. Process until finely chopped. Add the beans, orange juice, oil, tomato paste, coriander, cumin, and vinegar. Process until smooth and creamy. Season with salt and pepper to taste.

Makes 4 servings

Per serving: 140 calories, 6 g protein, 21 g carbohydrates, 4 g fat, 0 mg cholesterol, 6 g fiber, 253 mg sodium

Cocoa Thumbprints

Prep time: 15 minutes

Cooking time: 15 minutes

These little sconelike cookies can be filled with any flavor jam, jelly, preserves, or fruit spread. Our family's favorites include raspberry, strawberry, and orange. They make a nice after-school treat for both you and the kids.

1⅓   **cups whole-wheat pastry flour**

½   **cup sugar**

3   **tablespoons unsweetened cocoa powder**

2   **teaspoons baking powder**

4   **tablespoons unsalted butter or margarine, chilled**

⅓   **cup fat-free milk**

1   **teaspoon vanilla extract**

3   **tablespoons jam**

Preheat the oven to 350°F. Coat a baking sheet with cooking spray.

In a medium bowl, mix the flour, sugar, cocoa, and baking powder. Using a food processor, pastry blender, or two knives, cut in the butter or margarine until the mixture forms fine crumbs.

Make a well in the center of the flour mixture and pour in the milk and vanilla. Using a fork, stir just until the dough holds together. Knead in the bowl several times to make sure the dough is well-combined.

Roll the dough into 18 balls. Place on the prepared sheet. Using your thumb, make a deep well in the center of each ball. Smooth out the edges and fill each well with ½ teaspoon jam.

Bake for 15 minutes. Remove to a rack and cool.

Makes 18

Per cookie: 88 calories, 2 g protein, 15 g carbohydrates, 3 g fat, 7 mg cholesterol, 1 g fiber, 60 mg sodium

References

Chapter 1: Prime Yourself for Unparalled Energy

Brown, G. *The Energy of Life* (New York: Free Press, 2000).

Introduction to the Calm-Energy Switches

See, for example, Gleick, J. *Faster* (New York: Pantheon, 1999); and Loehr, J. E. *Stress for Success* (New York: Times Books, 1998).

Thayer, R. E. "Factor Analytic and Reliability Studies on the Activation-Deactivation Adjective Check List," *Psychological Reports* (42, 1978): 747–56.

Thayer, R. E., Takahashi, P. J., and Pauli, J. A.,"Multidimensional Arousal States, Diurnal Rhythms, Cognitive and Social Processes, and Extraversion," *Personality and Individual Differences* (9, 1988): 15–24; Thayer, R. E., *The Biopsychology of Mood and Arousal* (New York: Oxford University Press, 1991): 54, 149–51.

Thayer, *Biopsychology of Mood and Arousal*; Lazarus, R. S. *Emotion and Adaptation* (New York: Oxford University Press, 1991); Vincent, J. D. *The Biology of Emotions* (Cambridge, Mass.: Basil Blackwell, 1990); ed. Gray, J. A. *Psychobiological Aspects of Relationships between Emotions and Cognition* (Hillsdale, N.J.: Erlbaum, 1990).

Thayer, *Biopsychology of Mood and Arousal*: 9.

Csikszentmihalyi, M, *Flow: The Psychology of Optimal Experience* (New York: HarperCollins, 1991); Csikszentmihalyi, M. *The Evolving Self* (New York: HarperCollins, 1993).

See, for example,Csikszentmihalyi, *Flow*; Csikszentmihalyi, *The Evolving Self*; and Thayer, *Biopsychology of Mood and Arousal*: 9.

Csikszentmihalyi, M. *Finding Flow* (New York: Basic Books, 1997): 21.

See, for example, Thayer, *Biopsychology of Mood and Arousal* (London: Oxford University Press, 1991); and Thayer, R. E. *The Origin of Everyday Moods* (London: Oxford University Press, 1997).

Calm-Energy Switch #1: Launch the Day with High Energy and Low Tension

Zak, V., Carlin, C., and Vash, P. D. *The Fat-to-Muscle Diet* (New York: Berkley, 1988): 30.

Hager, D. L. "Why Breakfast Is Important," *Weight-Control Digest* 3 (1) (Jan.–Feb. 1993): 225–26.

Stamford, B. A., and Shimer, P. *Fitness without Exercise* (New York: Warner, 1990); Zak, Carlin, and Vash, *Fat-to-Muscle*: 30; Natow, A. B., and Heslin, J. *The Fat Attack Plan* (New York: Pocket Books, 1990): 42, 165.

Zak, Carlin, and Vash, *Fat-to-Muscle*: 30.

See, for example, Hauri, P., and Linde, S. *No More Sleepless Nights* (New York: Wiley, 1993).

Mark, V. H., with Mark, J. P. *Reversing Memory Loss* (Boston: Houghton Mifflin, 1992): 216–17; Mark, V. H., and Mark, J. P. *Brain Power: A Neurosurgeon's Complete Program to Maintain and Enhance Brain Fitness throughout Your Life* (Boston: Houghton Mifflin, 1989): 186–87; Benson, H., et al. *The Wellness Book* (New York: Birch Lane Press, 1992); Nathan, R. G., Staats, T. E., and Rosch, P. J. *The Doctors' Guide to Instant Stress Relief* (New York: Ballantine, 1987).

Sedlacek, K. *The Sedlacek Technique: Finding the Calm Within You* (New York: McGraw-Hill, 1989): 14.

Czeisler, C. H., et al. "Bright Light Induction of Strong (Type O) Resetting of the Human Circadian Pacemaker," *Science* 244 (June 16, 1989): 1328–33; Czeisler, C. H., et al. "Human Sleep: Its Duration and Organization Depend on Its Circadian Phase," *Science* 210 (Dec. 12, 1980); Kronauer, R., and Czeisler, C., quoted in "Jet Lag Breakthrough," *Conde Naste's Traveler* (Sept. 1989): 35–36.

Lamberg, L. *Bodyrhythms: Chronobiology and Peak Performance* (New York: Morrow, 1994): 42.

Sheats, C. *Lean Bodies* (Dallas: Summit Group, 1992): 25.

See, for example, Thayer, R. E., et al. "Mood and Behavior Following Moderate Exercise: A Test of Self-Regulation Theory," *Personality and Individual Differences*, 14 (1993): 97–104.

Zak, Calin, and Vash, *Fat-to-Muscle*; Stamford and Shimer, *Fitness without Exercise*: 41, 44.

Southwestern Health Institute in Phoenix. Study cited in Powell, D. R., American Institute for Preventive Medicine, *A Year of Health Hints* (Emmaus, Pa.: Rodale, 1990): 96.

See, for example, Moore-Ede, M. *The 24-Hour Society* (Reading, Mass.: Addison-Wesley, 1993); and Thayer, *The Origin of Everyday Moods*.

Moore-Ede, *24-Hour Society*: 55.

Vanderbilt University Study. Schlundt, D. G., et al. "The Role of Breakfast in the Treatment of Obesity," *American Journal of Clinical Nutrition*, 55 (1992): 645–51; *Obesity and Health*, 6 (12) (Nov.–Dec. 1992): 103.

Natow and Heslin, *Fat Attack Plan*: 42; Schlundt, et al. "The Role of Breakfast in the Treatment of Obesity," *American Journal of Clinical Nutrition* 55 (1992): 645–51; Hager, "Why Breakfast Is Important," *Weight-Control Digest* 3 (1) (Jan.–Feb. 1993): 225–26.

Zak, Carlin, and Vash, *Fat-to-Muscle*: 30.

Lamberg, *Bodyrhythms*: 42; *Prevention's Weight Loss Guide 1993* (Emmaus, Pa.: Rodale, 1993): 148.

See, Thayer, *The Origin of Everyday Moods*; and Jenkins, D. A., et al. *American Journal of Clinical Nutrition* 35 (1982): 1339–46.

Leibowitz, S. F., quoted in Marano, H. E. "Chemistry and Craving," *Psychology Today* (Jan.–Feb. 1993): 30–36, 74.

Stone, K. *Snack Attack* (New York: Warner, 1991): 169.

Levine, A. S., et al. "Effect of Breakfast Cereals on Short-Term Food Intake," *American Journal of Clinical Nutrition* 50 (1989): 1303–7.

Stone, *Snack Attack*: 33, 87.

Calm-Energy Switch #2: Find Instant Calmness

Thayer, *Biopsychology of Mood and Arousal*: 73.

Lazarus, R. S., quoted in *Executive Health Examiners. Coping with Executive Stress* (New York: McGraw-Hill, 1983): 169.

Gleick, J. *Faster* (New York: Pantheon, 1999).

Dossey, L., quoted in Fisher, A. B, "Welcome to the Age of Overwork," *Fortune* (Nov. 30, 1992): 71.

Kabat-Zinn, J., quoted in Ruben, D. "Pioneer Stress Reduction Clinic," *American Health* (Apr. 1991): 42–46.

I first wrote about the concept of the instant-calming sequence (ICS) in *Health and Fitness Excellence: The Scientific Action Plan* (Boston: Houghton Mifflin, 1989).

Lazarus, R. S. *American Psychologist*, 30 (1975): 553–61; DeLongis, A., et al. "Relationship of Daily Hassles, Uplifts, and Major Life Events to Health Status," *Health Psychology* 1 (1982): 119–36; Kanner, A. D., et al. "Comparison of Two Modes of Stress Measurement: Daily Hassles and Uplifts versus Major Life Events," *Journal of Behavioral Medicine* 4 (1981): 1–39.

Stone, A. A. *Journal of Personality and Social Psychology* 52 (1987): 988–93; "Mood Immunity," *Psychology Today* (Nov. 1987): 14.

Ibid.

Bandura, A., and Mahoney, M. J. "Maintenance and Transfer of Self-Reinforcement Functions," *Behaviour Research and Therapy* 12 (1974): 89–98; Denney, D. R. "Self-Control Approaches to the Treatment of Test Anxiety" in ed. Sarason, I. G., *Test Anxiety: Theory, Research, and Applications* (Hillsdale, N.J.: L. Erlbaum Associates, 1980): 209–43; Goldiamond, I. "Self-Reinforcement," *Journal of Applied Behavior* 9 (1976): 509–14; Stroebel, Luce, and Glueck, "Optimizing Compliance"; Stroebel, QR.

Ford, M. R., et al. "Quieting Response Training: Predictors of Long-Term Outcome," *Biofeedback and Self-Regulation* 8 (3) (1983): 393–408; Ford, M. R., et al. "Quieting Response Training: Long-Term Evaluation of a Clinical Biofeedback Practice," *Biofeedback and Self-Regulation* 8 (2) (1983): 265–78; Nathan, Staats, and Rosch, *The Doctors' Guide to Instant Stress Relief*; Stroebel, C. F., Ford, M. R., Strong, P., and Szarek, B. L. *Quieting Response Training: 5-Year Evaluation of a Clinical Biofeedback Practice* (Hartford, Conn.: Institute for Living, 1981); Stroebel, C. F., Luce, G., and Glueck, B. C. "Optimizing Compliance with Behavioral Medicine Therapies," *Current Psychiatric Therapies* (1983–84); Pribram, K. H. *Holonomic Brain Theory* (Hillsdale, N.J.: Erlbaum, 1988); Pribram, K. H., lecture at the Center for Health and Fitness Excellence, Bemidji, Minn. (June 13–14, 1987). For information on the 6-second quieting response, a method somewhat similar to the ICS, see Stroebel, C. F. *QR: The Quieting Reflex* (New York: Berkley, 1983; audiotape collection available from BMA, 200 Park Avenue South., New York, NY 10003); and Stroebel, E. *Kiddie QR* (QR Publications, 119 Forest Drive, Wethersfield, CT 06109). See also, Loehr, J. E. *Toughness Training for Life* (New York: Plume, 1993); and Loehr, J. E. *Stress for Success*.

Hendler, S. S. *The Oxygen Breakthrough* (New York: Pocket Books, 1989): 7, 8, 94.

Fried, *Breath Connection*; Hendler, *Oxygen Breakthrough*.

Snyder, G. "Just One Breath," *Tricycle Review* (Fall 1991): 55–61; Nathan, Staats, and Rosch, *The Doctors' Guide to Instant Stress Relief*: 6; Loehr, J. E., and McLaughlin, P. J. *Mentally Tough* (New York: Evans, 1986); Eliot, R. S., and Breo, D. L. *Is It Worth Dying For?* revised ed. (New York: Bantam, 1989); Harp, D. *The New 3–Minute Meditator* (Oakland, Calif.: New Harbinger, 1990); Fried, *Breath Connection*; Kabat-Zin, *Full-Catastrophe Living*.

Goleman, D., and Gurin, J. *Mind-Body Medicine: How to Use Your Mind for Better Health* (Yonkers, N.Y.: Consumer Reports Books, 1993).

"Breathing Linked to Personality," *Psychology Today* (July 1983): 109; Teich, M., and Dodeles, G. "Mind Control: How to Get It, How to Use It, How to Keep It," *Omni* (Oct. 1987): 53–60.

Ekman, P., Levenson, R. W., and Friesen, W. V. "Autonomic Nervous System Activity Distinguishes Among Emotions," *Science* (Sept. 16, 1983): 1208–10; Greden, J., et al. "University of Michigan," *Archives of General Psychiatry* 43 (1987): 269–74; Teich and Dodeles, "Mind Control"; Zajonc, R. B. "Emotion and Facial Efference: A Theory Reclaimed," *Science* 228 (4695) (Apr. 5, 1985): 15–21.

Stroebel, *QR*: 120.

See, for example, Cailliet, R., and Gross, L. *The Rejuvenation Strategy* (New York: Doubleday, 1987); Hendler, *Oxygen Breakthrough*; Fried, R. *The Breath Connection: How to Reduce Psychosomatic and Stress-Related Disorders* (New York: Plenum, 1990); and Sedlacek, *The Sedlacek Technique.*

Riskind, J. H., and Gotay, C. C. "Physical Posture: Could It Have Regulatory or Biofeedback Effects on Motivation and Emotion?" *Motivation and Emotion* 6 (3) (1982): 273–98; Weisfeld, G. E., and Beresford, J. M. "Erectness of Posture as an Indicator of Dominance or Success in Humans," *Motivation and Emotion* 6 (2) (1982): 113–31.

Montagu, A. *Growing Young* (New York: McGraw-Hill, 1983).

Loehr, J. E., and McLaughlin, P. *Mental Toughness Training* (Chicago: Nightingale-Conant, 1990): 18.

See, for example, Horn, J. "Models of Intelligence" in ed. Linn, R. *Intelligence: Measurement, Theory, and Public Policy* (Chicago: University of Illinois Press, 1989): 29–73; and Horn, J. "Cognitive Diversity: A Framework of Learning" in Ackerman, P. L., Sternberg, R. J., and Glaser, R. (eds.), *Learning and Individual Differences: Advances in Theory and Research* (New York: W. H. Freeman, 1989): 61–116.

Langer, E. J. *Mindfulness* (Reading, Mass.: Addison-Wesley, 1989): 137; Kabat-Zin, J. *Full-Catastrophe Living* (New York: Delacorte Press, 1990).

See, for example, Nadler, G., and Hibino, S. *Breakthrough Thinking* (Rocklin, Calif.: Prima Publishing, 1990); and Nadler, G., and Hibino, S., with Farrell, J. *Creative Solution Finding* (Rocklin, Calif.: Prima Publishing, 1995).

See, Csikszentmihalyi, *Flow*; and Csikszentmihalyi, *Finding Flow.*

Teich and Dodeles, "Mind Control"; Miller, E. E. *Software for the Mind* (Berkeley, Calif.: Celestial Arts, 1987); Otero, T. M. "Altering Your Inner Limits" in ed. Sheikh, A. A. *Anthology of Imagery Techniques* (Milwaukee, Wis.: American Imagery Institute, 1986): 289–311; Suinn, R. M. *Seven Steps to Peak Performance* (Lewiston, N.Y.: Hans Huber Publishers, 1986); Miller, E. E., lectures, Center for Health and Fitness Excellence, Bemidji, Minn. (May 1985, May 1986, and May 1987). Anchoring is an extension of holographic/holonomic theory of learning and memory. Pribram, *Holonomic Brain Theory*; Pribram, K. H. *Languages of the Brain* (New York: Brandon House, 1981). Variations of anchoring have been adapted from the systematic-desensitization approach of Joseph Wolpe, M.D.–Wolpe, J. *Psychotherapy by Reciprocal Inhibition* (Stanford, Calif.: Stanford University Press, 1958); Wolpe, J. *The Practice of Behavior Therapy* 2nd ed. (New York: Pergamin Press, 1973); Wolpe, J. *Life without Fear: Anxiety and Its Cure* (Oakland, Calif: New Harbinger, 1988).

Zilbergeld, B., and Lazarus, A. A. *Mind Power: Getting What You Want Through Mental Training* (Boston: Little, Brown, 1987): 19.

Teich and Dodeles, "Mind Control": 56.

See, for example, Rechtschaffen, S. *Time Shifting* (New York: Doubleday, 1996); Jaques, E., and Clement, S. D. *Executive Leadership: A Practical Guide to Managing Complexity* (Arlington, Va.: Cason Hall, 1991); and Jaques, E. *The Form of Time* (New York: Crane Russak, 1982).

See, for example, Childre, D., and Martin, H. *The HeartMath Solution* (New York: HarperCollins, 1999).

The Behavioral and Brain Sciences 8 (1986): 529–66; "Brain Shows Activation before Conscious Choice," *Brain/Mind Bulletin* (May 5, 1986): 1; Cattell, R. B. *Abilities: Their Structure, Growth, and Action* (Boston: Houghton Mifflin, 1971); Pribram, lecture (June 1987).

Winter, A., and Winter, R. *Build Your Brain Power* (New York: St. Martin's, 1986): 90.

Jaret, P. "Mind: Why Practice Makes Perfect," *Hippocrates* (Nov.–Dec. 1987): 90–91; Salthouse, T. *Scientific American* (Feb. 1984).

Jaret, "Mind."

See Csikszentmihalyi, *Flow*; Csikszentmihalyi, *Finding Flow*; Loehr, *Stress for Success*; Jaret, "Mind"; and Teich and Dodeles, "Mind Control."

Calm-Energy Switch #3: Hold Your Head High

Cailliet and Gross, *Rejuvenation Strategy*.

Imrie, with Dimson, *Goodbye Backache*.

Cailliet and Gross, *Rejuvenation Strategy*.

"Don't Be Slack about Good Posture," *University of California, Berkeley, Wellness Letter* (Oct. 1986): 6.

Cailliet and Gross, *Rejuvenation Strategy*.

Barlow, W. *The Alexander Technique* (New York: Knopf, 1972): 8.

Cailliet and Gross, *Rejuvenation Strategy*: 54.

Kraus, H. *Backache, Stress, and Tension* (New York: Pocket Books, 1969): 40; Imrie, D., with Dimson, C. *Goodbye Backache* (New York: Fawcett, 1983): 128–29.

Cailliet and Gross, *Rejuvenation Strategy*.

Bhatnager, V., et al. "Posture, Postural Discomfort, and Performance," *Human Factors* 27 (2) (Apr. 1985): 189–99; "Remedies for a Painful Case of Terminal-itis," *U.S. News and World Report* (Jan. 9, 1989): 60–61.

Riskind and Gotay, "Physical Posture."

Bhatnager, et al. "Posture, Posture Discomfort, and Performance."

Cailliet and Gross, *Rejuvenation Strategy*; Cailliet, R., quoted in "Good Posture: An Antidote for Aging," *Shape* (July 1987): 24.

Migdow, J. A., and Loehr, J. E. *Take a Deep Breath* (New York: Villard, 1986): 97.

Cailliet and Gross, *Rejuvenation Strategy*: 53.

Riskind, J. H., and Gotay, C. C. "Physical Posture: Could It Have Regulatory or Biofeedback Effects on Motivation and Emotion?" *Motivation and Emotion* 6 (3) (1982): 273–98; Weisfeld, G. E., and Beresford, J. M. "Erectness of Posture as an Indicator of Dominance or Success in Humans," *Motivation and Emotion* 6 (2) (1982): 113–31; Wilson, E., and Schneider, C. "Static and Dynamic Feedback in the Treatment of Chronic Muscle Pain," paper presented at the Biofeedback Society of American meeting (New Orleans, Apr. 16, 1985); Winter and Winter, *Build Your Brain Power, The Neuropsychology of Achievement* (Newark, Calif.: Sybervision Systems, 1985).

Astrand, P. O., and Rodahl, K. *Textbook of Work Physiology: Physiological Bases of Exercise* (New York: McGraw-Hill, 1986): 112; Hanna, T. *The Body of Life* (New York: Knopf, 1980).

Riskind and Gotay, "Physical Posture"; Weisfeld and Beresford, "Erectness of Posture"; Wilson, E., and Schneider, C. "Treatment of Chronic Muscle Pain"; Winter and Winter, *Build Your Brain Power, The Neuropsychology of Achievement*.

Ibid.

Cailliet and Gross, *Rejuvenation Strategy*.

Warfel, J. H. *The Head, Neck, and Trunk* 4th ed. (Philadelphia: Lea & Febiger, 1973): 46.

Binder, T. *Position Technic: The Science of Centering* (Boulder, Colo.: Binder: 1977).

Travell, J. G. *Office Hours: Day and Night* (New York: World Publishing, 1968): 270, 284, 285, 301, 302. Cited in Travell, J. G., and Simons, D. G. *Myofascial Pain and Dysfunction* (Baltimore: Williams and Wilkins, 1983): 112.

Gould, N. "Back-Pocket Sciatica," *New England Journal of Medicine* 290 (1974): 633.

Calm-Energy Switch #4: Do Less to Get Ahead

Hinton, E. "Steady As You Go," *Sports Illustrated* (Mar. 5, 1999): 72.

See, for example, Arnot, R. *The Biology of Success* (New York: Little, Brown, 2000).

Arnot, *Biology of Success*: 159–60.

Csiksyzentmihalyi, *Flow*.

See, for example, Loehr, *Stress for Success*.

Loehr, *Stress for Success*: 134.

Loehr, *Stress for Success*.

Calm-Energy Switch #5: Find Breathing Space

See, for example, Terr, L. *Beyond Love and Work: Why Adults Need to Play* (New York: Scribners, 1999); Schrage, M. *Serious Play* (Boston: Harvard Business School Press, 1999); and Montagu, A. *Neotony: Growing Young* (New York: McGraw-Hill, 1982).

Chafetz, M. D. *Smart for Life: How to Improve Your Brainpower at Any Age* (New York: Penguin, 1993): 64–65.

Rybcznski, W. *Waiting for the Weekend* (New York: Viking, 1991).

Langer, *Mindfulness*.

See, for example, Loehr, *Stress for Success*.

See, for example, De Bono, E. *Serious Creativity* (New York: HarperBusiness, 1992).

Grilo, C. M., Schiffman, S. "Longitudinal Investigation of the Abstinence Violation Effect in Binge Eaters," *Journal of Consulting and Clinical Psychology* 62 (1994): 611–19; Grilo, C. M., et al. "The Social Self, Body Dissatisfaction, and Binge Eating in Obese Females," *Obesity Research* 2 (1994): 24–27.

Ljungdahl, L. "Laugh If This Is a Joke," *New England Journal of Medicne* 261 (1989): 558; Dillon, K. M., et al. "Positive Emotional States and Enhancement of the Immune System," *International Journal of Psychiatry in Medicine* 15 (1) (1985–86): 13–18; Eckman, P., et al. "Autonomic Nervous System Activity Distinguishes among Emotions," *Science* 221 (1983): 1208–10; Berk, A. L. S., et al. *Clinical Research* 36 (1988): 121 and 435A; Berk, A. L. S., et al. *The Federation of American Societies for Experimental Biology (FASEB) Journal* 2 (1988): A1570.

Lefcourt, H. M., and Martin, R. A. *Humor and Life Stress* (New York: Springer-Verlag, 1986); Nezu, A. M., et al. "Sense of Humor as a Moderator of the Relation between Stressful Events and Psychological Distress: A Prospective Analysis," *Journal of Personality and Social Psychology* 54 (1988): 520–25.

Chapman, A., and Foot, H. *Handbook of Humor and Laughter: Theory, Research, and Applications* (New York: Wiley, 1982); "Laughing toward Longevity," *University of California, Berkeley, Wellness Letter* (June 1985): 1; "The Mind Fights Back," *Washington Post*; Brody, "Laughter," *New York Times*.

See, for example, Cooper, R. K., and Sawaf, A. *Executive EQ: Emotional Intelligence in Leadership and Organizations* (New York: Grosset/Putnam, 1997); Goleman, D. *Emotional Intelligence* (New York: Bantam, 1999); and Sternberg, *Successful Intelligence*.

For some great insights on this subject, see Vienne, V. *The Art of Doing Nothing* (New York: Potter, 1998).

See Nagler, W., and Androff, A. *The Dirty Half-Dozen: Six Radical Rules to Make Relationships Last* (New York: Warner, 1991).

Mackoff, B. *The Art of Self-Renewal* (Los Angeles: Lowell House, 1992).

Nagler and Androff, *The Dirty Half-Dozen*: 47–48.

Solomon, R. C. *About Love: Reinventing Romance for Our Times* (New York: Simon & Schuster, 1988): 264.

Nagler. *Dirty Half-Dozen*: 5–6, 17.

Ziv, A., and Gadish, O. *Journal of Social Psychology* 129 (1990): 759–68.

Seligman, M. E. P. *What You Can Change and What You Can't* (New York: Knopf, 1993): 132.

"Tokyoites More Tired, Stressed, Than Residents of N.Y. or L.A," *Montreal Gazette* (July 31, 1989).

Klesges, R. C. *Report to the Society of Behavioral Medicine*. Cited in *Environmental Nutrition* 15 (6) (June 1992): 1.

Flannery, R. B., Jr. "The Stress-Resistant Person," *Harvard Medical School Health Letter* (Feb. 1989): 5–7.

Diener, E. Quoted in *Psychology Today* (July–Aug. 1989): 39; Ornstein, R., and Sobel, D. *Healthy Pleasures* (Reading, Mass.: Addison-Wesley, 1989).

Introduction to the Active-Energy Switches

See, for example, Cailliet and Gross. *Rejuvenation Strategy*.

Moore-Ede. *24-Hour Society*: 53, 69.

Active-Energy Switch #1: Plan Your Time-Outs

See, for example, Loehr. *Stress for Success*; and Csikszentmihalyi, M. *Creativity* (New York: HarperCollins, 1996).

See, for example, Moore-Ede. *24-Hour Society*; and Lamberg. *Bodyrhythms*.

Dement, W. C. Foreword to Lamberg. *Bodyrhythms*: 8.

See, for example, Norfolk, D. *Executive Stress* (New York: Warner, 1986); Moore-Ede. *24-Hour Society*; and Grandjean, E. *Fitting the Task* 4th ed. (New York: Taylor and Francis, 1988).

Stellman, J., and Henifin, M. S. *Office Work Can Be Dangerous to Your Health* (New York: Ballantine, 1989): 28.

Heus, M., Heus, M., Heus, G., and Heus, J. *Low-Fat for Life* (Barneveld, Wis.: Micamar Publishing, 1994): 87; Batmanghelidj, F. *Your Body's Many Cries for Water* 2nd ed. (Falls Church, VA: Global Health Solutions, 1998.)

Darden, E. *A Day-by-Day 10-Step Program* (Dallas: Taylor Publishing, 1992): 43.

McArdle, Katch, and Katch. *Exercise Physiology*: 451; Hanson, P. G. *The Joy of Stress* (Kansas City: Andrews, McMeel & Parker, 1987): 27.

Thompson, D. Quoted in Roach, M. "Do You Fit in Your Office?" *Hippocrates* (July–Aug. 1989): 46.

McArdle, W. D., Katch, F. I., and Katch, V. L. *Exercise Physiology: Energy, Nutrition, and Human Performance* (Philadelphia: Lea & Febiger, 1986): 451; Swarth, J. *Stress and Nutrition* (San Diego: Health Media of America, 1986): 23; Brooks, G. A., and Fahey, T. D. *Exercise Physiology: Human Bioenergetics and Its Applications* (New York: Macmillan, 1985): 462.

Mark and Mark. *Brain Power*.

Goldman, R., and Hackman, R. M. *The "E" Factor* (New York: William Morrow, 1988); Goldman, R., Klatz, R., and Berger, L. *Brain Fitness* (New York: Doubleday, 1999).

McArdle, Katch, and Katch. *Exercise Physiology*: 451.

Hyman, J. W. *The Light Book* (Los Angeles: Tarcher, 1990); Ackerman, D. *A Natural History of the Senses* (New York: Random House, 1990).

Sobel and Ornstein. *Healthy Pleasures*.

Zajonc, A. *Catching the Light* (New York: Bantam, 1993); Moore-Ede. *24-Hour Society*: 60.

McIntyre, I., et al. *Life Sciences* 45 (1990): 327–32.; *Brain/Mind Bulletin* (Jan. 1990): 7.

Moore-Ede. *24-Hour Society*: 53, 69.

Active-Energy Switch #2: Reset Your Pace

For introductory reading, see Rossi, E. L., and Nimmons, D. *The 20-Minute Break* (New York: Tarcher, 1991); and Lamberg. *Bodyrhythms*.

Grandjean. *Fitting the Task*.

Janaro, R. E., et al. "A Technical Note on Increasing Productivity through Effective Rest-Break Scheduling," *Industrial Management* 30 (1)(Jan.–Feb. 1988): 29–33; Penc, J. "Motivational

Stimulation and System of Work Improvement," *Studia-Socjologiczne* 3 (102) (1986): 179–97; Foegen, J. H. "Super-Breaktime," *Supervision* 49 (Oct. 1988): 9–10; Bechtold, S. E., and Sumners, D. L. "Optimal Work-Rest Scheduling with Exponential Work-Rate Decay," *Management Science* 34 (Apr. 1988): 547–52; Krueger, G. P. "Human Performance in Continuous/Sustained Operations and the Demands of Extended Work/Rest Schedules: An Annotated Bibliography," *Psychological Documents* 15 (2) (Dec. 1985): 27–28; Boothe, R. S. "Optimization of Rest Breaks: A Productivity Enhancement," *Dissertation Abstracts International* 45 (9–A) (Mar. 1985): 2927; Gustafson, H. W. "Efficiency of Output in Self-Paced Work, Machine-Paced Work," *Human Factors* 24 (4) (Aug. 1982): 395–410; Janaro, R. E., and Bechtold, S. E. "A Study of the Reduction of Fatigue Impact on Productivity through Optimal Rest-Break Scheduling," *Human Factors* 27 (4)(Aug. 1985): 459–66; Okogbaa, O. G. "An Empirical Model for Mental Work Output and Fatigue," *Dissertation Abstracts International* 15 (2) (Dec. 1985): 27–28; Thatcher, R. E. *Journal of Personality and Social Psychology* 52 (1987): 119–25; Zarakovski, G. M., et al. "Psychophysiological Analysis of Periodic Fluctuations in the Quality of Activity within the Work Cycle," *Human Physiology* 8 (3) (May 1983): 208–20; Bechtold, S. E., et al. "Maximization of Labor Productivity through Optimal Rest-Break Schedules," *Management Science* 30 (12) (Dec. 1984): 1442–48.

Thayer. *Biopsychology of Mood and Arousal*; Globus, G. G., et al. "Ultradian Rhythms in Human Performance," *Perceptual and Motor Skills* 33 (1971): 1171–74; Kleitman, N. *Sleep and Wakefulness* rev. ed. (Chicago: University of Chicago Press, 1963); Kripe, D. F. "An Ultradian Rhythm Associated with Perceptual Deprivation and REM Sleep," *Psychosomatic Medicine* 34 (1972): 221–34; Lavie, P., and Scherson, A. "Evidence of Ultradian Rhythmicity in 'Sleep-Ability,'" *Electroencephalography and Clinical Neurophysiology* 52 (1981): 163–74; Gertz, J., and Lavie, P. "Biological Rhythms in Arousal Indicies," *Psychophysiology* 20 (1983): 690–95; Orr, W., et al. "Ultradian Rhythms in Extended Performance," *Aerospace Medicine* 45(1974): 995–1000.

Rossi and Nimmons. *20-Minute Break*: 35–36.

Rossi and Nimmons. *20-Minute Break*: 103.

Gallagher, W. *The Power of Place: How Our Surroundings Shape Our Thoughts, Emotions, and Actions* (New York: Poseidon Press, 1993).

Chafetz. *Smart for Life*.

Finke, R. *Creative Imagery: Discoveries in Visualization* (Hillsdale, N.J.: Erlbaum, 1990); Sedlacek. *The Sedlacek Technique*: 144.

Gallagher. *Power of Place*: 132.

Kaplan, R. "The Role of Nature in the Context of the Workplace," *Landscape and Urban Planning* 26 (1993).

Mental Medicine Update 2 (2) (Fall 1993).

Moore-Ede. *24-Hour Society*: 60.

Grilo, C. M., Wilfley, D. E., and Brownell, K. D. "Physical Activity and Weight Control: Why Is the Link So Strong?" *The Weight-Control Digest* 2 (3) (May–June 1992): 153–60; Grilo, C. M., Brownell, K. D., and Stunkard, A. J. "The Metabolic and Psychological Importance of Exercise in Weight Control," in eds. Stunkard, A. J., and Walden, T. A. *Obesity: Theory and Therapy* (New York: Raven Press, 1992); Piscatella, J. C. *Controlling Your Fat Tooth* (New York: Workman, 1991): 100–104.

"Muscles in a Minute," *USA Today* (Mar. 1, 2000): 9D.

Tkachuk, G., and Martin, G. *Professional Psychology: Research and Practice* (June 14, 1999).

Moore-Ede. *24-Hour Society*: 55–56.

See, for example, Loehr. *Stress for Success*: 159.

Cailliet, R. *Understand Your Backache* (Philadelphia: F.A. Davis, 1984): 118–21; Mensendieck, E. M. *Look Better, Feel Better* (New York: Harper and Row, 1954): 48.

Katch, F. I., et al. "Effects of Situp-Exercise Training on Adipose Tissue Cell Size and Activity," *Research Quarterly for Exercise and Sport* 55 (1984): 242–47; Clark, N. "Situps Don't Melt Ab Flab," *Runner's World* (Mar. 1985): 32.

Sharkey, B. J. *Physiology of Exercise* (Champaign, Ill.: Human Kinetics, 1984): 336; Cailliet. *Understand Your Backache*: 122–24; Cailliet and Gross. *Rejuvenation Strategy*.

Dienstbier, R., et al. "Catecholamine Training Effects from Exercise: A Bridge to Exercise-Temperament Relationships," *Motivation and Emotion* 2 (1987): 297–318.

Blair, S. N. *Living with Exercise* (Dallas: LEARN Education Center, 1991): 18.

Westcott, W. L. Quoted in *Shrink Your Stomach in Nothing Flat* (Emmaus, Pa.: Rodale, 1994): 15.

Daniels, L., and Worthingham, C. *Therapeutic Exercise for Body Alignment and Function* (Philadelphia: W. B. Saunders, 1977): 77; Yessis, M. "Kinesiology," *Muscle and Fitness* (Feb. 1985): 18–19, 142.

Lamb, L. E. *The Weighting Game* (Seacaucus, N.J.: Carol Publishing Group, 1991): 201.

Bailey, C. *Smart Exercise* (Boston: Houghton Mifflin, 1994): 28.

Grilo, Wifley, and Brownell. "Physical Activity and Weight Control."

Pavlou, K. N., et al. "Exercise as an Adjunct to Weight Loss and Maintenance in Moderately Obese Subjects," *American Journal of Clinical Nutrition* 49 (1989): 1115–23; Kayman, S., et al. "Maintenance and Relapse after Weight Loss in Women," *American Journal of Clinical Nutrition* 52 (1990): 800–807.

Kayman, et al. "Maintenance and Relapse after Weight Loss in Women."

Piscatella. *Controlling Your Fat Tooth*.

Tremblay, A. In *International Journal of Obesity* 13 (1989): 4.

National Institutes of Health Conference on Physical Activity and Obesity, held in Dec. 1992 in Bethesda, MD. Reported in *Obesity and Health* 8 (1) (Jan.–Feb. 1994): 10.

Walberg-Rankin, J. Quoted in *Men's Health* (Jan.–Feb. 1994): 83.

Pirie, L. *Getting Built* (New York: Warner Books, 1984): 146–48.

Duncan, J. Quoted in ed. Bricklin, M. *Prevention's Lose Weight Guidebook 1994* (Emmaus, Pa.: Rodale, 1994): 3.

Thompson: 42–46.

Kramer, J. "Biomechanische Veranderungen in Lumbalen Bewegungssegment," *Hippokrates* (1973).

Thompson: 46.

Stellman and Henifin. *Office Work*: 25–26.

Moore-Ede. *24-Hour Society*: 55.

Blackburn, G. L. Quoted in *Prevention* (Sept. 1992): 50.

Silverman, K., et.al. "Withdrawal Syndrome After the Double-Blind Cessation of Caffeine Consumption," *New England Journal of Medicine* 327 (16) (Oct. 15, 1992): 1109–14.

Dulloo, A. G., et al. "Normal Caffeine Consumption: Influence on Thermogenesis and Daily Energy Expenditure in Lean and Postobese Human Volunteers," *American Journal of Clinical Nutrition* 49 (1) (1989): 44–50.

Rodin, J. *Body Traps* (New York: Morrow, William, and Company, 1993)194.

Jenkins, D. A., et al. "Nibbling versus Gorging: Metabolic Advantages of Increased Meal Frequency," *New England Journal of Medicine* 321 (4) (Oct. 5, 1989): 929–34.

Jones, P. J., Leitch, C. A., and Pederson, R. A. "Meal-Frequency Effects on Plasma Hormone Concentrations and Cholesterol Synthesis in Humans," *American Journal of Clinical Nutrition* 57 (6) (1993): 868–74; Edelstein, S. L., et al. "Increased Meal Frequency Associated with Decreased Cholesterol Concentrations," *American Journal of Clinical Nutrition* 55 (1992): 664–69.

Edelstein, et al. "Increased Meal Frequency."

Lamb. *Weighting Game*: 95–96.

Leveille, T. "Adipose Tissue Metabolism: Influence of Eating and Diet Composition," *Federation Proceedings* 29 (1970): 1294–301; Lukert, B. "Biology of Obesity," in ed. Wolman, B. *Psychological Aspects of Obesity* (New York: Van Nostrand Reinhold, 1982): 1–14; Szepsi, B. "A Model of Nutritionally Induced Overweight: Weight 'Rebound' Following Caloric Restriction," in ed. Bray, G. *Recent Advances in Obesity Research* (London: Newman, 1978).

Leibowitz.

Miller, W. C. *The Non-Diet Diet* (Englewood, Colo.: Morton Publishing, 1991): 88.

Rossi and Nimmons. *20-Minute Break*: 122–23.

Blackburn, G. Cited in *Environmental Nutrition* 16 (2) (Feb. 1993): 1.

See, for example, Wurtman, J. J. *The Serotonin Solution* (New York: Fawcett, 1996); Wurtman, J. J. *Managing Your Mind and Mood through Food* (New York: HarperCollins, 1987); Spring, B., et al. "Carbohydrates, Tryptophan, and Behavior: A Methodological Review," *Psychological Bulletin* 102 (1987): 234–56; Benton. *Biological Psychiatry* 24 (1988): 95–100; Lieberman, H., et al. "Aging, Nutrient Choice, Activity, and Behavioral Responses to Nutrients," *Annals of the New York Academy of Science* 561 (1989): 196–208; Wurtman, R. J., and Wurtman, J. J. "Do Carbohydrates Affect Food Intake via Neurotransmitter Activity?" *Appetite* 11 (1988) (Suppl. 1): 42–47; Wurtman, J. J. "Recent Evidence from Human Studies Linking Central Serotoninergic Function with Carbohydrate Intake," *Appetite* 8 (3) (1987): 211–13; Wurtman, R. J. "Dietary Treatments That Affect Brain Neurotransmitters," *Annals of the New York Academy of Science* 499 (1987): 179–90; Leathwood, P. "Food Composition, Changes in Brain Serotonin Synthesis and Appetite for Protein and Carbohydrate," *Appetite* 8 (3) (1987): 202–5; Spring, B., et al. "Psychobiological Effects of Carbohydrates," *Journal of Clinical Psychiatry* 50 (Suppl) (May 1989): 27–34; Wurtman, J. J. "Carbohydrate Craving, Mood Changes, and Obesity," *Journal of Clinical Psychiatry* 49 (Suppl) (Aug. 1989): 37–39; Okuyama, H. "Does Food Affect Brain Function?" *Tanpakushitsu Kakusan Koso* 35 (3) (Mar. 1990): 275–79; Wurtman, R. J., and Wurtman, J. J. "Carbohydrates and Depression," *Scientific American* 260 (1) (Jan. 1989): 68–75.

Ibid.

Active-Energy Switch #3: Have a Vigorous Lunch

See, for example, Thayer. *The Origin of Everday Moods*; Rossi and Nimmons. *20-Minute Break*; and Grandjean. *Fitting the Task*.

See Wurtman J. J. *Managing Your Mind and Mood Through Food*.

See, for example, Langer. *Mindfulness*; and Langer, E. J. *The Power of Mindful Learning* (Reading, Mass.: Addison-Wesley, 1998).

Grandjean. *Fitting the Task*.

Craig, A. "Acute Effects of Meals on Perceptual and Cognitive Efficiency." presented at the conference *Diet and Behavior: A Multidisciplinary Evaluation* sponsored by the American Medical Association, November 27–29, 1984.

See, by way of introduction, Chafetz. *Smart for Life*.

"Better to Eat Ze Main Meal Earlier?" *Tufts University Diet and Nutrition Letter* 11 (4) (Jun. 1993): 1.

Schiffman, S. "The Use of Flavor to Enhance the Efficacy of Reducing Diets," *Hospital Practice* 21 (7) (1986): 44H–44R; Quebec studies cited in eds. Bricklin, M., and Imhoff, A. R. *Prevention's Lose Weight Guidebook 1992* (Emmaus, Pa.: Rodale, 1992): 64; Henry, C. J. K., and Emergy, B. "Effect of Spiced Food on Metabolic Rate," *Human Nutrition: Clinical Nutrition* 40C (1986): 165–68.

Ibid.

Weingarten, H. Quoted in Goldberg, J. "The Taste of Desire," *American Health* (Oct. 1990): 52.

See, for example, Rivlin, R., and Gravelle, K. *Deciphering the Senses* (New York: Simon & Schuster, 1984); and Sobel and Ornstein. *Healthy Pleasures*.

Wurtman, J. J. Quoted in "Peak-Performance Brain Food," *Omni Longevity* 2 (6) (Apr. 1988): 67.

Serafini, M., et al. "Invivo Antioxidant Effect of Green and Black Tea in Man," *European Journal of Clinical Nutrition* 50 (1996): 28–32.

Lieberman, H., and Spring, B. "Quantifying the Behavioral Effects of Food Constituents," Presented at the Conference *Diet and Behavior: A Multidisciplinary Evaluation* sponsored by the American Medical Association, November 27–29, 1984.

Rolls, B. J., et.al. "Foods with Different Satiating Effects in Humans," *Appetite* 15 (1990): 115–20.

National Cancer Institute and the USDA Human Nutrition Information Service Sept. 1992 press release.

Thayer. *The Origin of Everyday Moods*; Thayer, R. E., et al. "Mood and Behavior following Moderate Exercise: A Partial Test of Self-Regulation Theory," *Personality and Individual Differences* 14 (1993): 97–104.

Ed. American College of Sports Medicine. *Guidelines for Graded Exercise Testing Prescription* 4th ed. (Philadelphia: Lea & Febiger, 1991).

Cooper, K. H. *Controlling Cholesterol* (New York: Bantam, 1988): 219–243.

Astrand, P. *Health and Fitness* (New York: Walker, 1987): 12.

Tice, D. Study results reported in *New York Times* (Dec. 30, 1992): C6.

See, for example, Goldman, Klatz, and Berger. *Brain Fitness*: 76–79.

Marano, H. E. "Chemistry and Craving," *Psychology Today* (Jan.–Feb. 1993): 30–36, 74.

Stamford, B. A. "Meals and the Timing of Exercise," *The Physician and Sports Medicine* 17 (11) (Nov. 1989): 151.

Stamford and Shimer. *Fitness without Exercise*: 44, 128; Stamford. "Meals and the Timing of Exercise"; Davis, J. M., et al. "Weight Control and Calorie Expenditure: Thermogenic Effects of Pre-Prandial and Post-Prandial Exercise," *Addictive Behavior* 14 (3) (1989): 347–51; Poehlman, E. T., and Horton, E. S. "The Impact of Food Intake and Exercise on Energy Expenditure," *Nutrition Reviews* 47 (5) (May 1989): 129–37.

Stamford and Shimer. *Fitness without Exercise*: 44.

Myers, D. G. *The Pursuit of Happiness* (New York: Morrow, 1992): 76, 77–79, 206–207.

Cailliet and Gross. *Rejuvenation Strategy*: 9.

Hanson, D. Quoted in "Natural Weight Control," *Prevention* (Jan. 1994): 114.

Cooper, K. H. Personal communications (Aug. 21, 1986; May 15, 1988; Jan. 25, 1994).

Cooper, K. H. *The Aerobics Way* (New York: Bantam, 1977): 44.

Cooper, K. H. *The Aerobics Program for Total Well-Being* (New York: Bantam, 1988): 113.

McArdle, Katch, and Katch. *Exercise Physiology*.

Yessis, M. *Secrets of Soviet Sports Fitness and Training* (New York: M. Evans, 1987): 71–78; Lawrence, R. M., and Rosenzweig, S., *Going the Distance* (Los Angeles: Tarcher, 1987): 26–27; Shellock, F. G. "Physiological Benefits of Warmup," *Physician and Sports Medicine* 11 (10)(Oct. 1983): 134–39; Shyne, K. "To Stretch or Not to Stretch?" *Physician and Sports Medicine* 10 (9) (Sept., 1982): 137–40.

Sharkey, B. J. *New Dimensions in Aerobic Fitness* (Champaign, Ill.: Human Kinetics, 1991): 25–26.

France, K. "Competitive vs. Non-Competitive Thinking during Exercise: Effects on Norepinephrine Levels," paper presented at the annual meeting of the American Psychology Association, Toronto. (Aug. 1984).

Bailey, C. *Smart Exercise* (Boston: Houghton Mifflin, 1994): 129.

Schwartz, R. S., et al. "The Effect of Intensive Endurance-Exercise Training on Body Fat Distribution in Young and Older Men," *Metabolism* 40 (5) (May 1991): 545–51.

Stamford, B. A. Quoted in "Natural Weight Loss, "*Prevention* (May 1992): 35.

Ibid.

Active-Energy Switch #4: Go Home Feeling Better

Rossi and Nimmons. *20-Minute Break.*

Moore-Ede. *24-Hour Society.*

Thayer. *The Origins of Everyday Moods*: 209.

Mackoff. *The Art of Self-Renewal.*

Ehrbar, A. "Price of Progress: 'Re-Engineering' Gives Firms New Efficiency, Workers the Pink Slip," *Wall Street Journal* (Mar. 16, 1993): 1; Fisher, A. B. "Welcome to the Age of Overwork," *Fortune* (Nov. 30, 1992): 64–71; Huey, J. "Managing in the Midst of Chaos," *Fortune* (Apr. 5, 1993): 38–48.

Work/Family Directions, Inc. Research. Cited in *Achieving Balance* (Great Performance, Inc., Portland, OR, 1990).

Bolger, N., et al. "The Contagion of Stress Across Multiple Roles," *Journal of Marriage and the Family* 51 (Feb. 1989): 175–83; and "Marital Problems Affect Job," American Psychological Study reported in *USA Today* (Nov. 8, 1989).

Myers. *The Pursuit of Happiness*; House, J. S., et al. "Association of Social Relationships and Activities with Mortality: Prospective Evidence from the Tecumseh Community Health Study," *American Journal of Epidemiology* 116 (1) (1982): 123–40; Berkman, L. F., and Syme, L. O. "Social Networks, Host Resistance, and Mortality: A 9-Year Follow-Up of Alameda County Residents," *American Journal of Epidemiology* 102 (2) (1979): 186–204; Eisenberg, L. "A Friend, Not an Apple, A Day Will Keep the Doctor Away," *Journal of the American Medical Association* 66 (1979): 551–53; Cohen, S., and Wils, T. "Stress, Social Support, and Buffering Hypothesis," *Psychological Bulletin* 98 (1985): 210–57; Caplan, G. "Mastery of Stress: Psychological Aspects," *American Journal of Psychiatry* 138 (1981): 413–20; Lynch, J. J. *The Broken Heart: Medical Consequences of Loneliness* (New York: Basic Books, 1977); Jaffe, D. T., and Scott, C. D. *Take This Job and Love It* (New York: Simon & Schuster, 1988): 185.

Research by Princeton University psychologist John B. Jemmott III. Cited in Elias, M. "Friends May Help Keep Disease Away," *USA Today* (Oct. 11, 1989); Fassel, D. *Working Ourselves to Death* (New York: HarperCollins, 1990).

Fassel. *Working Ourselves to Death.*

Schor, J. B. *The Overworked American* (New York; Basic Books, 1991); Garden, A. M. *Journal of Occupational Psychology* 62 (1989): 223–224.

Crosby, F. J. Juggling (New York: Free Press, 1991); Schor. *The Overworked American;* Eckenrode, J., and Gore, S. (Eds.) *Stress between Work and Family* (New York: Plenum, 1990).

Miller, E. E. *Software for the Mind* (Berkley: Celestial Arts, 1988); ed. Sheikh, A. A. *Imagery: Current Theory, Research, and Application* (New York: Wiley Interscience, 1984); ed. Marks, D. F. *Theories of Image Formation* (New York: Brandon House, 1986); Suinn, R. M. *Seven Steps to Peak Performance* (Lewiston, N.Y.: Hans Huber Publishers, 1986).

Imber-Black, E., and Roberts, J. *Rituals for Our Times* (New York: HarperCollins, 1992); O'Neil, J. R. *The Paradox of Success* (New York: Tarcher, 1993).

Moore-Ede. *24-Hour Society;* Wyman. *The Light Book.*

Imber-Black, E., and Roberts, J. *Rituals for Our Times* (New York: HarperCollins, 1992); O'Neil, J. R. *The Paradox of Success* (New York: Tarcher/Putnam, 1993).

deBono, E. *Serious Creativity* (New York: HarperCollins, 1993).

Active-Energy Switch #5: Get Evening Relief

Imber-Black and Roberts. *Rituals for Our Times*; eds. Imber-Black, E., Roberts, J., and Whiting, R. *Rituals in Families and Family Therapy* (New York: Norton, 1988).

Imber-Black and Roberts. *Rituals for Our Times.*

Imber-Black and Roberts. *Rituals for Our Times*: 15, 45.

Nagler and Androff. *The Dirty Half-Dozen*: 47–48.

Stone. *Snack Attack*: 156.

Rolls, et al. "Foods with Different Satiating Effects in Humans."

"Better to Eat Ze Main Meal Earlier?"

Clouatre, D. *The Complete Guide to Anti-Fat Nutrients* (San Francisco: Pax Publishing, 1993): 106.

University of Minnesota study. Proceedings of the 10th International Congress on Nutrition.

Smith, A. F. Cited in DeAngelis, T. "On a Diet? Don't Trust Your Memory," *Psychology Today* (Oct. 1989): 12.

Brownell, K. D. *The LEARN Program for Weight Control* (Dallas: LEARN Education Center, 1991): 15.

Schiffman. "The Use of Flavor to Enhance the Efficacy of Reducing Diets."

Schiffman. "The Use of Flavor to Enhance the Efficacy of Reducing Diets"; Quebec studies cited in eds. Bricklin and Imhoff. *Prevention's Lose Weight Guidebook 1992*: 64.

Henry and Emergy. "Effect of Spiced Food on Metabolic Rate."

Wurtman, J. J. *Managing Your Mind and Mood through Food*; Chafetz. *Smart for Life*; Lamberg. *Bodyrhythms*.

Wolfe. *When He Has a Headache*.

Wurtman, J. J. *Managing Your Mind and Mood through Food*; Chafetz. *Smart for Life*; Lamberg. *Bodyrhythms*.

Rossi and Nimmons. *20-Minute Break*.

Darden. *Day-by-Day 10-Step Program*: 81–82.

Roffers, M. "Nutrition Myths," *Medical Self-Care* (Mar.–Apr. 1986): 52.

Stamford. Quoted in "Natural Weight Control."

Davis, et al. "Weight Control and Calorie Expenditure."; Gleeson, M. "Effects of Physical Exercise on Metabolic Rate and Dietary-Induced Thermogenesis," *British Journal of Nutrition* 47 (1982): 173; Bielinski, R., et al. "Energy Metabolism During the Postexercise Recovery in Man," *American Journal of Clinical Nutrition* 42 (1985): 69–82.

Stephens, T. "Physical Activity and Mental Health in the United States and Canada: Evidence from Four Population Surveys," *Preventive Medicine* 17 (1988): 35–47; Hogan, J. "Personality Correlates of Physical Fitness," *Journal of Personality and Social Psychology* 56 (1989): 284–88; Tucker, L. A. "Physical Fitness and Psychological Disorders," *International Journal of Sport Psychology* 21 (1990): 185–201.

Stamford, B. A. "What Time Should You Exercise?" *The Physician and Sports Medicine* 14 (8)(Aug. 1986): 162.

Stamford. "Meals and the Timing of Exercise"; Roffers. "Nutrition Myths."

"Natural Weight Control," *Prevention* (Apr. 1993): 67.

Clouatre. *Guide to Anti-Fat Nutrients*: 107; Davis, et al. "Weight Control"; Gleeson. "Effects of Physical Exercise on Metabolic Rate and Dietary-Induced Thermogenesis"; Bielinski, et al. "Energy Metabolism during the Postexercise Recovery in Man"; Darden. *Day-by-Day 10-Step Program*: 75.

Thayer, R. E. "Energy, Tiredness, and Tension Effects of a Sugar Snack versus Moderate Exercise," *Journal of Personality and Social Psychology* 52 (1987): 119–25.

Grilo, Wilfley, and Brownell. "Physical Activity and Weight Control: Why Is the Link So Strong?"; Grilo, Brownell, and Stunkard. "The Metabolic and Psychological Importance of Exercise in Weight Control"; Piscatella. *Controlling Your Fat Tooth*.

Introduction to the Sensory-Energy Switches

See, for example, Rivlin, R., and Gravelle, K. *Deciphering the Senses* (New York: Simon & Schuster, 1994).

Halleck, R. *The Education of the Nervous System* (New York: Macmillan, 1901).

Lapp, D. Quoted in University of Texas Lifetime Health Letter 3(12)(Dec., 1991): 7.

See, for example, Land, G. T. *Grow or Die: the Unifying Principle of Transformation* rev. ed. (New York: Wiley, 1986).

Montagu. *Growing Young.*

Diamond, M. C. *Enriching Heredity* (New York: Free Press, 1988); Diamond, M. C., and Hopson, J. *Magic Trees of the Mind* (New York: Plume, 1999).

See, for example, Winter and Winter. *Build Your Brain Power;* and Chafetz. *Smart for Life.*

Erickson, J. M. "Vital Senses: Sources of Lifelong Learning," *Journal of Education* 167 (3) (1985).

Justice, B. *Who Gets Sick? Thinking and Health* (Houston: Peak Press, 1987): 259.

Diamond, M. C. *How the Brain Grows in Response to Experience* (Los Altos, Calif.: Institute for the Study of Human Knowledge, 1983), audiocassette; *Brain/Mind Bulletin* 12 (7) (Mar. 1987): 1–5; Kiyono, S., et al. *Physiology and Behavior* 34: 431–35; Hwang, H. M., and Greenough, W. T. Paper presented at the annual meeting of the Society for Neuroscience (1986).

Rivlin and Gravelle. *Deciphering the Senses.*

Winter and Winter. *Build Your Brain Power.* 17.

Sensory-Energy Switch #1: Mix Up Your Habits

See, for example, Diamond. *Enriching Heredity;* Diamond and Hopson. *Magic Trees;* Montagu. *Growing Young;* and Bortz, W. M., II. *We Live Too Short and Die Too Long* (New York: Bantam, 1991).

See, for example, Sobel and Ornstein. *Healthy Pleasures.*

Beck, A., and Katcher, A. *Between Pets and People: The Importance of Animal Companionship* (New York: Putnam, 1983); Fitz-Gerald, F. T. "The Therapeutic Value of Pets," *Western Journal of Medicine* 144 (1986): 103–5; Friedmann, E., et al. "Animal Companions and 1-Year Survival of Patients after Discharge from a Coronary Unit," *Public Health Reports* 95 (1980): 307–12.

Montagu. *Growing Young.*

"Looking Forward to the Good Life at Age 100," *USA Today* (Dec. 21, 1992).

Bortz. *Live Too Short and Die Too Long:* 1.

Rowe, J. Quoted in "The Search for the Fountain of Youth," *Newsweek* (Mar. 5, 1990): 42.

Cutler, R. "Evolution of Longevity in Primates," *Journal of Human Evolution* 5 (1976): 169–202; Bortz. *Live Too Short and Die Too Long:* 1; Butler, R. N. Quoted in "Slowing Down the Clock," *20/20* (May 19, 1988).

Bortz. *Live Too Short and Die Too Long:* 47.

Langer. *Mindfulness:* 112–13.

Mulvey, A., and Langer, E. As discussed in Rodin, J., and Langer, E. "Aging Labels: The Decline of Control and the Fall of Self-Esteem," *Journal of Social Issues* 36 (1980): 12–29.

Katzman, P., and Carasu, T. "Differential Diagnosis of Dementia." In ed. Fields, W. S. *Neurological and Sensory Disorders in the Elderly* (Miami: Symposia Specialist Medical Books, 1975): 103–4.

Montagu. *Growing Young.*

See, for example, Sobel and Ornstein. *Healthy Pleasures;* Korbin, F. E., and Hendershot, G. E. "Do Family Ties Reduce Mortality?" *Journal of Marriage and the Family* 39(1977): 737–45.

For some excellent pioneering insights on this subject, see Masters, R. *NeuroSpeak* (Wheaton, Ill.: Quest Books, 1994).

Masters. *NeuroSpeak.*

Sime, W. E. "Psychological Benefits of Exercise," *Advances* (New York: Journal of the Institute for the Advancement of Health) 1 (4) (Fall 1984): 15–29; Roth, D. L., and Holmes, D. S. "Influence of Aerobic Exercise Training and Relaxation Training on Physical and Psychological Health Following Stressful Life Events," *Psychosomatic Medicine* (July–Aug. 1987); Morgan, W. P., and Goldston, S. E. *Exercise and Mental Health* (Washington, D.C.: Hemisphere Publishing, 1987).

Dustman, R., et al. "Aerobic Exercise Training and Improved Neuropsychologic Function of Older Individuals," *Neurobiology of Aging* 5 (1984): 35–42.

Bashore, T. "Age, Physical Fitness, and Mental-Processing Speed." In ed. Lawton, M. P. *Annual Review of Gerontology and Geriatrics Vol. IX Clinical and Applied Gerontology* (New York: Spring 1989).

Clarkson-Smith, L., and Hartley, A. A. "Relationships between Physical Exercise and Cognitive Abilities in Older Adults," *Psychology and Aging* 4 (2) (1989): 183–89.

Rogers, R. L., et al. "After Reaching Retirement Age, Physical Activity Sustains Cerebral Perfusion and Cognition," *Journal of the American Geriatrics Society* 38 (1990): 123–28.

Spriduso, W. W. *Journal of Gerontology* 35 (1980): 850.

"Mental Calisthenics to Keep Your Mind in Shape," *University of Texas Lifetime Health Letter* 3 (12) (Dec. 1991): 7.

Kandel, E. R., and Schwartz, J. H. "Molecular Biology of Learning: Modulation of Transmitter Release," *Science* 218 (4571) (1982): 433–43; Clark, G. "Cell Biological Analysis of Associative and Non-Associative Learning," paper presented at the annual meeting of the American Association for the Advancement of Science, New York (May 26, 1984); News feature, University of Illinois at Urbana (May 26, 1984).

In highlighting these mental activities, I've relied heavily on two primary references: Le Poncin, M. *Brain Fitness* (New York: Fawcett, 1990) and Chafetz. *Smart for Life.*

Chafetz. *Smart for Life*: 68.

Mark and Mark. *Brain Power*: 183.

Le Poncin. *Brain Fitness*: 38.

Chafetz. *Smart for Life*: 63–65.

Chafetz. *Smart for Life*: 64; Davis, B. *Perspectives in Biology and Medicine* 28 (1985): 457–64.

Chafetz. *Smart for Life*: 64.

Nelson, R. J., et al. "Variations in the Proportional Representations of the Hand in Somatosensory Cortex of Primates," paper presented at the Society for Neuroscience meeting, Boston, Mass. (Nov. 13, 1980); Jenkins, W. M., et al. Coleman Memorial Laboratories, University of California at San Francisco; Paper presented at the Society for Neuroscience meeting, Anaheim, Calif. (Oct. 13, 1984).

Winter and Winter. *Build Your Brain Power*: 17–43.

Le Poncin. *Brain Fitness*: 36–37.

Restak, R. *The Brain Has a Mind of Its Own* (New York: Crown, 1993): 60–61.

Shors, J. J., et al. "Unpredictable and Uncontrollable Stress Impair Neuronal Plasticity in the Hippocampus," *Brain Research Bulletin* 24 (5) (May 1990): 663–67; Thompson, R. F. Study cited in *Psychology Today* (Sep.–Oct. 1992): 44.

Yesavage, J., and Lapp, D., quoted in Toal, J. "The Fear of Forgetting," *American Health* (Oct. 1986): 77–86.

Sensory-Energy Switch #2: Stretch Your Senses

Diamond. *Enriching Heredity*; Diamond and Hopson. *Magic Trees.*

Diamond. *Enriching Heredity*: 114.

See, for example, Goertzel, V., and Goertzel, M. G. *Cradles of Eminence* (Boston: Little, Brown, 1962); Herrmann, D. *Helen Keller: A Life* (New York: Knopf, 1998); and Lash, J. P. *Helen and Teacher* (New York: Delacorte, 1980).

See, for example, Johnston, V. S. *Why We Feel* (Reading, Mass.: Perseus Books, 1999); Diamond. *Enriching Heredity*; Sobel and Ornstein. *Healthy Pleasures*; Erikson, J. M. *Wisdom and the Senses* (New York: Norton, 1988); Chafetz. *Smart for Life.*

Houston, J. The Possible Human (Los Angeles: Tarcher, 1982): 32.

Ornstein, R. *The Evolution of Consciousness* (New York: Prentice-Hall, 1991).

Diamond. *Enriching Heredity*; Hoffman, D. D. *Visual Intelligence* (New York: Norton, 2000); Winter and Winter. *Build Your Brain Power.*

Ackerman, D. *A Natural History of the Senses* (New York: Random House, 1990): xviii.

See Sobel and Ornstein. *Healthy Pleasures.*

Mental Medicine Update 2 (2) (Fall 1993).

Justice. *Who Gets Sick?*: 262.

Kaplan. "The Role of Nature in the Workplace": 193–201; Ulrich, R. S. "Natural versus Urban Scenes: Some Physiological Effects," *Environment and Behavior* 13 (5) (1981): 523–56; Ulrich, R. S. "View Through a Window May Influence Recovery from Surgery," *Science* 224 (4647) (1984): 420–21.

Sobel and Ornstein. *Healthy Pleasures*: 53.

Ulrich, R. S. "Human Responses to Vegetation and Landscapes," *Landscape and Urban Planning* 13 (1986): 29–44.

Weaver, R. A. "Characteristics of Circadian Rhythms in Human Functions," *Journal of Neural Transmission* 21 (Suppl) (1986): 351; Czeisler, C. A., et al. "Bright Light Induction of Strong (Type O) Resetting of the Human Circadian Pacemaker," *Science* 244 (1989): 1328–33; Czeisler, C. A. "Biological Rhythm Disorders, Depression, and Phototherapy: A New Hypothesis," *Psychiatric Clinics of North America* 10 (4) (Dec. 1987): 699; McIntyre, I., et al. *Life Sciences* 45 (1990): 327–32; *Brain/Mind Bulletin* (Jan. 1990): 7.

Thomas, L. Quoted in *Vis-a-Vis* (Apr. 1988): 28.

Moore-Ede. *24-Hour Society*: 61–62.

Kallan, C. "Probing the Power of Common Scents," *Prevention* (Oct. 1991): 39–43.

Torii, S. Studies cited in *The Futurist* (Sept.–Oct. 1990): 50.

Baron, R. A. Research paper presented at annual meeting of American Psychological Association. In *USA Today* (August 14, 1992).

Baron, R. A. Research cited in *The Futurist* (Sept.–Oct. 1990): 50.

Kallan. "Probing the Power of Common Scents."

Dember, W., and Warm, J. Studies reported at annual meeting of the American Association for the Advancement of Science (Washington, D.C., Jan. 1991).

"Accounting for Taste," *Universtiy of California at Berkeley Wellness Letter* 7 (2) (Nov. 1990): 7.

Lynch. *The Broken Heart.*

Goldstein, A. "Thrills in Response to Music and Other Stimuli," *Physiological Psychology* 8 (1) (1980): 126–29.

Arnot, *Biology of Success.*

Redd, W., and Badia, P. "Probing the Power of Common Scents," *Prevention* (Oct. 1991): 39–43.

Rosenfeld, A. H. "Music: The Beautiful Disturber," *Psychology Today* (Dec. 1985): 48–56; Karsh, S., and Merle-Fishman, C. *The Music within You* (New York: Simon & Schuster, 1985); ed. Hodges, A. *Handbook of Music Psychology* (Dubuque, Iowa: Kendall-Hunt, 1985).

Rider, M. S., et al. "The Effect of Music, Imagery, and Relaxation on Adrenal Corticosteroids," *Journal of Music Therapy* 22 (1) (1985): 46–58; Ryder, M. S., and Achterberg, J. "The Effect of Music-Mediated Imagery on Neutrophils and Lymphocytes," unpublished manuscript, 1987.

Tomatis, A. A. *The Conscious Ear* (Barrytown, N.Y.: Station Hill Press, 1991); eds. Gilmor, T. M., et al. *About the Tomatis Method* (Toronto: The Listening Centre, 1989).

Gilmor, et al. *The Tomatis Method*: 11.

"The Musical Brain," *U.S. News and World Report* (Jun. 11, 1990): 55–62.

Ackerman. *Natural History of the Senses*: 209.

Quoted in Ackerman. *Natural History of Senses*: 212.

Winter and Winter. *Build Your Brain Power*: 30.

Reinisch, J. Kinsey Institute for Research in Sex, Gender, and Reproduction. In "Communication Counters Misconceptions," *USA Today* (May 22, 1992): 9D.

Markman, H. and Notarius, C. *We Can Work It Out* (New York: Putnam, 1993).

Zilbergeld, B. *The New Male Sexuality* (New York: Bantam, 1992): 4.

Rossi and Nimmons. *20-Minute Break*: 174–75.

Cutler, W. D. *Love Cycles* (New York: Random House, 1995): 20.

Scantling, S., and Browder, S. *Ordinary Women, Extraordinary Sex* (New York: Dutton, 1993): 198–99.

Alperstein, L. P. Quoted in Castleman, M. "Pillow Talk," *Medical Self-Care* (Spring 1985): 45–55.

Gottman, J, and Silver, N. *Why Marriages Succeed or Fail* (New York: Simon & Schuster, 1994): 154–55.

Barchach, L., and Geisinger, D. L. *Going the Distance* (New York: Doubleday, 1991); Rosenthal. *Sex after 40.*

Schreiner-Engle, P. Quoted in Siegel, P. M. "Can You Psych Yourself into Sex?" *Self* (Dec. 1990): 145.

Gottman and Silver. *Why Marriages Succeed or Fail*: 155.

Zilbergeld, B. quoted in Wade, C. "Self-Help for Lovers: Relaxing for Romance," *American Health* (May 1985): 41–44.

Brooks, M. *Instant Rapport* (New York: Warner, 1989): 210.

Sensory-Energy Switch #3: Imagine or Invent

Bach, M. *I, Monty* (Honolulu: Island Heritage Ltd., 1977).

See, for example, Lynch, J. J. *The Language of the Heart* (New York: Basic Books, 1985); Diamond. *Enriching Heredity*; Johnson, G. *The Palaces of Memory* (New York: Knopf, 1991); and Childre, D., and Martin, H. *The HeartMath Solution* (New York: HarperCollins, 1999).

Picasso, P. *Picasso's One-Liners* (New York: Artisan, 1997).

Rodgers, W. L., and Hertzog, A. R. "Interviewing Older Adults," *Journal of Gerontology* 42 (1987): 387–94.

Rowe, J. W., and Kahn, R. L. "Human Aging: Usual and Successful," *Science* 237 (1987): 143–49.

Spence, J. D. *The Memory Palace of Matteo Ricci* (New York: Viking, 1984).

Journal of the American Medical Association (Apr. 6, 1994).

Kra, S. *Aging Myths* (New York: McGraw-Hill, 1986); Le Poncin. *Brain Fitness*; Chafetz. *Smart for Life*; "Building a Better Brain," *Omni Longevity* 1 (1) (Nov. 1986): 1–2; ed. Schaie, K. W. *Longitudinal Studies of Adult Psychological Development* (New York: Guildford Press, 1983); "Senility Reconsidered: Treatment Possibilities for Mental Impairment in the Elderly," Task force sponsored by the National Institute on Aging, Bethesda, Md., *Journal of the American Medical Association* (July 18, 1980): 259–60; Duara, R., et al. "Cerebral Glucose Utilization as Measured with Positron Emission Tomography in 21 Resting, Healthy Men Between the Ages of 21 and 83 Years," *Brain* 106 (1983): 761–75; Rosenzweig, M. R. "Experience, Memory, and the Brain" *American Psychologist* (Apr. 1984).

Le Poncin. *Brain Fitness*: 65; Zhang, M. Y., et al. "The Prevalence of Dementia and Alzheimer's Disease in Shanghai, China: Impact of Age, Gender, and Education," *Annals of Neurology* 27 (4) (Apr. 1990): 428–37; Research by Robert Katzman of the University of California, San Diego, and Richard Mayeux of Columbia University. Cited in *Psychology Today* (Sept.–Oct. 1992): 45.

Chafetz. *Smart for Life*: xii–xiii.

Schaie, K. W. "Late-Life Potential and Cohort Differences in Mental Abilities," in ed. Perlmutter, M. *Late-Life Potential* (Washington, D.C.: The Gerontological Society of America, 1990): 43.

Stevens, C. Quoted in *Psychology Today* (Sept.–Oct. 1992): 46.

Raichle, M. Quoted in *Psychology Today* (Sept.–Oct. 1992): 46.

Mark with Mark. *Reversing Memory Loss*: 1–3.

See, for example, Schnak, R. C. *Tell Me a Story* (New York: Scribners, 1990); Coles, R. *The Call of Stories* (Boston: Houghton Mifflin, 1989); Remen, R. N. *Kitchen Table Wisdom* (New

York: Riverside, 1996); and Beach, B. K. "Learning with Roger Schank," *Training and Development* (Oct. 1993): 39–44.

Williams, W. C. in Cole. *The Call of Stories*: 30.

Locke, J. L. *The De-Voicing of Society: Why We Don't Talk to Each Other Anymore* (New York: Simon & Schuster, 1998).

See, for example, Lynch. *The Language of the Heart*; Pribram, K. H. *Brain and Perception: Holonomy and Structure in Figural Processing* (Hillsdale, N.J.: Lawrence Erlbaum, 1991); Talbot, M. *The Holographic Universe* (New York: HarperCollins, 1991); Pinker, S. *The Language Instinct* (New York: William Morrow, 1994); Ornstein. *Evolution of Consciousness*; Diamond. *Enriching Heredity*; Dossey, L. *Healing Words* (New York: HarperCollins, 1993); Coles. *The Call of Stories*; Schank. *Tell Me a Story*.

Amabile, T. M. *The Social Psychology of Creativity* (New York: Springer-Verlag, 1983).

Sternberg. *Successful Intelligence*: 219.

See, for example, Clifton, D. O., and Nelson, P. *Soar with Your Strengths* (New York: Delacorte, 1992); and Buckingham, M., and Coffman, C. *First, Break All the Rules* (New York: Simon & Schuster, 1999).

See Buckingham, M., and Coffman, C. *First, Break All the Rules* (Simon & Schuster, 1999).

See Clifton and Nelson. *Soar with Your Strengths*: 36; and Sternberg. *Successful Intelligence*: 49.

Clifton and Nelson. *Soar with Your Strengths*: 43–61.

Maslow, A. *Toward a Psychology of Being* (New York: Harper & Row, 978).

See, for example, Jacobs, R. W. *Real Time Strategic Change* (San Francisco: Berrett-Koehler, 1994).

Sensory-Energy Switch #4: Strengthen Your Sight Skills

See, for example, Anderson, J., and Reder, L. "An Elaborate Processing of Depth of Processing" in eds. Cerrick, L., and Craik, F. *Levels of Processing in Human Memory* (Hillsdale, N.J.: Erlbaum, 1979): 385–403; Noice, H. "The Role of Explanations and Plan Recognition in Learning," *Cognitive Science* 15 (1991): 425–60; and Hilgard, E., and Marquis, D. G. *Conditioning and Learning* (New York: Appleton-Crofts, 1961).

See, for example, Raudenbush, S. W., et al. "Higher-Order Instructional Goals," *American Educational Research Journal* 20 (3) (1993): 523–53.

See, for example, Langer. *The Power of Mindful Learning*: 14.

Le Poncin. *Brain Fitness*: 40, 60.

Black, I. B., et al. "Neurotransmitter Plasticity at the Molecular Level," *Science* 225 (4668) (1984): 1266–70; Kandel, E. R., and Schwartz, J. H. "Molecular Biology of Learning: Modulation of Transmitter Release," *Science* 218 (4571) (1982): 433–43; World Health Organization. *Treatise on Neuroplasticity and Repair in the Central Nervous System* (Geneva, Switzerland, 1983).

Nightingale, E. "Our Changing World" radio program (Chicago: Nightingale-Conant Corporation, 1974).

Ed. Holton, G. "Albert Einstein Autobiographical Notes," translated by ed. Schilpp, P. A. *Albert Einstein: Philosopher-Scientist* (Evanston, Ill.: Library of Living Philosophers, 1949); Erikson. *Wisdom and the Senses*: 30–33.

Erikson, E. H. *Psychoanalytic Reflections of Einstein's Centenary* (Princeton, N.J.: Princeton University Press, 1982).

Cox, C. M. "The Early Mental Traits of 300 Geniuses," *Genetic Studies of Genius Vol. II* (Stanford, Calif.: Stanford University Press, 1926).

Richter, I. A. *The Notebooks of Leonardo Da Vinci* (New York: Oxford University Press, 1952).

See, for example, Baldwin, N. *Edison: Inventing the Century* (New York: Hyperion, 1997).

See, for example, Frank, S. D. *Remember Everything You Read* (New York: Times Books, 1990); McCarthy, M. J. *Mastering the Information Age* (New York: Tarcher, 1991); Princeton Language

Institute. *Twenty-First-Century Guide to Increasing Your Reading Speed* (New York: Dell, 1995); Wenger, W., and Poe, R. *The Einstein Factor* (Rocklin, Calif.: Prima, 1996).

See, for example, Rogers, T., et al. "Self-Reference and the Encoding of Personal Information," *Journal of Personality and Social Psychology* 35 (1977): 677–88.

Dryden, G., and Vos, J. *The Learning Revolution* (Torrance, Calif.: Jalmar Press, 1994); Wenger, W. *Beyond Teaching and Learning* (Gaithersburg, Md.: Project Renaissance, 1992); Gross, R. *Peak Learning* (Los Angeles: Tarcher, 1991); Berg, H. S. *Super Reading Secrets* (New York: Warner, 1992); Siler, T. *Breaking the Mind Barrier* (New York: Simon & Schuster, 1990); Herrmann, D. J. *Super Memory* (Emmaus, Pa.: Rodale, 1990); Frank. *Remember Everything You Read*; Rose, C. *Accelerated Learning* (New York: Dell, 1985).

Cailliet and Gross. *Rejuvenation Strategy*: 52; Hendler. *The Oxygen Breakthrough*.

Moore-Ede. *24-Hour Society*: 54–55.

Ed. Holton, G. "Albert Einstein Autobiographical Notes"; Erikson. *Wisdom and the Senses*: 30–33.

See, for example, Mark with Mark. *Reversing Memory Loss*.

Chafetz. *Smart for Life*: 63–65.

Sensory-Energy Switch #5: Sleep Deeper

National Sleep Foundation survey. *USA Today* (Mar. 23, 1999): 1A.

Dement, W. Series of *USA Today* articles, 1992 and 1993; Dotto, L. *Losing Sleep* (New York: Morrow, 1991): 179.

Dement, W. Quoted in Friend. *USA Today* (Jan. 3, 1993).

Davis, B. *Perspectives in Biology and Medicine* 28 (1985): 457–464.

Chafetz. *Smart for Life*: 64.

Here are several excellent resources on overcoming insomnia and getting great sleep: Hauri and Linde. *No More Sleepless Nights*; Perl, J. *Sleep Right in 5 Nights* (New York: Morrow, 1993); and Dement, W. C. *The Promise of Sleep* (New York: Delacorte Press, 1999).

Lamberg, L. "The Boy Who Ate His Bed . . . and Other Mysteries of Sleep," *American Health* (Nov. 1990): 56.

Williams, G. III. "Early Morning Dangers: Why Your Body Hates to Wake Up," *American Health* (Dec. 1986): 56–59; Arnot, R. B. *CBS News* (Jan. 13, 1987).

Shapiro, C. M., et al. "Fitness Facilitates Sleep," *European Journal of Applied Physiology* 53 (1984): 1–4; Baekland, F. Downstate Medical Center, New York, 1966 study, and Shapiro, C., and Zloty, R. B., University of Manitoba studies, both reported in Mirkin, G., *Dr. Gabe Mirkin's Fitness Clinic* (Chicago: Contemporary Books, 1986).

Sewitch, D. "Slow-Wave Sleep-Deficiency Insomnia: A Problem in Thermo-Down Regulation at Sleep Onset," *Psychophysiology* 24 (1987): 200–215; Perl. *Sleep Right in 5 Nights*: 232–33.

Hauri and Linde. *No More Sleepless Nights*: 130–31.

Horne, J. A., et al. *Sleep* 10 (1987): 383–92; Willensky, D. "Hints for Sound Sleep," *American Health* (May 1992): 50.

Hauri, P. In "Sleepless in America," *USA Today* (Mar. 23, 1999): A2.

Perl. *Sleep Right in 5 Nights*: 213.

Eds. Van Toller, S., and Dodd, G. H. *Perfumery: The Psychology and Biology of Fragrance* (London: Chapman and Hall, 1991); Krier, B. A. "Scents of Health," *Los Angeles Times* (Mar. 27, 1991): E1; O'Neill, M. "Taming the Frontier of the Senses," *New York Times* (Nov. 27, 1991): B1.

Kallan, C. "Probing the Power of Common Scents."

Redd, W., Memorial Sloan-Kettering Cancer Center in New York City, and Badia, P., Bowling Green State University of Ohio. Studies cited in Kallan. "Probing the Power of Common Scents."

Schwart, G., University of Arizona in Tucson. Studies cited in Kallan. "Probing the Power of Common Scents."

Lamberg. *Bodyrhythms*: 46; Wurtman. *Managing Your Mind and Mood through Food*.

Perl. *Sleep Right in 5 Nights*: 205.

Broughton, R. "Performance and Evoked Potential Measures of Various States of Daytime Sleepiness," *Sleep* 5 (Suppl. 2) (1982); Dott, L. C. *Asleep in the Fast Lane* (Toronto: Stocklart, 1990: 138; Hauri, P. "Behavioral Treatment of Insomnia," *Medical Times* 107 (6) (1986): 36–47; Regestein, Q. R. "Practical Ways to Manage Insomnia," *Medical Times* 107 (6) (1986): 19–23.

Winget, C. Quoted in Dolnick, E. "Snap Out of It," *Health* (Feb.–Mar. 1992): 87; ". . . can produce a state of 'time confusion' in the body that is identical to jet lag." Perls. *Sleep Right in 5 Nights*: 206.

Hauri. "Behavioral Treatment of Insomnia."; Regestein. "Practical Ways to Manage Insomnia."

Perl. *Sleep Right in 5 Nights*: 195, 209.

Introduction to the Heartfelt-Energy Switches

McCraty, R., et al. "The Effects of Emotions on Short-Term Heart Rate Variability Using Power Spectrum Analysis," *American Journal of Cardiology* 76 (14) (1995): 1089–93.

See, for example, eds. Armour, J., and Ardell, J., *Neurocardiology* (New York: Oxford University Press, 1994); Childre and Martin. *The HeartMath Solution*; Institute of HeartMath Web site.

See, for example, Song, L., Schwartz, G., and Russek, L. "Heart-Focused Attention and Heart-Brain Synchronization: Energetic and Physiological Mechanisms," *Alternative Therapies in Health and Medicine* 4 (5) (1998): 44–62.

McCraty, et al. "The Effects of Emotions on Short-Term Heart Rate Variability Using Power Spectrum Analysis."

See, for example, Song, Schwartz, and Russek. "Heart-Focused Attention and Heart-Brain Synchronization."

See, for example, McCraty, R., Atkinson, M., and Tiller, W. A. "New Electrophysiological Correlates Associated with Intentional Heart Focus," *Subtle Energies* 4 (3) (1995): 251–68; and Lynch. *The Language of the Heart*.

Drucker, P. In *Creative Living* (Fall 1997).

Battery of studies on success at work; contact Jodi Taylor, vice president, Center for Creative Leadership; Colorado Springs, CO; April 1998.

Heartfelt-Energy Switch #1: Engage People Eye to Eye

Lynch. *Language of the Heart*: 310.

Josselson, R. *The Space between Us* (San Francisco: Jossey-Bass, 1992): 99.

See, for example, Bathurst, B. *The Lighthouse Stevensons* (New York: HarperCollins, 1999).

See, for example, Rossi. *20-Minute Break*.

Heartfelt-Energy Switch #2: Ask Openly and Listen Deeply

Myers. *The Pursuit of Happiness*; see also Locke. *The De-Voicing of Society*.

Lynch. *Language of the Heart*.

Stafford, W. "A Ritual to Read to Each Other," *Stories That Could Be True* (New York: HarperCollins, 1977): 52.

Locke. *The De-Voicing of Society*.

See Langer. *The Power of Mindful Learning*.

Lynch. *Language of the Heart.*

See, for example, Locke. *The De-Voicing of Society.*

See, for example, Zajonc, R. B. "Styles of Explanation in Social Psychology," *The European Journal of Social Psychology* (Sept.–Oct. 1989).

See, for example, Muller, W. *How, Then, Shall We Live?* (New York: Bantam, 1996).

See Cooper, R. K., and Sawaf, A. *Executive EQ: Emotional Intelligence in Leadership and Organizations* (New York: Grosset/Putnam, 1997).

Lynch. *Language of the Heart* (New York: Basic, 1985): 3–4.

Lynch. *Language of the Heart*: 243.

See, for example, Thayer. *The Origin of Everday Moods*; Locke. *The De-Voicing of Society*; and Lynch. *Language of the Heart.*

For an excellent book on this subject, see Stone, D., Patton, B., and Heen, S. *Difficult Conversations: How to Discuss What Matters Most* (New York: Viking, 1999).

Lynch. *Language of the Heart*; Childre and Martin. *The HeartMath Solution.*

Heartfelt-Energy Switch #3: Empathize

Coles, R. *The Moral Intelligence of Children* (New York: Random House, 1999).

See, for example, Thayer. *The Origin of Everyday Moods.*

See, for example, Sober, E., and Wilson, D. S. *Unto Others: The Evolution and Psychology of Unselfish Behavior* (Boston: Harvard University Press, 1999); and Kohn, A. *The Brighter Side of Human Nature* (Boston: Houghton Mifflin, 1993).

House, et al. "The Association of Social Relationships and Activities with Mortality."

Maurois, A. *Prometheus—The Life of Balzac* (New York: Harper & Row, 1965): 57–58.

A similar story is told by Irving Cramer, executive director of MAZON: A Jewish Response to Hunger, in Dosick, W. *Golden Rules* (New York: HarperCollins, 1995).

Rein, G., Atkinson, M., and McCraty, R. "The Physiological and Psychological Effects of Compassion and Anger," *Journal of Advancement in Medicine* 8 (2) (1995): 87–105.

House, J. S., et al. "Association of Social Relationships and Activities with Mortality: Prospective Evidence from the Tecumseh Community Health Study," *American Journal of Epidemiology* 116 (1) (1982): 123–40; Berkman and Syme. "Social Networks, Host Resistance, and Mortality"; Eisenberg. "A Friend, Not an Apple, A Day Will Keep the Doctor Away"; Syme, L. "People Need People," *American Health* (July–Aug. 1982): 49–51; Cohen and Wils. "Stress, Social Support, and Buffering Hypothesis"; Russell, D. W., and Cutrona, C. E. "Social Support, Stress, and Depressive Symptoms among the Elderly: Test of a Process Model," *Psychology and Aging* 6 (2) (1991): 190–201; Oslon, R. B., et al. "Social Networks and Longevity: A 14-Year Follow-Up Study among Elderly in Denmark," *Social Science and Medicine* 33 (10) (1991): 1189–95.

House, J. S., et al. "Social Relationships and Health," *Science* 241 (1988): 540–45.

Study cited in Kerman, A. *The H.A.R.T. Program* (New York: HarperCollins, 1991): 228.

See, for example, Childre and Martin. *The HeartMath Solution.*

Gottman. *Why Marriages Succeed or Fail*: 195.

Gray, J. *Men Are from Mars, Women Are from Venus* (New York: HarperCollins, 1992): 177.

Nagler. *Dirty Half-Dozen*: 113.

Lawrence, J. "Excuse Me, But . . . Whatever Happened to Manners?" *USA Today* (Dec. 16, 1996): 1.

Renick, Blumberg, and Markman, H. J. "Prevention"; and Markman, H. J. Quoted in Blau. "Can We Talk?": 45.

Bartolome, F., and Evans, P. *Must Success Cost So Much?* (New York: Basic Books, 1988); Kaplan, R. F. *Beyond Ambition: How Driven Managers Can Lead Better and Live Better* (San Francisco: Josey-Bass, 1991).

Gottman. *Why Marriages Succeed or Fail*; Notarius and Markman. We Can Work It Out.

Gottman, J. M., and Krokoff. "Marital Interactions"; Levenson, R. W., and Gottman, J. M. "Physiological and Affective Predictors of Change in Relationship Satisfaction," *Journal of Personality and Social Psychology* 49 (10) (July 1985): 85–94; Gottman, J. M., and Levenson, R. W. "Assessing the Role of Emotion in Marriage," *Behavioral Assessment* 8 (1) (1986): 31–48.

Gray. *Men Are from Mars*: 67–68.

Levenson and Gottman. "Physiological and Affective Predictors."

Gray. *Men Are from Mars*: 68.

Locke. *The De-Voicing of Society*.

Pennebaker, J. W. *Opening Up: The Healing Power of Confiding in Others* (New York: Morrow, 1990).

Burt, R. S. *Strangers, Friends, and Happiness* GSS Technical Report No. 72 (Chicago: National Opinion Research Center, University of Chicago, 1986).

Francis, M. E., and Pennebaker, J. W. "Talking and Writing as Illness Prevention," *Medicine, Exercise, Nutrition, and Health* 1 (1) (Jan.–Feb. 1992): 27–33.

Pennebaker, J. W., et al. "Accelerating the Coping Process," *Journal of Personality and Social Psychology* 58 (1990): 528–37.

Francis and Pennebaker. "Talking and Writing."

Pennebaker, J. W. *Opening Up* (New York: Morrow, 1990): 50.

Pennebaker. *Opening Up*: 51.

Heartfelt-Energy Switch #4: Discover Your Passion

See, for example, Solomon, R. C. *The Passions: Emotions and the Meaning of Life* (Indianapolis: Hackett Publsihing, 1993); and Butler, T., and Waldroop, J. "Job Sculpting," *Harvard Business Review* (Sept.–Oct. 1999): 144–52.

Ray, M., and Myers, R. *Creativity in Business* (New York: Doubleday, 1987).

See, for example, Pennebaker. *Opening Up*; and Francis and Pennebaker. "Talking and Writing as Illness Prevention."

Nerburn, K. *Small Graces* (Novato, Calif.: New World Library, 1998).

I am grateful to Esther M. Orioli for the insights on this kind of simple, successful behavior-change process. See, for example, Orioli, E. M. *The StressMap 21-Day-Rule Action-Planning Workbook* (San Francisco: Essi Systems, 1993).

See, for example, Damasio, A. R. *Descartes' Error: Emotion and Reasoning* (New York: Grosset/Putnam, 1994); Cooper and Sawaf. *Executive EQ*; Damasio, A. R. *The Feeling of What Happens* (New York: HarcourtBrace, 1999).

Butler and Waldroop. "Job Sculpting."

Ibid.

Heartfelt-Energy Switch #5: Leave Your Imprint

Adapted from a report on CBS News Radio; WWJ 950 Detroit; (Aug. 2, 1999): 8:45 A.M.

Heschel, A. *What Is Man?* (Stanford: Stanford University Press, 1965).

See, for example, Leider, R. J. *The Power of Purpose* (San Francisco: Berrett-Koehler, 1997).

Index

Underscored references indicate boxed text.

A

Abdomen
    fat loss in, 212–13
    forced exhalation for, <u>174</u>
    one-touch relaxation and, 34–36
Abdominal exercises, 173
    Abdominal Curl, 178–80
    Trans-Pyramid Exercise, 175, 178
Abdominal fat, 212–213
Action, active energy and, 11
Active energy, 11–12, 147–51
    action and, 11
    benefits of, <u>150</u>
    breaking point and, 215
    energy-boosting activities for, <u>182–83</u>
    in evening, 227–43
    fat loss and, 11, 148
    foods for, 433–36
    forced exhalation for, <u>174</u>
    hot and spicy food for, <u>198</u>
    ice-cold water for, <u>160–61</u>
    in late afternoon, 215–25
    light aerobics after lunch for, <u>206–7</u>
    metabolism and, 11, 30
    vs. reserved energy, 11–12, 148
    shifting between tasks for, <u>196–97</u>
    smart pacing for, 153–63
    tracking evening eating for, <u>235</u>
    transition to home for, <u>221</u>
    water balance and, 159
    youthfulness and, 147

Active relaxation, 143–44
    health benefits of, 143
Adaptability, 79
Adenosine triphosphate (ATP), health
    problems and, 60
Adrenaline, fat loss and, 213
Aerobic capacity, 180
Aerobic exercise, 203–14, <u>206–7</u>
    for burning body fat, 212–14
    cardiovascular endurance and, 208
    competition and stress during, 211–12
    cooldown after, 214
    easy speedups during, 212
    fat loss and, 212–14
    heart rate and, 209, 210
    intensity of, 210
    predicted maximal heart rate and, 210
    scheduling, 211
    warmup before, 210
Afternoon slump, 215–16
    exercises for, 220
    importance of humor during, 224–25
    reversing, with light, 219–20
    transition to evening after, 221–24
Aging
    accelerated by
        poor posture, 87, 90
        routine, 252
        stress, <u>55</u>
    maintaining cerebral efficiency while,
        <u>323</u>
    mental sharpness and, 308

synchronizing, 366, 368
ultradian, 165–69
   in close relationships, 365–66
   essential breaks and, 166–71, 180–82,
      185–87
   love life and, 166–71, 366
Biscotti
   Chocolate–Chocolate Chip Biscotti,
      449
   Orange–Poppy Seed Biscotti, 446–47
Blackberries
   Mixed-Berry Pie, 439
Bloodflow, reduced, 65–66
Blood pressure
   breakfast and, 43
   decreasing, by drinking water, 158
   human dialogue and, 382
   medical checkup before exercising and,
      205
   stress and, 54
Blood sugar
   arguments and, 230
   breakfast and, 43
   eating and, 185–86
   energy and, 185–87
   fatigue and, 186
   giant-size sodas and, 202
   glycogen and, 38–39, 45
   overeating caused by low, 186
   tension and, 186
Blueberries
   Blueberry-Cream Fruit Dip, 447
   Mixed-Berry Pie, 439
Body fat
   adrenaline and, 213
   caffeine and, 185
   losing, through
      active energy, 11
      exercise, 177, 212–14
      sleeping in cool environment, 240
      snacking, 186
   water intake and, 158
Body temperature
   sleeping and, 342
   weight loss and, 240
Brain
   amygdala, 253
   facial expression and bloodflow to,
      62–64
   fatigue, 196

function
   aging and, 308, 323
   breakfast and, 45
   mental exercise for, 307–8
   dehydration and, 160
   sleep and, 272, 337–39
   water balance and, 160
Brainpower, 251
   improving, 308
   vocabulary and, 270
Breakfast
   benefits of, 42–43
   Bircher-Benner muesli, 48–49
   brain function and, 45
   calm energy and, 42–43
   Cinnamon Scones with Walnut Cream,
      444–45
   while commuting, 48
   Fresh Cranberry Loaf, 443
   Fruit Smoothy, 47
   Lemon Lift Muffins, 440–41
   metabolism and, 30–31
   60-second, 46–47
   skipping, 46–49
      pitfalls of, 30–31, 44
   suggestions for, 47–49
   sympathetic nervous system and,
      43–44
   ultimate energy and, 48
   weight-loss benefits and, 45
   whole-grain cereal, 46, 47, 48, 49
   Whole-Grain English Muffin Cheese
      Melt, 47
Breaking point, 215
Breaks, 126–127, 166–171, 180–182,
   185–187, 193–194
   finding time for, 126–27
   physical, 98, 181
   productivity and, 168
   for reducing fatigue, 168
   timing, 168–69
Breathing
   for calm energy, 33, 61
   exercise
      forced exhalation, 174
      for posture, 95
   health benefits of proper, 59–60
   in instant-calming sequence, 56–62
   interruption of, due to stress, 60–62
   relaxed, 61

Environment, value of natural setting and, 171, 286–87
Enzymes, fat-burning, _177_, 213
Essential breaks, 166–70
  disengaging during, 170–71
  exercise during, 172, _174_
  fluid intake during, 181–84
  food for, 169–70, 185–89, _190–91_
  inspiration during, 192
  length and timing of, 167, 169
  recognizing need for, 168–69
  releasing muscle tension during, 180–81
  vs. strategic pauses, 167
  ultradian rhythm and, 166–70
Essential oils, 290
ETT, _205_
Eucalyptus scent, for sensory fatigue, 290
Evening. _See also_ Dinner
  family rituals during, 227, _228_, 229
  increased energy for, 229–43
  putting day into perspective during, 242–43
  transition from work in, 221–24
Evening slump, 195–96, 196
Excelling vs. competing, 106–9
Exercise. _See also_ Aerobic exercise
  Abdominal Curl, 178–80
  for afternoon energy, 203–12
  benefits of, _150_
    enhanced brain function, _265_
    energy-boosting, _182–83_
    health, 180–81
    improved cholesterol/HDL ratio, 209
    increased alertness, 39, _40–41_
    mental agility, _265_
    sensory energy, _265_
    slowed aging, _265_
    tension relief, 180
    weight loss, _176–77_
  for better sleep, 342
  breathing exercise, for
    calm energy, _61_
    midsection, _174_
  calm energy and, 39
  checking with doctor before, _205_
  after eating, _206–7_, 237–38
  getting dressed for, 41–42
  habit, 30–40
  head-nod exercise, _97_
  intensity of, 180

  for late-afternoon energy, 220
  memory exercise, _305_
  metabolism and, 30–31
  moderate, 172, 180–81
  in morning, 38–42
  one-touch relaxation, 34–36, _34–36_
  for posture, _95_
  reducing body fat with, 148, _176–77_
  shifting between tasks during, _197_
  stretching, 220
  stroke risk and, _265_
  Trans-Pyramid Exercise, 175, 178
Exercise-tolerance test (ETT), _205_
Expression, facial, 62–64, _63_
Eye contact
  as expression of heartfelt energy, 360–61, 365–68
  feelings of intimacy and, 366
  personal relationships and, 367
Eyes
  effect of reading on, _331_
  response of, to heartfelt energy, 370
Eyestrain
  avoiding, 157, 158
  contact lenses and, 159

F

Facial expression, 62–64, _63_
Family rituals, 227–29, _228_
Fat. _See_ Abdominal fat; Body fat; Dietary fat, in
Fat cravings. _See_ Cravings, fat
Fatigue
  blood sugar and, 186
  breakfast and, 43
  eucalyptus scent for, 290
  from eyestrain, 157
  high-fat food and, 198
  inactivity, _207_
  late-afternoon, 215–25
  midday, 195–96
  music for, 292–93
  natural scenes and, 171
  posture and, 90
  calm energy and, 51
  short breaks for relieving, 168
  tendency toward, 23
  water and, _158_

positive feelings and, 393–94
snacking and, 186
water balance and, 159, _159_, 160–61,
    162
Hearing, 292–93
Heart, electromagnetic field of, 352
Heart attacks, value of pets for preventing,
    _256_
Heart disease
    diet and, 231–32
    medical checkup before exercising and,
        _205_
    snacking to reduce risk of, 186
    stress and, 54
    timing of meals and, 231–32
Heartfelt energy, 13–14, 231, 351–430
    avoiding verbal battles and, 365
    being a good listener and, 369–85
    character building and, 14
    communication and, 357–85, 399–401
    constancy and, 362–63
    emotional honesty and, 362
    empathy and compassion and, 387–95
    expressing feelings and, 401
    expressions of appreciation and,
        396–98
    eye contact and, 357–68
    feeling valued and, _376_
    health and, 354
    leaving imprint and, 413–23
    passion and, 403–12
    personal interactions and, 359–65
    questions about life and, 374–75
    recognizing other perspectives and, 380
    respecting people and, 364
    sharing views and, 380
    vs. surface energy, 15
Heart rate monitor, exercise and, 210–11
Helplessness, feelings of
    poor posture and, 90
    somatic retraction and, 66
High-density lipoprotein (HDL), 209
Home
    as buffer zone, 139
    relaxation time and, 222–24
    transition from work to, 137–42, _221_,
        297
Hopes, charting, with LifeMap, 318–20
Hostility, 141–42
Housework, male sexuality and, 297

Humor. _See also_ Laughter
    cosmic, _134–35_
    cultivating, 129–32
    to defuse tension and anger, 140–41
    evening relaxation and, 224
    library of, 132
    in marriage, 140
Hunger
    arguments and, 139
    diet drinks and, 185
    irritability and, 139, 230
    thirst mistaken for, 181
"Hurry sickness," 54
Hypertension. _See_ Blood pressure

I

ICS. _See_ Instant-calming sequence
Ideas, charting, with LifeMap, 318–20
Imagination
    enhancing sensory energy with,
        301–20
    invoking good memories with, 171
Immune system
    emotional experiences and, 393–94
    laughter and, 130
    mood fluctuations and, _55_
Impatience, carbohydrate-rich foods and,
    188
Inactivity fatigue, _207_
Insomnia, 337–47
Inspiration
    during breaks, 192
    empathy and, 392–93
    of passion, 403–12
Instant-calming sequence (ICS), 56–84
    as automatic response, 80–81
        acknowledging reality and, 73
        recalling your best and, 73–78
    in crisis management, _70–71_
    fluid intelligence and, 82
    lightening facial expression for, 62–64
    ongoing training and, 80–81
    opportunities to use, 83
    overcoming criticism with, _74–75_
    posture and, 98
    relaxed breathing and, 59–62
    releasing tension through, 65–67
    speeding up, 81–83

Instant-calming sequence (ICS) *(continued)*
  in strategic pause, 157
  in streamlining, 113, 115
  visual reminders for, <u>77</u>
Instant calmness, 51–53, 82
  frustration and, 54, <u>55</u>, 56
  recognizing tense tiredness and, 53–54
Insulin production, caffeine and, 185
Intellectual interest, aging and, 308
Intelligence, fluid vs. crystallized, 68
Interests, evaluating, <u>316</u>
Intimacy
  establishing feelings of, 366
  vitality and well-being from, 297, 298
Irritability
  breakfast and, 43
  caused by
    hunger, 139
    tense tiredness, 53

J

Jasmine, as relaxing scent, 290
Jaw, one-touch relaxation for, 34–36
Journals, 326, 401–2. *See also* Notebooks,
    Note making
Joy, laughter and, 130

K

Kidney stones, water intake and, <u>158</u>
Kindness, 360–61

L

Language, brain capacity and, <u>270</u>
Laughter, 224. *See also* Humor
  brain chemicals and, 130
  cosmic humor and, <u>134–35</u>
  immune system and, 130
Learning, 397. *See also* Reading
  creative imagination and, 322
  importance of continued, 321–36
  importance of observation in, 322–25
  information packages and, 321
  without memorization, 321–22
  training senses and, 325–26

Legumes, 199
Lemon
  Lemon Lift Muffins, 440–41
  scent, <u>289</u>
  tea, for energy, 291
Life, questions about, 374–75
LifeMap, for building sensory energy,
    318–20
Light
  as energy booster, 37–38, 162, 171
  late-afternoon energy and, 219–20
  morning energy and, 37–38
  sensory energy and, 287–88
Limbic system, 62
Lime
  Chili-Lime Pita Crisps, 458
Liming, 120–34
Linear subvocalization, 330
Listening, 369–85
Longevity, sensory energy and, 251
Lounging, 135
Love. *See also* Marriage; Partners; Sex
  family activities and, <u>238</u>
Lunch
  avoiding fried foods for, 202
  effect of skipping, 194, 195
  food choices for, 201–203
  ice water or iced tea with, 198–99
  low-fat, 198
  suggestions for, 198–203
Lunch break
  as breathing space, 194–95
  exercise during, 203–14, <u>206–7</u>
Lung capacity
  aerobic exercise and, 209
  posture and, 88, 90

M

Manners, value of, 398
Marriage. *See also* Partners; Relationships;
    Sex
  conflict in, 399
  confrontation in, 399
  humor in, 140
  men's expressiveness and happiness of,
    399
  nurturing intimate relationships and,
    366

open communication in, 399–401
relaxing together and, 140
stonewalling in, 400
Massage
sensory energy and, 291–92
for stress relief, 223–24
Maximal graded exercise test,
(MAxGXT), <u>205</u>
Mayonnaise, 200–201
Meals. *See also* Appetizer(s); Breakfast;
Dessert(s); Dinner; Food; Lunch;
Snacks
pitfalls of skipping, 30–31, 44, 194,
195
timing of, 434–36
Medical checkup, prior to exercising,
<u>205</u>
Meditation, passive, 55
Memory
aging and, <u>305</u>
impairment, from overwork,
273–74
loss of
preventing, 307–8
due to stress, 274
physical exercise to improve, 204
reinforced by sleep, <u>272</u>, 339
rosemary for enhancing, 290
vital, 308–10
Mental agility
effect of exercise on <u>265</u>
mental calisthenics for, 269, 271–73
Mental attitude, posture and, 85–100,
<u>86</u>
Mental exercise
sensory cross-training for, 268
for sensory energy, <u>260–61</u>, 269,
271
for sensory experiences, 280–81
Metabolism
active energy and, 11, 30
breakfast and, 30–31
caffeine and, 185
effect of taste on, 196
morning exercises for increasing,
30–31
production of water by, <u>161</u>
snacking to increase, 186
thermic effect of food and, 234
water intake and, <u>158</u>

Mexican food, 198, 202
Midsection, exhalation exercise for,
<u>174</u>
Mood
bright light and, 38
caffeine and, 184
effect of foods on, 189
facial expressions and, 62
fluctuations and immune functioning,
55
posture and, 87–88, 90
Morning
exercise in, 30, 38–42
for fat-burning, 30–31, 38
for increasing metabolism, 38–39
for reducing tension, 39
waking-up habits in, 29–49
easing out of sleep, 32–33
generating calm energy through, 33,
37
getting extra light, 37–38
one-touch relaxation, 34–36
physical activity, 38–42
water deficit in, 161
Muesli, Bircher-Benner, 48–49
Muscle tension, releasing, 180–81
Musculoskeletal loading, 181
Music
sensory energy and, 271, 292–93
streamlining and, 112–13
waking to, 341

N

Nachos, fat content of, 202
Natural scenes
benefits of, 286–87
energizing effects of, 171
Neck exercise for posture, <u>97</u>
Neotony, 257
Nervous system, 249
Neufchâtel cheese
Blueberry-Cream Fruit Dip, 447
Neurocardiology, 351
Neuromuscular coordination, water
balance and, <u>160</u>
Neuroplasticity, <u>323</u>
Noiception sensory system, 248
Notebooks, 317, 326

Scones
  Cinnamon Scones with Walnut Cream,
    444–45
Secondhand experiences, 282–83
Seeds, as protein source, 441
Self-awareness, sensory energy and,
  285–86
Senility. *See also* Aging
  fear of, 258
Senses, 247–48
  educating the nervous system and, 249
  hearing, 292–93
  sex and, 294–95
  sight, 248, 321–36
  smell, 248, 288, 289, 290–91
  taste, 196–97, 234–35, 290–91, 435
  touch, 248, 291–92, 367
  training, with note making, 325–26
Sensory cues, one-touch relaxation for,
  34–36
Sensory-emotional bond, 298
Sensory energy, 12–13, 247–347
  benefits of, 250
  children as source of, 262–64
  cross-training for, 268
  evaluating interests and, 316
  exercise and, 265
  expanding, 275–99
  extending senses for, 254
  growing young and, 12
  healthy pleasures and, 283–85
  imagination and, 301–20
  language skills and, 270
  learning and, 258–59, 321–36
  LifeMap and, 318–20
  light and, 287–88
  longevity and, 12, 251
  memory and, 305, 306–10
  mental agility and, 269, 271–73
  music and, 291–92
  nature and, 286–87
  new experiences and, 316
  pets as source of, 256
  physical fitness and, 271–73
  reading for, 329
  vs. routine energy, 13, 252
  scents for, 288–289, 291
  secondhand senses and, 282–83
  self-awareness and, 285–86
  sensory engagement and, 260–61

sensory stimulation and, 275–99
sex and, 293–99
sleep and, 272, 337–47
storytelling and, 309, 310, 312
technological communications and, 312
touch and, 291–92
visuospatial activity and, 269, 271
vocabulary and, 270
Zeigarnick Effect and, 317–18
Sensory experience, 280–81
  energy and, 283–84
  memory and, 306–7
Sensory stimulation, 275–99
  increasing, 281–82
  secondhand experience and, 282–83
  to slow aging, 275
  storytelling and, 310–13
Sensory systems, 248
Sex. *See also* Love; Marriage; Partners
  aging and, 294
  avoiding routine in, 296
  biological rhythms and, 366
  body tour and, 296–97
  breathing rhythm and, 299
  emotional closeness and, 298
  improving, 294
  making time for, 241
  sensory-emotional bond and, 298
  as source of stress, 293–94
  use of senses in, 294–95
Sexuality, male, and housework, 297
Shoulders, one-touch relaxation for,
  34–36
Sight, 321–36
  sensory systems associated with, 248
Sitting, 91–98
  adjusting chair for, 98
  bending at hips while, 94, 96
  chairs with adjustable armrests for, 94
  crossing legs while, 96
  emptying pockets before, 94
  head-nod exercise for, 96
  instant-calming sequence and, 98
  keeping feet flat while, 96
  reading at proper height while, 96–97
  short breaks for, 98
  squarely, 94–95
  torso shift exercise for, 96
  using telephone while, 97–98
Skillpower vs. willpower, 425–30

Online Help

www.100percentalive.com

Visit this Web site featuring links to many of Dr. Robert Cooper's seminars and educational programs as well as a variety of his favorite books, articles, music CDs, and other products related to high-energy living.

www.LessonsinLeadership.com

See Dr. Robert Cooper at a live half-day or full-day seminar near you, and order related products from his pioneering work on 21st-century leadership, emotional intelligence, and excelling under pressure.

www.LeighBureau.com

Schedule Dr. Robert Cooper to talk to your group or organization.